Current Clinical Urology

Current Clinical Urology

Edited by Clark Hardy

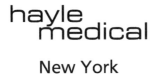

New York

Hayle Medical,
750 Third Avenue, 9th Floor,
New York, NY 10017, USA

Visit us on the World Wide Web at:
www.haylemedical.com

ISBN: 978-1-64647-550-6

Cataloging-in-Publication Data

Current clinical urology / edited by Clark Hardy.
 p. cm.
Includes bibliographical references and index.
ISBN 978-1-64647-550-6
1. Urology. 2. Genitourinary organs--Diseases. 3. Clinical medicine. I. Hardy, Clark.
RC871 .C55 2023
616.6--dc23

Table of Contents

Preface

Urology, also known as genitourinary surgery, is a study of the diseases related to the urinary-tract system. It also involves the study of the disorders associated with the male reproductive organs. The organs which come under the scope of urology include the bladder, kidneys, urethra, ureters, prostate, seminal vesicles, vas deferens, epididymis, adrenal glands, testes and penis. Some of the sub-disciplines of this field are endourology, neurourology, reconstructive urology, urologic oncology and female urology. Endourology is a subfield within urology which involves the application of minimally invasive techniques for examining the urinary tract and performing surgery. Neurourology focuses on urinary tract dysfunction which is caused by neuropathy disorders. This book is a valuable compilation of topics, ranging from the basic to the most complex advancements in the field of clinical urology. It brings forth some of the most innovative concepts and elucidates the unexplored aspects of this field of medicine. As this field is emerging at a fast pace, this book will help the readers to better understand the upcoming concepts in urology.

Various studies have approached the subject by analyzing it with a single perspective, but the present book provides diverse methodologies and techniques to address this field. This book contains theories and applications needed for understanding the subject from different perspectives. The aim is to keep the readers informed about the progresses in the field; therefore, the contributions were carefully examined to compile novel researches by specialists from across the globe.

Indeed, the job of the editor is the most crucial and challenging in compiling all chapters into a single book. In the end, I would extend my sincere thanks to the chapter authors for their profound work. I am also thankful for the support provided by my family and colleagues during the compilation of this book.

Editor

Hydronephrosis Classifications: Has UTD Overtaken APD and SFU?

Santiago Vallasciani[1]*, Anna Bujons Tur[2], John Gatti[3], Marcos Machado[4], Christopher S. Cooper[5], Marie Klaire Farrugia[6], Huixia Zhou[7], Mohammed El Anbari[8] and Pedro-José Lopez[9,10]

[1] Division of Urology, Department of Surgery, Sidra Medicine, Doha, Qatar, [2] Division of Pediatric Urology, Puigvert Foundation, Barcelona, Spain, [3] Division of Pediatric Urology, Children's Mercy Hospital, Kansas City, MO, United States, [4] Division of Pediatric Urology, University of São Paulo, São Paulo, Brazil, [5] Department of Urology, University of Iowa Hospitals and Clinics, Iowa City, IA, United States, [6] Division of Pediatric Urology, Chelsea and Westminster Hospital NHS Foundation Trust, London, United Kingdom, [7] Department of Pediatric Urology, Bayi Children's Hospital, Affiliated of the Seventh Medical Center of PLA General Hospital, Beijing, China, [8] Division of Clinical Informatics, Sidra Medicine, Doha, Qatar, [9] Hospital Exequiel Gonzalez Cortes & Clinica Alemana, Santiago, Chile, [10] University of Chile, Santiago, Chile

*Correspondence:
Santiago Vallasciani
santiago.vallasciani@gmail.com

Objective: To collect baseline information on the ultrasonographic reporting preferences.

Method: A 13-multiple choice questionnaire was designed and distributed worldwide among pediatric urologists, pediatric surgeons, and urologists. The statistical analysis of the survey data consisted of 3 steps: a univariate analysis, a bivariate and a multivariate analysis.

Results: Three hundred eighty participants responded from all the continents. The bivariate analysis showed the significant differences in the geographical area, the years of experience and the volume of cases. Most of the physicians prefer the SFU and APD systems because of familiarity and simplicity (37 and 34%, respectively). Respondents noted that their imaging providers most often report findings utilizing the mild-moderate-severe system or the APD measurements (28 and 39%, respectively) except for North America (SFU in 50%). Multivariate analysis did not provide significant differences.

Conclusion: Our study evaluates the opinions regarding the various pediatric hydronephrosis classification systems from a large number of specialists and demonstrates that there is no single preferred grading system. The greatest reported shortcoming of all the systems was the lack of universal utilization. The observations taken from this study may serve as basis for the construction of a common worldwide system. As APD and SFU are the preferred systems and the UTD a newer combination of both, it is possible that with time, UTD may become the universal language for reporting hydronephrosis. This time, based on the result of this survey, seems not arrived yet.

Keywords: hydronephrosis, classification, survey, pediatric urology, ultrasound, pediatric radiology

INTRODUCTION

Ultrasound reports serve as an instrument to communicate anatomic findings to health care providers permitting the patient's physician to make therapeutic decisions and counsel families. In the specific case of hydronephrosis, the report can be generated from the maternal-fetal specialist in the prenatal period or the pediatric radiologist postnatally. To communicate the results of the ultrasound study reliably and accurately, several classifications have been developed. Initially the anterior-posterior diameter of the renal pelvis (APD) was developed. Subsequently, additional systems that included other anatomical details regarding the calyces, renal parenchyma, ureters, and/or bladder were developed. These classification systems included the Society of Fetal Urology (SFU), Onen, UTD (Urinary Tract Dilatation), and European Society of Pediatric Radiology system (ESPR).

To date, there is no clear consensus on which of these systems offer better categorization of the dilatations, the best inter/intra-rater reliability, or the best prognostic value at the time of its assessment in cases of suspected or diagnosed urinary tract obstruction or vesicoureteric reflux. Even among pediatric urologists and surgeons, the individuals who will utilize these reports to make therapeutic and surgical decisions, no apparent consensus exists on which system is preferable. To advance communication and subsequent research in this area, a clear consensus among pediatric urologists regarding the preferable system for categorization and reporting of hydronephrosis is needed.

We hypothesize that there is no single preferred hydronephrosis grading system among pediatric surgeons and urologists. The aim of this study was to collect baseline information on the ultrasonographic reporting preferences among pediatric urologists and surgeons evaluating hydronephrosis and correlate it with the reporting system utilized in their localities.

MATERIALS AND METHODS

A 13-multiple choice questionnaire was designed by the authors (Appendix 1 in **Supplementary Material**). It was comprised of 4 questions on surgical specialty and type of practice, 4 on classification preferences, 3 related to communication with report providers, and 2 on future perspectives (Appendix 1 in **Supplementary Material**).

Institutional Review Board of the Institution of the first author waived the review by them as considered not a requirement for the present research. The participation of the responders was voluntary and considered as consent. The responders were also able to decide whether to provide their names and email contact or remain anonymous.

From November 2018 to February 2019, the questionnaire was accessible online through GoogleForm(R) platform and publicized through mailing lists (peds-urology@lists.it.uab.edu, novo-uroped@googlegroups.com, European Society for Pediatric Urology roster members database) and social media groups (Sociedad Iberoamericana de Urologia Pediatrica, Argentinian, Chilean, and Brazilian Society for Pediatric Urology). The Society for Fetal Urology advertised it through their members. Colleagues in China had an alternative link to the same survey through SurveyMonkey(R). Duplicate respondents were avoided as these survey platforms identify the respondent before allowing them to submit the survey. A secondary assessment of potential duplicated responses was performed manually by the authors reviewing case by case the answers.

The statistical analysis of the survey data consists of 3 steps: a univariate analysis by providing the frequencies and representing graphically each variable alone; a bivariate analysis by measuring dependence of each variable from a first group with each variable from a second group, this is done using a G-test which is more general than a chi-square test; and a multivariate analysis using Multiple Correspondence Analysis (MCA) to form groups of the surveyed people depending on their answers to all the questions. All the statistical analyses are performed using the R statistical software version 3.5.0.

RESULTS

Three hundred and eighty physicians participated to the questionnaire. The univariate analysis results are depicted in the **Figures 1**, **2**.

Globally, the two most preferred systems were the SFU system and the renal Pelvic AP diameter with 37 and 34%, respectively (140/380 and 129/380). The more recently developed UTD system ranked third in terms of overall preference with 18% choosing it as their preference. A minority of participants (8%) choose the mild-moderate-severe system and only 1% chose the Onen or the ESPR system (**Figure 2**, right).

The classification systems most utilized by providers was based on an open question (question 11) that permitted the participant to choose more than one classification system. Globally there were 601 responses to this question, averaging nearly 2 study systems per respondent. This resulted in an increase of the popularity of the mild-moderate-severe (28%) and a net reduction on SFU and UTD (25 and 7). The Pelvic AP diameter was slightly increased (39%) while the Onen and ESPR remained uncommon (0.3 and 1%) (**Figure 2**, left).

The bivariate analysis (**Table 1**) showed significant differences in the type of responses. Three main variables affected these differences: The geographical area for favorite classification system, communication with providers, system used by providers and attempt to build a common system, the years of experience attempting to build a common system and willingness to change the preferred system, and the volume of cases per provider.

There were significant differences in preferred grading system related to the geographical area (**Supplementary Table 1**). Asia, Europe and Oceania prefer the Pelvic AP diameter (47, 45, and 57%) whereas Middle East/North Africa and North America prefer the SFU system (63 and 59%). South America did not show a marked difference among the Pelvic AP diameter and SFU (38 and 30%). Within geographic areas, there were major differences in communication with providers. The majority of

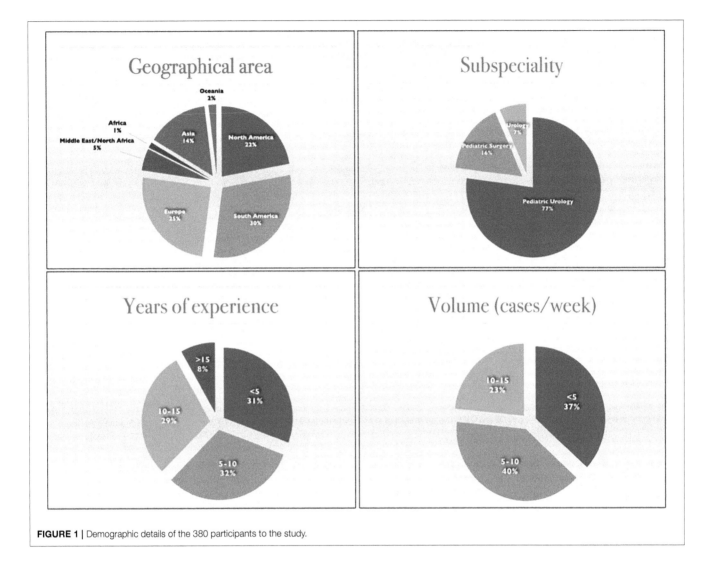

FIGURE 1 | Demographic details of the 380 participants to the study.

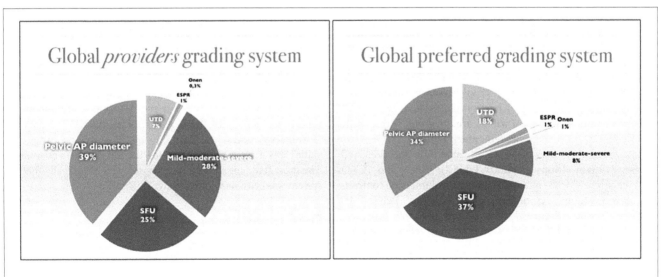

FIGURE 2 | Graphic representation of the differences between Grading systems provided and Grading systems preferred.

TABLE 1 | *P*-values corresponding to a G-test of independence between the variables Q5, Q7, Q8, …Q13 and the demographic variables Q1, …, Q4.

	Q1. What is your subspecialty?	Q2. What is your geographical area?	Q3. Years of experience in Pediatric Urology	Q4. How many cases of hydronephrosis you manage in a typical week?
Q5. When you deal with a case of hydronephrosis, which is your favorite classification system?	0.05201	**0.00000007**	0.3287	**1.955e-06**
Q7. Why do you prefer the system you use? (you can choose more than one)	0.4818	0.07535	0.7218	0.2789
Q8. What are the shortcomings of the system you use? (you can choose more than one)	0.9644	0.3354	0.6167	0.6515
Q9. Do you have direct communication with your radiology report providers?	0.3372	**0.001802**	0.1221	0.1835
Q10. If yes, how often?	0.4125	**0.00004**	0.938	0.257
Q11. Which is the most frequently used classification system you see in your practice (the one most used by your providers)? (you can choose more than one)	0.9974	**0.0000005**	0.2386	**0.0004758**
Q12. Did you attempt to build a common language for description of hydronephrosis among your own team?	0.1706	**0.001403**	**0.008423**	0.4134
Q13. Are you available to change your preference in case the majority of Pediatric Urologist prefers another grading system?	0.586	0.1987	**0.0403**	0.6104

We see that the responses to question Q5 depend on the demographic variables Q2 and Q4. Q9 is dependent on Q2. Q10 depends on Q2. The answers to Q11 depend on Q2 and Q4 while the answers to Q12 are associated with Q2 and Q3. Finally, the categories taken by Q13 depends on the categories taken by Q3. Bolded P values < 0.005.

the participants described direct communication to varying degrees (**Supplementary Table 2**). In Europe, North America and Oceania this is more common than in the rest of the world. The frequency of this contact is also different with the higher frequency in Europe and Oceana. The grading system used by providers also varied geographically (**Supplementary Table 3**). In all the regions except North America the most utilized system by the providers is the Pelvic AP diameter. In North America, the SFU system is the most frequently used. In most areas, there was an attempt to build a common system, but more common in Europe, South America, and Oceania (**Figure 3** and **Supplementary Table 4**).

Years of experience was associated with an increased attempt to build a common system (**Supplementary Table 5**). The willingness to change the preferred system (91%, range 88–98) revealed that those who most willing are the group with middle experience (10–15 years) (**Supplementary Table 6**).

The volume of cases also had an impact on the preferred grading system (**Supplementary Table 7**). SFU and UTD preference grew with increasing patient volume. In contrast, the low volume responders preferred the Pelvic AP diameter system (**Figure 3**). The system used by providers (**Supplementary Table 8**) was similar to the preferred grading system. Higher volumes correlated with preference for SFU and UTD and lower volumes with the mild-moderate-severe system.

The multivariate analysis revealed no statistically significant correlations between all the variables studied (two-dimensional correspondence analysis plot of the questionnaire data using the package ade4 in R with data points labeled by continents is available in the complementary documents of this manuscript).

The participants were able to express their opinions regarding the utility of each system by grading it from "very useful" to "useless" (question 6). This was also an open question permitting multiple responses. Scores were given according to the number of responses in each category except for "not known" which was not scored. In order to assign a numeric value to this answer, each category had a weighted multiplying factor as shown in **Table 2**. The highest scores for utility were obtained by the Pelvic AP diameter and the SFU systems. The systems categorized as "not known" by most of the participants were the ESPR and the Onen (112 and 127, respectively).

Participants were invited to express their opinion regarding the strengths of their preferred systems. Points of strength for mild-moderate-severe, Pelvic AP diameter, and SFU systems was "Familiarity" and "Simplicity." In addition, "Good prognostic value" was a strength reported for the SFU and UTD systems. The most frequent shortcomings noted were principally that the system was "Not used universally."

DISCUSSION

Prenatal and postnatal hydronephrosis is a very common condition affecting approximately 1% of pregnancies. In many countries/areas the role of pre and postnatal counseling and care for hydronephrosis is provided by Pediatric Urologist or by either Pediatric Surgeons or Adult Urologists dedicated to pediatric

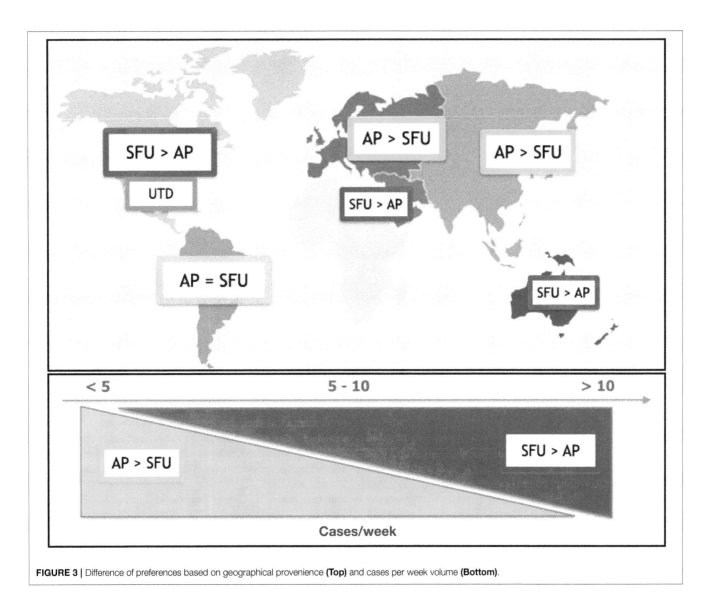

FIGURE 3 | Difference of preferences based on geographical provenience **(Top)** and cases per week volume **(Bottom)**.

patients. The goal of a common and objective language in the description of the degree and characteristics of hydronephrosis along with prognostic clinical correlation has been attempted since the wide use of ultrasound as first line investigation in both the prenatal and postnatal period. Dhillon et al. published a detailed report correlating the degree of dilatation with the clinical outcome in terms of need for surgical intervention (5). Although many experienced physicians prefer to independently assess the radiological images rather than rely on reports, the images are not always available adding delays in management decision and timing of intervention.

Grading systems have evolved in complexity over time beginning with the simpler, classic "mild-moderate-severe" system (6) and the anterior-posterior diameter (7). In 1993 the Society for Fetal Urology proposed the SFU classification system for postnatal hydronephrosis (1), followed by the European Society for Pediatric Radiology which proposed its modified system by adding the anterior-posterior diameter (2). In 2007,

Onen presented his individual experience with a modified system aimed to better stratify the ultrasound characteristics of the hydronephrotic kidney and its clinical significance (3). Finally, a consensus among several societies of Pediatric Urology, Nephrology and Radiology was accomplished in 2014 and resulted in the Urinary Tract Dilatation system (4). This system introduced additional characteristics of the urinary tract not considered in the previous systems including ureteric dilation and bladder abnormalities and can be considered an integration of the SFU and anterior-posterior diameter systems.

The evolution of classification systems has attempted to improve prognostic ability by combining additional sonographic findings. The use of multiple different classification systems makes communication and translation of research findings difficult. Over the last 30 years, multiple studies have been done evaluating the strengths and challenges of the various classification systems. Considering multiple specialities, Zanetta et al. (8) demonstrated lack of agreement within different

TABLE 2 | Opinion of the responders of each system.

	Very useful (x4)	Somewhat useful (x3)	Minimally useful (x2)	Useless (x1)	SCORE	Not known
Mild-moderate-severe system	46 (184)	125 (375)	129 (258)	53	**870**	5
Pelvic AP Diameter measurements	184 (736)	137 (411)	31 (62)	4	**1,213**	2
Society of Fetal Urology system (1)	191 (764)	125 (375)	24 (48)	2	**1,189**	8
ESPR Pediatric Uroradiology Working Group grading (2)	29 (116)	138 (276)	63 (126)	10	**528**	**112**
Onen grading system (3)	22 (88)	120 (360)	64 (128)	17	**593**	**127**
Urinary Tract Dilation (UTD) classification system (4)	113 (452)	142 (426)	51 (102)	4	**984**	**44**

Bolded values of higher significance.

specialities involved in the management of hydronephrosis both in grading system and management. Our study uniquely evaluates opinions regarding the various pediatric hydronephrosis classification systems from a large number of surgical specialists from throughout the world.

Our study supports our hypothesis that that there is no single preferred hydronephrosis grading system among pediatric surgeons and urologists. The geographical differences were subtle in some areas while particularly marked in others. This may reflect agreement between regional societies or presence of leadership opinions that influence preferences toward a particular system.

Our study is not without limitation. Although we had 380 respondents, it is not known how representative this group is of the global census of physicians that manage fetal and pediatric hydronephrosis. Currently there is no estimation of the number of physicians (pediatric urologists, pediatric surgeons) practicing worldwide. Based on the organization with the highest number of physicians dedicated to Pediatric Urology, the European Society for Pediatric Urology whose roster is of 790 members from different areas of the world (www.espu.org website) plus another 450 certified by SPU and SFU, it can be hypothesized that the number of respondents to the present survey represents a significant portion of the physicians managing cases of children with hydronephrosis. The utilization of multiple sources of engagement and repetition of the invitations was a strategy to enhance inclusion and representation as recommended by Ponto in the paper on surveys as a research tool (9).

The heterogeneity in "years of experience," "subspeciality," and "geographic area" are also limitations of the study. The lack of an overriding organization for physicians treating hydronephrosis necessitated broad solicitation of voluntary participation by physicians of differing backgrounds. Another limitation is that the opinions were expressed anonymously [although 284/380 (73%) participants voluntarily disclosed their identity] making it impossible to assess the validity of all responses.

CONCLUSION

The present survey demonstrates that there is no single preferred hydronephrosis grading system among pediatric surgeons and urologists. Despite a clear favorite, even with regional variations,

most of the physicians charged with the management of pediatric hydronephrosis prefer the SFU and APD systems because of familiarity and simplicity with these systems (37 and 34%, respectively). Respondents noted that their imaging providers most often report findings utilizing the mild-moderate-severe system or the APD measurements (28 and 39%, respectively) except for North America where the SFU system is more seen (50%). The greatest reported shortcoming of all the systems was the lack of universal utilization. Nearly all respondents were optimistic that if a consensus regarding a classification system was determined, they would be able to have this new system implemented at their institution. The observations taken from this study may serve as basis for the construction of a common worldwide system among physicians managing hydronephrosis and imaging providers. As APD and SFU are the preferred systems and the UTD a newer combination of both, it is possible that with time, UTD may become the universal language for reporting hydronephrosis. The result of this survey, however, shows that this time has not come yet.

AUTHOR CONTRIBUTIONS

SV, AB, JG, MM, CC, and P-JL: conception and design. SV, AB, JG, MM, CC, MF, HZ, and P-JL: acquisition of data. SV and ME: analysis and interpretation of data. SV, ME, JG, and CC: drafting of the manuscript. JG, CC, MF, and P-JL: critical revision of the manuscript for important intellectual content. ME: statistical analysis. All authors contributed to the article and approved the submitted version.

SUPPLEMENTARY MATERIAL

Supplementary Figure 1 | Two-dimensional correspondence analysis plot of the questionnaire data using the package ade4 in R. The data points are labeled by continents.

Supplementary Table 1 | Preferred system by geographical area.

Supplementary Table 2 | Communication with providers by geographical area.

Supplementary Table 3 | System by providers by geographical area.

Supplementary Table 4 | Attempt to build a common system by geographical area.

Supplementary Table 5 | Attempt to build a common system by years of experience.

Supplementary Table 6 | Availability to change the preferred system by years of experience.

Supplementary Table 7 | Preferred system by number of cases seen by week.

Supplementary Table 8 | System by providers by number of cases seen by week.

REFERENCES

1. Fernbach SK, Maizels M, Conway JJ. Ultrasound grading of hydronephrosis: introduction to the system used by the Society for Fetal Urology. *Pediatr Radiol.* (1993) 23:478–80.

2. Riccabona M, Avni FE, Blickman JG, Dacher JN, Darge K, Lobo ML, et al. Imaging recommendations in paediatric uroradiology: minutes of the ESPR workgroup session on urinary tract infection, fetal hydronephrosis, urinary tract ultrasonography and voiding cystourethrography, Barcelona, Spain, June 2007. *Pediatr Radiol.* (2008) 38:138–45. doi: 10.1007/s00247-007-0695-7

3. Onen A. An alternative grading system to refine the criteria for severity of hydronephrosis and optimal treatment guidelines in neonates with primary UPJ-type hydronephrosis. *J Pediatr Urol.* (2007) 3:200–5. doi: 10.1016/j.jpurol.2006.08.002

4. Nguyen HT, Benson CB, Bromley B, Campbell JB, Chow J, Coleman B, et al. Multidisciplinary consensus on the classification of prenatal and postnatal urinary tract dilation (UTD classification system). *J Pediatr Urol.* (2014) 10:982–98. doi: 10.1016/j.jpurol.2014.10.002

5. Dhillon HK. Prenatally diagnosed hydronephrosis: the Great Ormond Street experience. *Br J Urol.* (1998) 81(Suppl. 2):39–44.

6. Ellenbogen PH, Scheible FW, Talner LB, Leopold GR. Sensitivity of gray scale ultrasound in detecting urinary tract obstruction. *Am J Roentgenol.* (1978) 130:731–3.

7. Grignon A, Filion R, Filiatrault D, Robitaille P, Homsy Y, Boutin H, et al. Urinary tract dilatation *in utero*: classification and clinical applications. *Radiology.* (1986) 160:645–7.

8. Zanetta VC, Rosman BM, Bromley B, Shipp TD, Chow JS, Campbell JB, et al. Variations in management of mild prenatal hydronephrosis among maternal-fetal medicine obstetricians, and pediatric urologists and radiologists. *J Urol.* (2012) 188:1935–9. doi: 10.1016/j.juro.2012.07.011

9. Ponto J. Understanding and evaluating survey research. *J Adv Pract Oncol.* (2015) 6:168–71.

2

Prenatal Diagnosis and Findings in Ureteropelvic Junction Type Hydronephrosis

Recep Has* and Tugba Sarac Sivrikoz

Division of Perinatology, Department of Obstetrics and Gynecology, Istanbul Faculty of Medicine, Istanbul University, Istanbul, Turkey

*Correspondence:
Recep Has
recephas@gmail.com

The widespread use of obstetric ultrasonography has increased the detection rate of antenatal hydronephrosis. Although most cases of antenatal hydronephrosis are transient, one third persists and becomes clinically important. Ultrasound has made differential diagnosis possible to some extent. Ureteropelvic junction type hydronephrosis (UPJHN) is one of the most common cause of persistent fetal hydronephrosis and occurs three times more in male fetuses. It is usually sporadic and unilateral. However, when bilateral kidneys are involved and presents with severe hydronephrosis, the prognosis may be poor. Typical ultrasound findings of UPJHN is hydronephrosis without hydroureter. The size and appearance of the fetal bladder is usually normal without thickening of the bladder wall. Several grading systems are developed and increasingly being used to define the severity of prenatal hydronephrosis and provides much more information about prediction of postnatal renal prognosis. If fetal urinary tract dilation is detected; laterality, severity of hydronephrosis, echogenicity of the kidneys, presence of ureter dilation should be assessed. Bladder volume and emptying, sex of the fetus, amniotic fluid volume, and presence of associated malformations should be evaluated. Particularly the ultrasonographic signs of renal dysplasia, such as increased renal parenchymal echogenicity, thinning of the renal cortex, the presence of cortical cysts, and co-existing oligohydramnios should be noticed. Unfortunately, there is no reliable predictor of renal function in UPJHN cases. Unilateral hydronephrosis cases suggesting UPJHN are mostly followed up conservatively. However, the cases with bilateral involvement are still difficult to manage. Timing of delivery is also controversial.

Keywords: fetal hydronephrosis, ureteropelvic junction obstruction, fetal pelviectasia, pediatric urinary tract dilation, ultrasound

KEY CONCEPTS

- UPJHN is the most common cause of persistent antenatal hydronephrosis. It is usually unilateral and three times more in male fetuses.
- UPJHN may be 10–30% bilateral and should be managed cautiously for the deterioration of renal functions.
- In all cases with prenatal UPJHN, AP renal pelvis diameter, presence and localization of calyx dilation, renal parenchymal features, presence of urinoma and oligohydramnios should be assessed.

- Patients in the high-risk group should be monitored during the prenatal period with an interval of 2–4 weeks, however patient monitoring should be customized according to the other negative findings.
- When UPJHN is detected during the prenatal period, consulting with pediatric urologists before delivery may contribute the postnatal management plans.

INTRODUCTION

Congenital hydronephrosis is one of the most common anomalies encountered at the prenatal ultrasound evaluation. It is observed in 1–4% of all pregnancies (1, 2).

Prenatal urinary system evaluation should preferably follow an anatomical sequence in order to identify the cause of the dilation. Therefore, urinary system examination in the prenatal period should demonstrate position of bilateral kidneys, dilation of renal pelvis and presence of calyx dilation (central and peripheral), echogenicity of kidney parenchyma, both ureters, bladder size and wall thickness, and anatomy of the external genitalia.

Detection of urinary system malformations are related to the week of gestation when the screening has been performed. Urinary system is usually assessed at 19–21 weeks of gestation, and late onset hydronephrosis is commonly missed during this period. Therefore, urinary system anomalies are not infrequently identified in the third trimester up to a rate of 5% (3).

URINARY SYSTEM EVALUATION WITH PRENATAL ULTRASOUND

Examination of the urinary system in fetal ultrasound scan begins with identifying the presence of kidneys and bladder. From the 11–12 weeks of gestation, fetal kidneys can be visualized by transvaginal ultrasonography as hyperechogenic structures (4) (**Figure 1a**). Fetal kidneys are imaged in the abdomen at both sides of vertebral column on axial, longitudinal and coronal planes (**Figures 1b–d**). Kidneys appear as two round paravertebral structures on axial views and renal pelvis oriented toward the midline (**Figure 1b**). The appearance of normal kidney looks bean-like on longitudinal and coronal planes. At coronal plane, both kidneys can be visualized on the same section and can be compared to each other (**Figure 1d**). Size of the kidneys can be evaluated by measuring the renal length and comparing it to normal charts. Normal kidneys have the same echogenicity with liver and spleen (**Figure 1c**). When kidney echogenicity is higher than spleen or liver, it is considered to be hyperechogenic. The cortex and medulla of the kidneys also become differentiable in fetuses older than 18 weeks and difference becomes more significant toward the third trimester (**Figures 1c,d**, **2c**). The renal cortex is slightly echogenic at the periphery of medulla. The adrenal glands are located cranial to the kidneys as more hypoechogenic structures (**Figures 1c, 2d**).

After evaluation of the location of both kidneys, parenchymal features, the assessment of the dilation (pelviectasis) of the renal pelvis should be made. From the beginning of the second trimester, renal pelvis becomes detectable and the kidneys generally lose their previous hyperechogenic appearance. Renal pelvis always appears as a sonolucent area in the medial of the kidneys (**Figure 1b**). Pelviectasis or hydronephrosis is evaluated in the sections of the fetal abdominal transverse planes, by measuring the anteroposterior diameter (APD) of the renal pelvis, where possible the fetal back is perpendicular to the probe (**Figure 2a**). Dilation of the renal pelvis may differ by gestational week, maternal hydration, or bladder distension (5–7).

The bladder can be visualized into the fetal pelvis from the 10th week of pregnancy, however from the 12th week on the pelvis it should be visible as a sonolucent cystic structure between both umbilical vessels (**Figure 2b**). Ideal position to measure bladder wall thickness is near the umbilical arteries in axial plane of the fetal pelvic area. Bladder wall thickness does not exceed 2 mm in prenatal period regardless of gestational week (8, 9). Fetal bladder empties and refills every 25–30 min during second and third trimester. Although nomogram charts to check the bladder size may be used, subjective assessment is usually gives

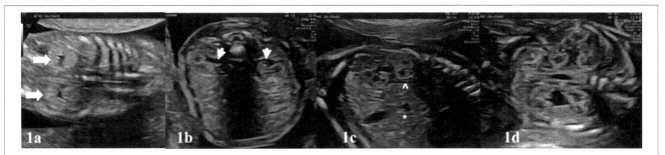

FIGURE 1 | In **(a)**, kidneys of a 12-week fetus. The best visualization of kidneys (white bold arrows) can be obtained in coronal plane with transvaginal ultrasound at this gestational age. **(b)** Transabdominal ultrasound shows the normal appearance of both kidneys on the axial plane at 20 + 6 weeks of gestation. Kidneys are located both sides of vertebra and renal pelvis (white arrow-heads) oriented toward the midline. **(c)** Longitudinal plane, echogenicity of the kidney is comparable to the liver (*). Hypoechoic adrenal gland (∧) is located cranial to the kidney. Cortico-medullary differantiation (white chevron) can be noticed. **(d)** Coronal plane shows two bean-like kidneys in the same section. This plane is useful to compare the kidneys. The corticomedullary differantiation can be noticed easily on the coronal plane.

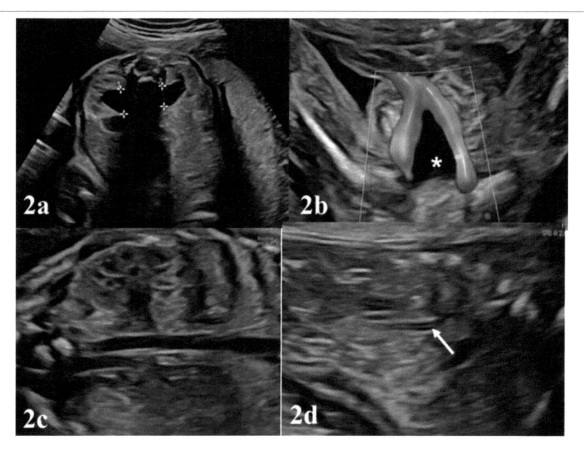

FIGURE 2 | (a), the normal appearance of the fetal bladder (white asterisk) in the pelvis between both umbilical vessels. (b) The appearance of kidneys in the 22 weeks with mild renal pelvis diameter. Antero-posterior diameter (APD) of pelvis renalis should be measured in the axial plane, better if fetus in dorso-anterior position. (c) Note the corticomedullary differentiation in a normal appearing fetal kidney. In (d), white arrow depicts the surrenal gland lying on the kideny, shown as echogenic medulla and hypoechogenic cortex.

satisfactory information. Ureters and urethra are not typically visible structures in the prenatal period. These structures may be visualized when dilated in case of bladder outlet obstruction or vesicoureteral reflux.

Fetal urine is the primary source of the amniotic fluid after 14–16 weeks of gestation. Normal volume of amniotic fluid is not only the predictor of normal renal function, but also needed for proper development of fetal lungs. Therefore, the assessment of urinary system should also include evaluation of amniotic fluid volume.

To summarize, when antenatal hydronephrosis (ANH) is diagnosed, the following parameters should be examined in a certain order by ultrasound:

- Severity and progress of hydronephrosis: As the APD increases, the possibility of concomitant congenital urinary system anomalies increases. Presence of calyx dilation and involvement of central or peripheral calices should be assessed. Repeat ultrasound examinations in the second and third trimesters will guide to determine neonatal prognosis. In the presence of severe pelviectasis, the need for surgical intervention may significantly increase in the neonatal period (10).

- Laterality: Such as, if UPJHN is bilateral, the risk for additional congenital kidney anomalies and renal function impairment is increased.
- Parenchymal appearance: An echogenic renal cortex suggests abnormal change of the renal parenchyma. The presence of parenchyma thinning or cortical cyst is associated with impaired renal function. These changes are often observed as consequence of UPJHN, and other lower urinary tract obstructions such as posterior urethral valve (PUV) or VUR.
- Urinoma/urinary ascites: Urinoma is an encapsulated paranephric pseudocyst confined to the Gerota's fascia. It often develops secondary to obstructive pathologies. Although it is rare, it co-exists with dysplastic non-functional kidney on the same side in 80% of cases (11). Urinary ascites develops in cases with lower urinary tract obstruction following to spontaneous or iatrogenic rupture of the kidney or bladder.
- Ureter: Ureter dilation is not observed with UPJHN. It is typically associated with obstructions distal to the uretero-pelvic junction, such as PUV and other infravesical obstructions or vesico-ureteral reflux (VUR) (Figures 4a,b).
- Bladder/ureterocele: Bladder size, appearance, and wall thickness are normal in UPJHN. If increased bladder wall thickness and trabeculation is detected, obstruction distal to

the bladder neck (PUV) should be considered (**Figures 4a,b**). Ureterocele is a cystic dilation of ureter detected inside the bladder. It is usually seen with duplication of the collecting system anomalies, secondary to distended ureters.
- Amniotic fluid volume: Oligohydramniosis develops after decreased urine output due to the urinary tract obstruction or decreased urine production as a result of impaired renal function. It is usually predictor of poor prognosis and implicates severe renal disease, where both kidneys are affected.

EVALUATION OF ANTEROPOSTERIOR PELVIS DIAMETER (APD) AND CLASSIFICATION

Fetal hydronephrosis is usually detected by ultrasound in the second trimester and defined as a renal pelvis diameter measurement above ≥4 mm. As gestational week progresses, definition of threshold values for dilation of the renal pelvis increases in the prenatal period (7) (**Table 1**). A measurement of ≤ 3 mm is considered normal in all gestational weeks (12). Mild hydronephrosis (APD 4–10 mm) may be a transient finding, or rarely associated with renal or chromosomal abnormalities. More severe dilation increases the risk of congenital anomalies of the kidney and urinary tract (CAKUT). Nguyen et al. reported that 50–70% of the urinary system dilations detected in antenatal period are temporary (7). Determining specific limit values for each trimester of the pregnancy is important for the frequency, follow-up and management of the pelviectasis in both prenatal and postnatal period. Among the prenatal mild pelviectasis cases, only a small proportion have a serious problem in the postnatal period. Renal pathology is confirmed in postnatal period in 12–14% of mild, 45% of moderate and 90% of severe pelviectasis cases detected in the second and third trimesters of pregnancy (13). Presence of calyx dilation and identification of parenchymal echogenicity is important for the prediction of clinically significant ANH cases (14). When calyx dilation (pelvicaliectasis) is accompanied to the renal pelvis dilation, the location should also be defined as central or peripheral. This is important for the classification and prediction of prognosis.

In order to plan postnatal follow-up, several classification systems for the urinary tract dilation (UTD) have been proposed based on ultrasonographic findings. The most common used classification systems are the Society for Fetal Urology (SFU) Hydronephrosis Grading System and the Urinary Tract Dilation (UTD) Classification System (1, 7). SFU system has five grades (0–4) (7). In this classification system, intra and extra-renal dilation of the renal pelvis is defined subjectively. Dilation of central and peripheral calyces is assessed and parenchymal thickness is described subjectively (**Table 2**).

In UTD classification system, measurement of renal pelvis antero-posterior diameter, presence of calyx dilation, subjective definition of parenchymal thickness and parenchymal appearance are specified. Dilation of ureters, assessment of

TABLE 1 | Stage of antenatal hydronephrosis (ANH) based on renal pelvis APD in relation to gestational age.

Degree of ANH	APD at 2nd trimester	APD at 3rd trimester
Mild	4–7 mm	7–9 mm
Moderate	7–10 mm	9–15 mm
Severe	>10 mm	>15 mm

TABLE 2 | The sonographic SFU Grading system for fetal urology (https://www.uab.edu/images/peduro/SFU).

	Pattern of renal sinus
SFU grade 0	No splitting
SFU grade 1	Urine in pelvis barely splits sinus
SFU grade 2	Urine fills intrarenal pelvis
SFU grade 2	Urine fills extrarenal pelvis, major (central) calyces dilated
SFU grade 3	SFU G2 and minor (peripheral) calyces uniformly dilated and parenchyma preserved
SFU grade 4	SFU G3 and parenchyma thin

bladder (wall thickness, ureterocele, and dilated posterior urethra) and presence of oligohydramnios are also considered (**Table 3**) (1). The most important difference of this classification is, quantitative assessment of urinary system (1). Patients are monitored in the prenatal period by separating them into low-risk and high-risk groups according to the severity of the features determined in the UTD classification. As the grade advances prognostic significance increases in UTD system. For example, a fetus has 9 mm renal pelvis AP diameter with increased echogenicity of the kidneys is classified in high-risk group. UTD system may be used also for postnatal cases. This system can evaluate antenatal and postnatal hydronephrosis simultanously, therefore, some studies stated that it is the classification system with the highest correlation with neonatal results (15).

An alternative classification system for primary UPJHN was proposed by Onen in 2007 (14). According to Onen's grading system (AGS), isolated pelvic dilation was classified as grade 1. Grade 2 is the presence of calyx dilation in addition to renal pelvis dilation. Grade 3 includes <50% loss in renal parenchyma and grade 4 has severe parenchymal loss. AGS covers essentially neonatal period and is used only for primary UPJHN. Using AGS grading system may simplify the follow-up and treatment plan in postnatal patients with UPJHN. However, it may be difficult to assess the thinning of medulla and cortex separately in the fetus particularly before the third trimester and this system needs to be studied in prenatal period to make a statement on it. UTD system is actually combination of APD classification and SFU and provides more information for the diagnosis. More studies are needed to be done in the prenatal period to compare the SFU, UTD, and AGS classification systems for UPJHN. A comparison of all three grading systems and radiological assessment is demonstrated in **Table 4** (16).

TABLE 3 | Urinary Tract Dilation Classification System.

Ultrasound findings	Time at presentation		
	16–27 weeks	≥28 weeks	Postnatal (>48 h)
Anterior-posterior renal pelvis diameter (APRPD)	<4 mm	<7 mm	<10 mm
Calyceal dilatation	No	No	No
Central	No (if yes high risk)	No (if yes high risk)	No (if yes high risk)
Peripheral			
Parenchymal thickness	Normal	Normal	Normal
Parenchymal appearance(echogenicity, corticomedullar differentiation, pericortical cysts, urinoma)	Normal	Normal	Normal
Ureter(s)	Normal	Normal	Normal
Bladder	Normal	Normal	Normal
Oligohydramnios	No	No	NA

TABLE 4 | Prenatal and postnatal evaluation systems used in UPJHN classification (Courtesy of Onen A, 2020, in press).

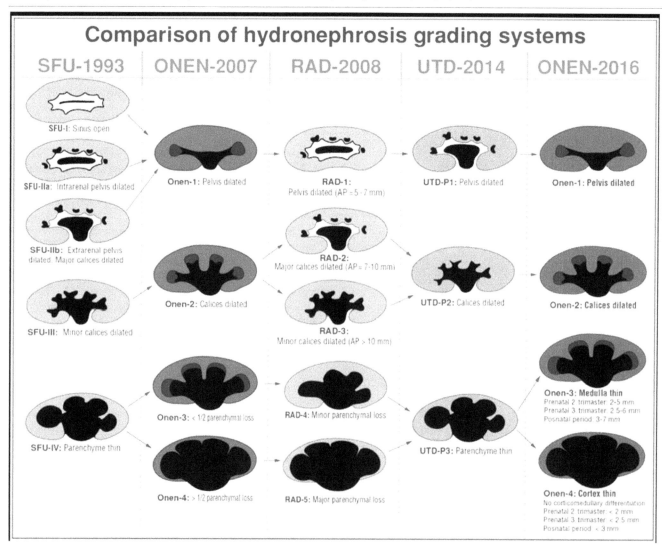

ULTRASONOGRAPHIC FINDINGS OF UPJHN IN THE PRENATAL PERIOD

The main cause of hydronephrosis is obstruction at any level of the urinary system. Some obstructive changes may develop very early in fetal life and may cause cystic-dysplastic pathology in the fetal kidney. Therefore, the initial time of obstruction and its consequences are as important as the severity of the dilation. UPJHN is the most common reason of ANH Other causes include vesico-ureteral reflux, uretero-vesical junction obstruction, posterior urethral valve, and other rare incidents (1). Each is caused by different levels of obstruction and carries different ultrasonographic features. Accurate prenatal diagnosis will not only provide appropriate follow-up and prenatal interventions, but also help to prepare for the postnatal management.

The most common pathological cause of antenatal hydronephrosis UPJHN constitutes 10–30% of antenatal hydronephrosis (7). It is reported in 1/750–1/1,500 live births (17). UPJHN is three times more common in males than in females particularly in the neonatal period (18). It is usually sporadic, unilateral and mostly the left side (68%) is affected (19, 20). The etiology of uretero-pelvic junction obstruction is obscure with an adynamic narrow segment causing the obstruction (21).

Typical finding in UPJHN in prenatal ultrasound is unilateral renal pelvis dilation with or without caliectasis, while the ureter is not dilated (**Figures 3a,b**, **Video S1**). Bladder dimensions and bladder wall thickness are normal in UPJHN. Presence and localization of caliectasis as central or peripheral, is important for grading systems of SFU and UTD, particularly in prenatal period. Evaluation of appearance of the parenchyma is also essential. As the pelviectasia/caliectasia advances, the parenchyma thickness decreases and echogenicity increases on the affected kidney.

Assessment of the severity of the dilation is essential for the grading systems in all cases of hydronephrosis detected in prenatal ultrasound. For example, in SFU grade 3 dilation, pelvis and peripheral calyces are dilated, but parenchymal thickness is normal (**Table 2**) (7). However, in SFU grade 4, the parenchyma gets thinner. The difference between SFU grade 1 and 2 is the presence of central calyx dilation in grade 2, independent of the measurement of pelvic dilation. Similar to the UTD system, the SFU grading system can be used both in the pediatric and in the prenatal period.

Most of the urinary system anomalies can be diagnosed by prenatal ultrasound. However, with maternal obesity, advanced gestational week or presence of oligohydramniosis, visualization of the structures may be challenging. Fetal magnetic resonance

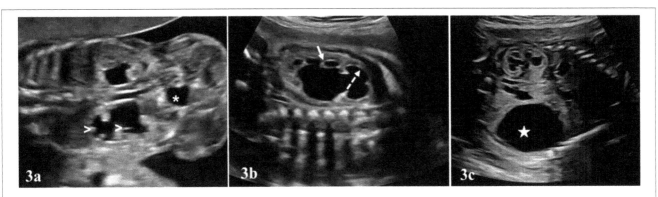

FIGURE 3 | In **(a)**, bilateral UPJHN is seen in a fetus at 22 weeks of pregnancy. Renal pelvis dilated in both kidneys. There is also dilated calyces in the lower kidney (white arrow heads). The size and appearence of the bladder (asterisk *) is normal, and ureters are not visible. **(b)** Central (dashed arrow) and peripheral calyces (short arrow) in the renal pelvis are dilated. Renal parenchyma is also thinned. **(c)** Increased echogenicity in the renal parenchyma (upper kidney). A large urinoma (white star) was seen in the lower kidney.

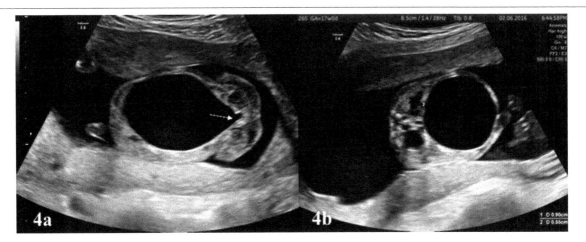

FIGURE 4 | **(a)** Large bladder with "key hole" appearance (white colored dashed arrow) is typical finding of infravesical obstruction, mostly due to PUV in male fetuses. **(b)** The affected kidneys in the same fetus **(a)** showing increased renal pelvis diameter and parenchymal echogenicity.

imaging (MRI) is an important adjunct to ultrasound in evaluation of fetal urogenital system. While ultrasound remains the primary diagnostic modality, MRI helps in more complicated cases or where ultrasound is limited due to technical factors such as poor acoustic window (22). Prenatal MRI may also be useful in differential diagnosis of VUR from UPJHN, particularly in positions where the fetal pelvis is difficult to visualize the ureter dilation (23). Imaging in T1-T2-weighted MRI sequences is rather guiding to evaluate the functional status of fetal kidneys (24). Kajbafzadeh et al. reported that the sensitivity of prenatal MRI in differential diagnosis of urinary system anomalies was 92% in their study (24). Particularly, MRI is informative when type of calyx dilation is difficult to distinguish in cases with prenatal UPJHN (24).

OTHER URINARY SYSTEM ULTRASOUND FINDINGS IN PRENATAL UPJHN

The excessively dilated collection system rarely ruptures spontaneously in UPJHN. As a result, an encapsulated paranephric pseudocyst (urinoma) confined to the Gerota's fascia is formed (25, 26). The urinoma is located on the affected kidney side as an elliptical or crescentric cystic mass adjacent to the kidney and vertebral column (**Figure 3c**). Similar to in UPJHN, urinoma can occur in the cases with PUV, where the intrarenal pressure can be high enough to cause rupture. PUV can be differentiated more easily with the presence of large bladder which typically looks like a key hole and coexist with bilateral hydroureteronephrosis (**Figures 4a,b**).

Urinoma is often detected at 19–30 weeks of gestation in UPJHN. Other cystic structures such as lymphangioma, neuroblastoma and ureteric duplication, which are located in this region, should also be considered in differential diagnosis (27). Modifying the time of delivery or interventions such as shunt placement to the urinoma is not necessary in the prenatal period. Urinomas may regress spontaneously before birth, but this does not imply better prognosis. The presence of urinoma with the dysplastic changes in the kidney parenchyma is associated with a poor prognosis (25, 27). Postnatal normal kidney function in UPJHN cases affected by ipsilateral urinoma is only 7% (28, 29). Another study reported that the prognosis is more morbid in the presence of urinoma with prenatal UPJHN than other urinary tract obstructions (11).

Oligohydramniosis is one of the most important prognostic parameters in evaluating kidney functions in fetal life. Single vertical pocket (SVP) or amniotic fluid index (AFI) are the most frequently used methods in the evaluation of oligohydramniosis. The threshold used to define oligohydramniosis is SVP ≤ 2 cm or AFI ≤ 5 cm. Bilateral UPJHN with dysplastic changes in kidneys and subsequent oligohydramniosis indicates poor prognosis (18, 30). Since chronic oligohydramniosis is associated with fetal lung hypoplasia, it affects neonatal prognosis directly.

Bilateral UPJHN is detected 10–30% in prenatal ultrasound (20) (**Figure 3a**, **Video S1**) and it is frequently detected in <6 month old infants in neonatal period (8, 20). The most diagnostic challenge is differentiation of bilateral UPJHN cases

with VUR. VUR is more common in girls, and hydronephrosis is typically presented with ureter dilation (**Video S2**). Since postnatal management of VUR cases is different from UPJHN, its differentiation in the prenatal period is also important for follow up and management.

Another factor determining the prognosis in prenatal and postnatal period is the appearance of the contralateral kidney. Additional urinary system anomalies are present in 50% of UPJHN. The most common condition which is seen in contralateral kidney is UPJHN. Among the other urinary system anomalies, multicystic dyplastic kidney (MCDK) (**Figure 5a**), VUR, duplication of the collecting system, rotation and fusion anomalies in the other kidney are reported in conjunction with UPJHN (18). The actual incidence of MCDK with UPJHN is unknown, and its frequency has been reported to range between 2 and 27% (31). Since monitoring and management changes in the presence of other kidney anomalies, the anatomy and location of the contralateral kidney should be carefully evaluated.

OTHER SYSTEM ANOMALIES CO-EXISTING WITH UPJHN IN PRENATAL ULTRASONOGRAPHY

The incidence of chromosome anomalies accompanying prenatal UPJHN obstruction is relatively low and reported around 1–3%. Karyotype analysis is not crucial in isolated cases when other parameters are favorable. However, in the presence of associated anomalies, prenatal diagnostic invasive procedures should be offered (32). Congenital heart disease, VA(C)TER(L) association, Schinzel-Giedon syndrome and Camptomelic dysplasia are among the most common other system anomalies associated with UPJHN in the prenatal period (33, 34). A comprehensive fetal anatomy scan should be carried out for other systems, particularly including fetal heart, gastrointestinal tract and spine (8, 18).

PARAMETERS DETERMINING POOR PROGNOSIS IN PRENATAL UPJHN

Prenatal management of UPJHN primarily depends on the APD, taken into account by the gestational week. Progression of the obstruction, presence of dilation in calyx system and parenchymal condition of the affected kidney guides the follow-up. Gestational age at presentation, presence of unilateral or bilateral involvement, and other coexisting anomalies are important to determine the prognosis. If there is bilateral UPJ obstruction, associated anomaly in the contra-lateral kidney and/or oligohydramniosis, the prognosis will be negatively affected.

Jiang et al. reported a spontaneous regression rate of 61%, and persistence rate of 23% in cases diagnosed with antenatal bilateral UPJHN (35). Probability of postnatal surgery was 15% in cases where renal pelvis AP diameter was ≥ 15 mm (35). When calyx dilatation is ≥ 10 mm, spontaneous resolution is 37%, the possibility of persistence is 29% and the surgical requirement is around 33% (35). However, in cases where calyx dilatation

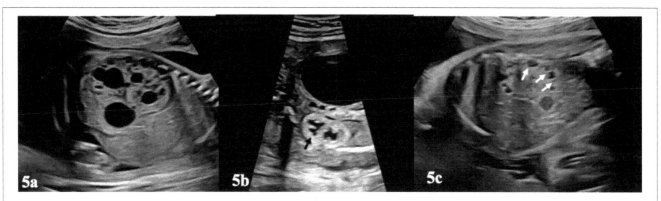

FIGURE 5 | (a) Depicts a multicystic-dysplastic kidney, which can be seen in the contralateral kidney in a fetus with prenatal UPJHN in other kidney. Notice the difference between **(a,c)** and **Figure 3**. **(b)** This figure shows increased echogenicity of the lower kidney and loss of cortico-medullary differentiation of renal parenchyma (blac arrow). **(c)** Pericortical cysts (white arrows) and echogenic parenchyma was shown on **(b)**.

was <5 mm and AP diameter was <10 mm, 90–100% regression was reported, and there is virtually no need for surgery (0–3.7%) (35). This study has shown that pelvic AP diameter plays a primary role along with calyx dilation in determining the follow-up process and the need for intervention. Perlman et.al. analyzed the outcome of 35 fetuses diagnosed with severe isolated hydronephrosis (AP diameter >15 mm) and 48 fetuses with associated with congenital anomalies of the kidney and urinary tract (CAKUT) (10). The CAKUT group was associated with a significantly increased incidence of postnatal need for surgery (17.6 vs. 44.2%, $P = 0.014$), dysplastic kidney (0 vs. 14%, $P = 0.023$), and total abnormal outcome (52.9 vs. 86%, $P = 0.001$). A recent meta-analysis assessed the diagnostic value of APD of the fetal renal pelvis in predicting postnatal surgery. Diagnostic OR of antero-posterior diameter for predicting postnatal surgery was 13.3 mm. The authors suggested 15 mm AP diameter of APD may be used as a cut-off for the prediction of surgery (36). Elmaci et al. emphasized that spontaneous resolution rate was 71%, especially in cases with UPJHN-type antenatal hydronephrosis, where APD was ≤ 20 mm (37).

Regardless of etiology of hydronephrosis, abnormal parenchyma (thin and/or echogenic) appearance is a common parameter used in both SFU (grade 4) and UTD (high risk) classifications. The thickness and echogenicity of parenchyma affected by UPJHN is particularly important to predict renal function (**Figures 3c, 5b**). However, there is no consensus regarding the location of the assessment of parenchymal thickness prenatally. Moreover, subjective determination of parenchymal thickness may cause more conflicting results. Correlation between parenchymal thickness and prognosis is not clear even in postnatal studies (38). Nevertheless, loss of uniform structure of the renal parenchyma, presence of peri-cortical renal cysts (**Figure 5c**) and increased renal parenchymal echogenicity in prenatal ultrasound are associated with impaired renal function (**Figures 3b, 5b**) (39).

Despite all efforts, the contribution of SFU and UTD systems to prediction of prognosis in antenatal hydronephrosis is still uncertain (40). Both is proposed to be used regardless of etiology of hydronephrosis. Several studies have shown that inter-observer reliability of UTD classification is superior to SFU classification (41, 42). The use of other urinary system ultrasound parameters (kidney echogenicity, ureter dilation, ureterocele, oligohydramnios) in UTD classification increases its reliability. Renal pelvis AP diameter is the only quantitative criteria in UTD classification. However, other studies have shown that AP diameter does not make any significant predictive impact in terms of prognosis compared to other parameters (40, 41). A comparison of UTD and SFU grading system for their ability to predict time to hydronephrosis resolution showed that cumulative resolution rate at 3 years was higher in SFU grades (43). Among 401 patients 328 (82%) had resolution in 24 ± 18 months in study population (43). The lower the grade the better the resolution in both grading systems.

PRENATAL FOLLOW-UP AND MANAGEMENT OF DELIVERY

Fetuses with UPJHN should be followed up with ultrasound at regular intervals in prenatal period. Observation of regression, stable continuation or progression should be noted. Spontaneous resolution is often associated with mild dilated renal pelvis AP diameter. Of the 80% cases of the dilation between 4 and 8 mm are resolved, whereas only <15% of the >9 mm cases are regressed in the second trimester (44). Low-risk group includes patients with mild APD with normal kidney echogenicity, normal cortico-medullary differentiation, absence of peripheral calyx dilation. Therefore, it may be appropriate to re-evaluate the low-risk cases only for a second time in the third trimester. The unfavorable prognostic findings are; severe AP dilation (≥7 mm before 28 week or ≥10 mm after), increased kidney echogenicity, parenchymal thinning, peripheral calyx dilatation, presence of oligohydramnios, abnormality in the contra-lateral kidney and presence of bilateral UPJHN. Prenatal ultrasound follow-up examination in 2 week intervals is recommended by most authors in cases with unilateral severe UPJHN, bilateral

UPJHN or contra-lateral kidney anomaly (7, 30). Other mild cases should be followed up with 4–6 week intervals until birth (1, 7, 45).

It is recommended to evaluate these cases together with pediatric urologists during the prenatal period, where possible. Multidisciplinary management of the cases will contribute positively to the postnatal outcome (46).

Several studies have shown that the timing or type of delivery does not affect the postnatal course in cases with UPJHN. Benjamin et al. investigated the impact of gestational age on urologic outcomes for the fetuses with hydronephrosis and concluded that late preterm/early term delivery resulted in worse short-term postnatal renal outcomes. They recommended delivery at 39 weeks (47). However, the cases with oligohydramniosis (bilateral UPJHN or contralateral kidney anomaly) are associated with loss of renal function in the third trimester, and earlier delivery may be considered for this group, although the benefit is questionable.

CONCLUSION

Ultrasonography has the essential place in prenatal diagnosis, and has a key role in the antenatal diagnosis of kidney anomalies. Hydronephrosis is the most frequently diagnosed urinary system anomaly in the prenatal period. UPJHN is the most common pathological finding of the fetal genitourinary system. Although it is usually unilateral and have a favorable postnatal prognosis, outcome may be poor when bilateral or when associated with severity indicators. Unfavorable prognostic factors which indicate loss of kidney function are; increase in kidney echogenicity, loss of cortico-medullary differentiation, presence of pericortical cysts, and oligohydramniosis. Ultrasound follow up of the findings in the urinary system at certain intervals is important for the management of pre and postnatal period. Adaption of one of the classification systems such as UTD or SFU or AGS may contribute to the objective assessment of both prenatal and postnatal management. In the absence of obstetric risk factors such as presence of oligohydramnios, positive contribution of delivery timing to the prognosis has not been demonstrated yet.

AUTHOR CONTRIBUTIONS

RH: drafting the work and revising it. TS: providing images, drafting the work, and revising it. All authors listed on manuscript have participated in the present work.

REFERENCES

1. Nguyen HT, Benson CB, Bromley B, Campbell JB, Crow J, Coleman B, et al. Multidisciplinary consensus on the classification of prenatal and postnatal urinary tract dilatation (UTD Classification system). *J Pediatr Urol.* (2014) 10:982–99. doi: 10.1016/j.jpurol.2014.10.002

2. Chiodini B, Ghassemi M, Khelif K, Ismaili K. Clinical outcome of children with antenatally diagnosed hydronephrosis. *Front Pediatr.* (2019) 7:103. doi: 10.3389/fped.2019.00103

3. Odibo AO, Marchiano D, Quinones JN, Riesch D, Egan JF, Macones GA. Mild pyelectasis: evaluating the relationship between gestational age and renal pelvic anterior-posterior diameter. *Prenat Diagn.* (2003) 23:824–7. doi: 10.1002/pd.709

4. Bronshtein M, Kushnir O, Ben-Rafael Z, Shalev E, Nebel L, Mashiach S, et al. Transvaginal sonographic measurement of fetal kidneys in the first trimester of pregnancy. *J Clin Ultrasound.* (1990) 18:299–301. doi: 10.1002/jcu.1870180413

5. Anderson N, Clautice-Engle T, Allan R, Abbott G, Wells JE. Detection of obstructive uropathy in the fetus: predictive value of sonographic measurements of renal pelvic diameter at various gestational ages. *Am J Roent.* (1995) 164:719–23. doi: 10.2214/ajr.164.3.7863901

6. Odibo AO, Raab E, Elowitz M, Merril JD, Macones GA. Prenatal mild pyelectasis: evaluating the thresholds of renal pelvic diameter associated with normal postnatal renal function. *J Ultrasound Med.* (2004) 23:513–7. doi: 10.7863/jum.2004.23.4.513

7. Nguyen HT, Herndon CD, Cooper C, Gatti J, Kirsch A, Kokorowski P, et al. Society for urology consensus statement on the evaluation and management of antenatal hydronephrosis. *J Pediatr Urol.* (2010) 6:478–80. doi: 10.1016/j.jpurol.2010.02.205

8. Paladini D, Volpe P. *Ultrasound of Congenital Anomalies,* 2nd ed. New York, NY: CRC Press (2014). p. 307–309. doi: 10.1201/b16779

9. Leung VY, Rasalkar DD, Liu JX, Sreedhar B, Yeung CK, Chu WC. Dynamic ultrasound study on urinary bladder in infants with antenatally detected fetal hydronephrosis. *Pediatr Res.* (2010) 67:440–3. doi: 10.1203/PDR.0b013e3181d22b91

10. Perlman S, Roitman L, Lotan D, Kivilevitch Z, Pode-Shakked N, Pode-Shakked B, et al. Severe fetal hydronephrosis: the added value of associated congenital anomalies of the kidneys and urinary tract (CAKUT) in the prediction of postnatal outcome. *Prenat Diagn.* (2018) 38:179–83. doi: 10.1002/pd.5206

11. Oktar T, Salabas E, Kalelioglu I, Atar A, Ander H, Ziylan O, et al. Fetal urinoma and prenatal hydronephrosis: how is renal function affected? *Turkish J Urol.* (2013) 39:96–100. doi: 10.5152/tud.2013.016

12. Pates JA, Dashe JS. Prenatal diagnosis and management of hydronephrosis. *Early Human Dev.* (2006) 82:3–8. doi: 10.1016/j.earlhumdev.2005.11.003

13. Ismaili K, Avni F, Martin WK, Hall M. Brussels free university perinatal nephrology study group. Long term clinical outcome of infants with mild and moderate fetal pyelectasis: validation of neonatal ultrasound as a screening tool to detect significant nephrouropathies. *J Pediatr.* (2004) 144:759–65. doi: 10.1016/j.jpeds.2004.02.035

14. Onen A. An alternative grading system to refine the criteria for severity of hydronephrosis and optimal treatment guidelines in neonates with primary UPJ-type hydronephrosis. *J Pediatr Urol.* (2007) 3:200–5. doi: 10.1016/j.jpurol.2006.08.002

15. Zhang H, Zhang L, Guo N. Validation of "urinary tract dilation" classification system: correlation between fetal hydronephrosis and postnatal urological abnormalities. *Medicine.* (2020) 99:18707. doi: 10.1097/MD.0000000000018707

16. Onen A. Grading of hydronephrosis: an ongoing challenge. *Front Pediatr.* (in press).

17. Dias CS, Silva JMP, Pereira AK, Marino VS, Silva LA, Coelho AM, et al. Diagnostic accuracy of renal pelvic dilatation for detecting surgically managed ureteropelvic junction obstruction. *J Urol.* (2013) 190:661–6. doi: 10.1016/j.juro.2013.02.014

18. Karnak I, Woo LL, Shah SN, Sirajuddin A, Kay R, Ross JH. Prenatally detected ureteropelvic junction obstruction: clinical features and associated urologic abnormalities. *Pediatr Surg Int.* (2008) 24:395–402. doi: 10.1007/s00383-008-2112-1

19. Churchill BM, Feng WC. Ureteropelvic junction anomalies: congenital UPJ problems in children. In: Gearhart JP, Rink RC, Mouriquand PDE, editors. *Pediatric Urology.* Philedelphia, PA: WB Saunders Company (2001). p. 318–46.

20. Leo CFT, Lakshmanan Y. Anomalies of the renal collecting system: ureteropelvic junction obstruction (pyelocalyectasis) and infundibular stenosis. *Clinical Ped Urol. Martin Dunitz, London.* (2002) 168:559–631. doi: 10.1097/00005392-200212000-00114

21. Babu R, Vittalraj P, Sundaram S, Shalini S. Pathological changes in ureterovesical and ureteropelvic junction obstruction explained by fetal ureter histology. *J Pediatr Urol.* (2019) 15:240e1–e7. doi: 10.1016/j.jpurol.2019.02.001

22. Faghihimehr A, Gharavi M, Mancuso M, Sreedher G. Fetal MR imaging in urogenital system anomalies. *J Matern Fetal Neonatal Med.* (2019) 32:3487–94. doi: 10.1080/14767058.2018.1465039

23. Cassart M, Massez A, Metens T, Rypens F, Lambot MA, Hall M, et al. Complementary role of MRI after sonography in assessing bilateral urinary tract anomalies in the fetus. *Am J Roent.* (2004) 182:689–95. doi: 10.2214/ajr.182.3.1820689

24. Kajbafzadeh AM, Payabvash S, Elmi A, Jamal A, Hantoshzadeh Z, Mehdizadeh M. Comparison of magnetic resonance urography with ultrasound studies in detection of fetal urogenital anomalies. *J Pediatr Urol.* (2008) 4:32–39. doi: 10.1016/j.jpurol.2007.07.005

25. Stathopoulos L, Merrot T, Chaumoitre K, Bretelle F, Michel F, Alessandrini P. Prenatal urinoma related to ureteropelvic junction obstruction: poor prognosis of affected kidney. *J Urology.* (2010) 76:190–4. doi: 10.1016/j.urology.2010.03.030

26. Kleiner B, Callen PW, Filly RA. Sonographic analysis of the fetus with ureteropelvic junction obstruction. *Am J Roent.* (1987) 148:359–63. doi: 10.2214/ajr.148.2.359

27. Ghidini A, Strobelt N, Lynch L, Berkowitz RL. Fetal urinoma: a case report and review of its clinical significance. *J Ultrasound Med.* (1994) 13:989–91. doi: 10.7863/jum.1994.13.12.989

28. Benacerraf BR, Peters CA, Mandell J. The prenatal evaluation of a non-functioning kidney in the setting of obstructive hydronephrosis. *J Clin Ultrasound.* (1991) 19:446–50. doi: 10.1002/jcu.1870190716

29. Gorincour G, Rypens F, Toiviainen-Salo S, Grignon A, Lambert R, Audibert F, et al. Fetal urinoma: two new cases and a review of the literature. *Ultrasound Obstet Gynecol.* (2006) 28:848–52. doi: 10.1002/uog.2830

30. Liu DB, Armstrong WR, Maizels M. Hydronephrosis: prenatal and postnatal evaluation and management. *Clin Perinatol.* (2014) 41:661–78. doi: 10.1007/s11934-014-0430-5

31. Mathiot A, Liard A, Eurin D, Dacher JN. Prenatally detected multicystic renal dysplasia and associated anomalies of the genito-urinary tract. *J Radiol.* (2002) 83:731–5.

32. Bornstein E, Barnhard Y, Donnenfeld AE, Ferber A, Divon MY. The risk of a major trisomy in fetuses with pyelectasis: the impact of an abnormal maternal serum screen or additional sonographic markers. *Am J Obstet Gynecol.* (2007) 196:24–6. doi: 10.1016/j.ajog.2007.01.011

33. Evans JA. Urinary tract. In: Stevenson RE, Hall JG, editors. *Human Malformations and Related Anomalies.* 2nd ed. Oxford: Oxford University Press (2006). p. 1161–1190.

34. Tough H, Fujinaga T, Okuda M, Aoshi H. Schinzel-giedion syndrome. *Int J Urol.* (2001) 8:237–41. doi: 10.1046/j.1442-2042.2001.00291.x

35. Jiang D, Chen Z, Lin H, Xu M, Geng H. Predictive factors of contralateral operation after initial pyeloplasty in children with antenatally detected bilateral hydronephrosis due to ureteropelvic junction obstruction. *J Urol Int.* (2018) 100:322–26. doi: 10.1159/000487196

36. Zhang L, Li Y, Liu C, Li X, Sun H. Diagnostic value of anteroposterior diameter of renal pelvis for predicting postnatal surgery: a systematic review and meta-analysis. *J Urol.* (2018) 200:1346–53. doi: 10.1016/j.juro.2018.06.064

37. Elmaci MA, Donmez MI. Time to resolution of isolated antenatal hydronephrosis with anteroposterior diameter ≤ 20 mm. *Eur J Ped.* (2019) 178:823–8. doi: 10.1007/s00431-019-03359-y

38. Arora S, Yadav P, Kumar M, Singh SK, Sureka SK, Mittal V, et al. Predictors for need of surgery in antenatally detected hydronephrosis due to UPJ obstruction – A prospective multivariate analysis. *J Ped Urol.* (2015) 11:248e1–e5. doi: 10.1016/j.jpurol.2015.02.008

39. Chi T, Feldstein VA, Nguyen HT. Increased echogenicity as a predictor of poor renal function in children with grade 3 to 4 hydronephrosis. *J Urol.* (2006) 175:1898–901. doi: 10.1016/S0022-5347(05)00930-4

40. Chalmers DJ, Meyers ML, Brodie KE, Palmer C, Campbell JB. Inter-rater reliability of the APD, SFU and UTD grading systems in fetal sonography and MRI. *J Pediatr Urol.* (2016) 12:305e1–5. doi: 10.1016/j.jpurol.2016.06.012

41. Han M, Kim HG, Lee JD, Park SY, Sur YK. Conversation and reliability of two urological systems in infants: the society for fetal urology and the urinary tract dilatation classification system. *Pediatr Radiol.* (2017) 47:65–73. doi: 10.1007/s00247-016-3721-9

42. Nelson CP, Heller HT, Benson CB, Asch EH, Durfee SM, Logvinenko T, et al. Interobserver reliability of the antenatal consensus classification system for urinary tract dilatation. *J Ultrasound Med.* (2019) 39:551–57. doi: 10.1002/jum.15133

43. Braga LH, McGrath M, Farrokhyar F, Jegatheeswaran K, Lorenzo AJ. Society for fetal urology classification vs urinary tract dilation grading system for prognostication in prenatal hydronephrosis: a time to resolution analysis. *J Urol.* (2018) 199:1615–21. doi: 10.1016/j.juro.2017.11.077

44. Feldman DM, DeCambre M, Kong E, Borgida A, Jamil M, McKenna P, et al. Evaluation and follow-up of fetal hydronephrosis. *J Ultrasound Med.* (2001) 20:1065–9. doi: 10.7863/jum.2001.20.10.1065

45. Zanetta VC, Rosman BM, Bromley B, Shipp TD, Chow JS, Campbell JB, et al. Variation in management of mild prenatal hydronephrosis among maternal-fetal medicine obstetricians, and pediatric urologists, and radiologists. *J Urol.* (2012) 188:1935–9. doi: 10.1016/j.juro.2012.07.011

46. Gong Y, Xu H, Li Y, Zhou Y, Zhang M, Shen Q, et al. Exploration of postnatal integrated management for prenatal renal and urinary tract anomalies in China. *J Matern Fetal Neonatal Med.* (2019) 29:1–6. doi: 10.1080/14767058.2019.1608176

47. Benjamin T, Amodeo RR, Patil AS, Robinson BK. The impact of gestational age at delivery on urologic outcomes for the fetus with hydronephrosis. *Fetal Pediatr Pathol.* (2016) 35:359–68. doi: 10.1080/15513815.2016.1202361

3

Using Deep Learning Algorithms to Grade Hydronephrosis Severity: Toward a Clinical Adjunct

Lauren C. Smail [1,2], *Kiret Dhindsa* [3,4,5], *Luis H. Braga* [6,7,8]*, *Suzanna Becker* [1,5,9] *and*
Ranil R. Sonnadara [1,2,3,4,5,9]

[1] Department of Psychology, Neuroscience & Behaviour, McMaster University, Hamilton, ON, Canada, [2] Office of Education Science, McMaster University, Hamilton, ON, Canada, [3] Department of Surgery, McMaster University, Hamilton, ON, Canada, [4] Research and High Performance Computing, McMaster University, Hamilton, ON, Canada, [5] Vector Institute for Artificial Intelligence, Toronto, ON, Canada, [6] Division of Urology, Department of Surgery, McMaster University, Hamilton, ON, Canada, [7] Division of Urology, Department of Surgery, McMaster Children's Hospital, Hamilton, ON, Canada, [8] McMaster Pediatric Surgery Research Collaborative, McMaster University, Hamilton, ON, Canada, [9] Centre for Advanced Research in Experimental and Applied Linguistics, McMaster University, Hamilton, ON, Canada

Correspondence:
Luis H. Braga
braga@mcmaster.ca

Grading hydronephrosis severity relies on subjective interpretation of renal ultrasound images. Deep learning is a data-driven algorithmic approach to classifying data, including images, presenting a promising option for grading hydronephrosis. The current study explored the potential of deep convolutional neural networks (CNN), a type of deep learning algorithm, to grade hydronephrosis ultrasound images according to the 5-point Society for Fetal Urology (SFU) classification system, and discusses its potential applications in developing decision and teaching aids for clinical practice. We developed a five-layer CNN to grade 2,420 sagittal hydronephrosis ultrasound images [191 SFU 0 (8%), 407 SFU I (17%), 666 SFU II (28%), 833 SFU III (34%), and 323 SFU IV (13%)], from 673 patients ranging from 0 to 116.29 months old ($M_{age} = 16.53$, $SD = 17.80$). Five-way (all grades) and two-way classification problems [i.e., II vs. III, and low (0–II) vs. high (III–IV)] were explored. The CNN classified 94% (95% CI, 93–95%) of the images correctly or within one grade of the provided label in the five-way classification problem. Fifty-one percent of these images (95% CI, 49–53%) were correctly predicted, with an average weighted F1 score of 0.49 (95% CI, 0.47–0.51). The CNN achieved an average accuracy of 78% (95% CI, 75–82%) with an average weighted F1 of 0.78 (95% CI, 0.74–0.82) when classifying low vs. high grades, and an average accuracy of 71% (95% CI, 68–74%) with an average weighted F1 score of 0.71 (95% CI, 0.68–0.75) when discriminating between grades II vs. III. Our model performs well above chance level, and classifies almost all images either correctly or within one grade of the provided label. We have demonstrated the applicability of a CNN approach to hydronephrosis ultrasound image classification. Further investigation into a deep learning-based clinical adjunct for hydronephrosis is warranted.

Keywords: hydronephrosis, machine learning, deep learning, ultrasound, diagnostic imaging, grading, diagnostic aid, teaching aid

INTRODUCTION

Machine learning is a field of research with far reaching applications that is generating considerable interest in medicine (1, 2). Deep learning, a subset of machine learning, is a general term for an algorithm that trains a many layered network to learn hierarchical feature representations from raw data. Due to the hierarchical nature of deep learning models, complex functions can be learned to solve difficult classification problems that were previously unsolvable by classic machine learning algorithms (3). Deep convolutional neural networks (CNNs) are a type of deep learning algorithm that are well-suited to computer vision tasks (3) due to their ability to take advantage of the multi-scale spatial structure of images (4). This makes CNN models an attractive candidate architecture for tackling medical imaging problems. In particular, they offer a promising avenue for creating clinical adjuncts to help train physicians, and flag/grade challenging diagnostic cases.

Prenatal hydronephrosis (HN) is a condition that involves accumulation of urine with consequent dilatation of the collecting system in fetuses. It is the most frequent neonatal urinary tract abnormality, occurring in 1–5% of all newborn babies (5). HN is detected by prenatal ultrasound (US) imaging and can be caused by several underlying conditions, such as uteropelvic junction obstruction or vesico-ureteral reflux (6). Although many cases eventually resolve on their own, in severe forms, afflicted infants may require surgical intervention (7, 8), and failure to intervene can result in loss of renal function (9, 10).

All patients with prenatal HN are normally evaluated after birth by postnatal renal ultrasonography to determine HN severity and the best course of treatment. Appropriate HN grading is important, as misclassification of any patient into the inappropriate HN category can lead to incorrect management and unnecessary testing since treatment is directly dependent on HN severity. Given the need for accurate and unambiguous classification of HN, numerous HN grading systems have been developed (11). However, poor inter-rater reliability (12, 13), particularly for intermediate HN grades, suggests that grading still relies on subjective interpretation of ultrasound images, as clear and objective criteria have not been fully established.

Owing to the ability of deep learning algorithms to classify images into diagnostic categories based solely on data-driven pattern recognition, the main purpose of this study was to extend on our previous work (14) to investigate whether deep learning algorithms can effectively grade the severity of HN using a prospectively collected HN database and separate them into 5 main classes. Secondary investigations were also conducted to assess whether the same model can effectively discriminate between low and high HN grades (SFU 0, I, II vs. III, IV), and between moderate (SFU II vs. III) cases. The results of this study may provide important insights into whether deep learning is a promising avenue of future study for discriminating different grades of HN, and developing clinical adjuncts. Given that our models were trained on images with human expert-generated training labels, we hypothesized that our deep learning model would perform at or very close to that of a human expert at HN grading. This would validate our method as a potential training tool for medical students and as an adjunctive tool for clinical experts.

MATERIALS AND METHODS

Study Population and Exclusion Criteria

Our database consists of 2-dimensional renal B-mode US images from an ongoing large prospective cohort study involving all patients diagnosed with prenatal HN who were referred to a tertiary care pediatric hospital. The database contains one sagittal US image per patient visit, spanning 687 patients. Each image was assigned a grade according to the Society for Fetal Urology (SFU) system, one of the most widely adopted HN classification systems (15), ranging from 0 (normal kidney) to IV (severe HN with parenchymal thinning). Grades were provided by three separate physicians (2 fellowship trained pediatric urologists and 1 fellowship trained pediatric radiologist—agreement $K = 90\%$) with discrepancies resolved by consensus. From these 687 patients, 2,492 sagittal renal US images were collected. Seventy-two images from 14 patients were excluded due to poor image quality (e.g., blurry, large annotation overlaid, no visible kidney), leaving 2,420 sagittal US images from 673 patients ($N_{female} = 159$, $N_{male} = 514$) ranging from 0 to 116.29 months old ($M_{age} = 16.53$, $SD = 17.80$) to be included in the analysis. Of these, 191 were labeled as SFU 0, 407 as SFU I, 666 as SFU II, 833 as SFU III, and 323 as SFU IV. Ethics clearance for this study was obtained through the Research Ethics Board.

Preprocessing

Preprocessing is a crucial step in machine learning, as standardizing images and taking simple steps to reduce noise and non-discriminative variability improves the ability of models to learn relevant information. In this study, all images were cropped to remove any annotations and blank space in the margins. The images were then despeckled using the bi-directional FIR-median hybrid despeckling filter to remove speckle noise from the images (16). Despeckling is a standard preprocessing technique for US images since speckle noise is caused by interference between the US probe and reflecting US waves. Finally, the image pixel values were normalized between 0 and 1, and all images resized to 256 × 256 pixels to provide a consistent image input size into our network. The final image size was chosen based on the smallest dimension of the cropped images to ensure that images were not stretched.

Data augmentation is a common approach to reducing overfitting and improving classification performance for small datasets (3, 17). It works by introducing variations on each image during training so as to build robustness into the model. In this study, we augment the data by rotating each image up to 45°, performing horizontal and vertical flips with a 50% probability, and shifting the image vertically and horizontally up to 20%.

Model Architecture

A CNN is a type of neural network that has been particularly successful in computer vision applications. CNNs are constructed from alternating convolutional layers and pooling layers. The structure of a CNN is inspired by that of the mammalian visual system, where earlier cortical areas receive input from small regions of the retina and learn simple local features such as edges, while regions at progressively higher levels in the visual system have correspondingly broader receptive fields, and learn complex features such as shape detectors. In a CNN, convolutional layers learn multiple local features of an image by processing it across many overlapping patches, while pooling layers summate the filter responses from the previous layer, thereby compressing the representations learned by the preceding convolutional layer to force the model to filter out unimportant visual information. As in the visual system, successive convolutional layers have progressively larger receptive fields, permitting more complex, and abstract image features to be learned in higher layers of the network. In classification models a standard multilayer perceptron, made up of a few fully connected layers of neurons (called dense layers) receives the learned image representation from the convolutional layers and attempts to classify the image. The entire network is trained using backpropagation, a neural network learning procedure which iteratively updates the strengths of the connections between layers of neurons in order to minimize classification error on the training data. For a detailed explanation of how CNNs work and are designed, see Le Cun et al. (18).

The CNN model used in the current study was developed using the Keras neural network API with Tensorflow (19, 20). The final architecture contained five convolutional layers, a fully connected layer of 400 units, and a final output layer where the number of units was equal to the number of classes for the given task (i.e., five or two) (**Figure 1**). The architecture was determined by experimenting with five-way SFU HN classification. The output unit/class with the highest overall final activation was used as the model's prediction and was compared against the provided label to assess performance. See **Supplementary Materials** for a description of all technical details.

Model Training and Evaluation

Five-way (all SFU grades) and binary classification tests were conducted using 5-fold cross validation. See **Supplementary Materials** for a description of this process. The binary classification tests were selected due to their clinical relevance and included distinguishing between mild (0, I, and II) and severe (III and IV) HN grades, and between moderate grades (II vs. III). Layer-wise relevant propagation (21) was used to visualize model output.

RESULTS

Our model achieved an average five-way classification accuracy of 51% (95% CI, 49–53%), and an average weighted F1 score of 0.49 (95% CI, 0.47–0.51). Furthermore, 94% (95% CI, 93–95%) of images were either correctly classified or within one grade of the provided label (**Figure 2**).

Our model classified mild vs. severe HN with an average accuracy of 78% (95% CI, 75–82%), and an average weighted F1 of 0.78 (95% CI, 0.74–0.82). When differentiating between moderate grades (SFU II and III), our model achieved an average accuracy of 71% (95% CI, 68–74%) and an average weighted F1 score of 0.71 (95% CI, 0.68–0.75). See **Table 1** for a comprehensive overview of model performance.

		Predicted				
		0	I	II	III	IV
Actual	0	20 (0.83%)	114 (4.71%)	50 (2.10%)	7 (0.29%)	0 (0%)
	I	20 (0.83%)	159 (6.57%)	190 (7.85%)	34 (1.40%)	4 (0.17%)
	II	8 (0.33%)	121 (5.00%)	357 (14.75%)	179 (7.40%)	1 (0.04%)
	III	0 (0%)	21 (0.87%)	198 (8.18%)	540 (22.31%)	74 (3.06%)
	IV	2 (0.08%)	6 (0.25%)	7 (0.29%)	160 (6.61%)	148 (6.12%)

FIGURE 2 | The confusion matrix of the CNN model. Boxes along the diagonal in gray represent the number (percentage) of cases where the CNN made the correct classification decision. Light gray boxes represent the cases where the CNN was incorrect by one grade, and white boxes indicate cases where the CNN was incorrect by two or more grades.

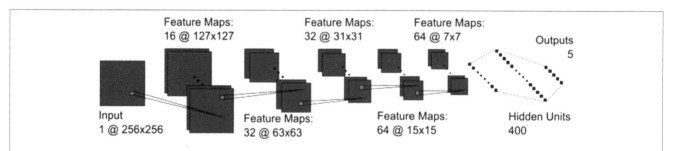

FIGURE 1 | The CNN architecture containing all convolutional (dark gray) and fully connected (black) layers. The convolutional kernels (light gray squares) were 3 × 3 pixels in all layers.

TABLE 1 | CNN model classification results averaged across the 5-folds.

Classification problem	Accuracy (%)	Sensitivity	Specificity	PPV	F1
Five-way (0 to IV)	51 (49–53)				0.49 (0.47–0.51)[a]
SFU 0		0.11 (0–0.21)	0.99 (0.97–1.00)	0.26 (0.05–0.47)	0.15 (0.01–0.29)
SFU 1		0.39 (0.35–0.43)	0.87 (0.84–0.90)	0.39 (0.34–0.44)	0.38 (0.35–0.42)
SFU II		0.54 (0.43–0.65)	0.75 (0.72–0.79)	0.45 (0.42–0.49)	0.48 (0.43–0.53)
SFU III		0.65 (0.60–0.70)	0.76 (0.74–0.78)	0.59 (0.53–0.65)	0.61 (0.56–0.66)
SFU IV		0.46 (0.29–0.62)	0.96 (0.94–0.98)	0.65 (0.54–0.75)	0.52 (0.38–0.66)
Mild (0, I, II) vs. Severe (III, IV)	78 (75–82)				0.78 (0.74–0.82)[a]
Mild		0.89 (0.82–0.96)	0.66 (0.51–0.81)	0.75 (0.69–0.81)	0.81 (0.78–0.84)
Severe		0.66 (0.51–0.81)	0.89 (0.82–0.96)	0.87 (0.80–0.94)	0.73 (0.64–0.82)
SFU II vs. SFU III	71 (68–74)				0.71 (0.68–0.75)[a]
SFU II		0.76 (0.60–0.92)	0.67 (0.52–0.82)	0.67 (0.59–0.75)	0.69 (0.63–0.75)
SFU III		0.67 (0.52–0.82)	0.76 (0.60–0.92)	0.80 (0.73–0.87)	0.71 (0.65–0.77)

The 95% confidence intervals are given in parentheses.
[a] Weighted average.

DISCUSSION

We investigated the potential of deep CNN to create clinical adjuncts for HN. This was achieved by testing our model's ability to classify HN US images. We tested our model's performance on three different classification tasks that are relevant to clinical practice. These results, along with their potential clinical implications, are discussed below.

Five-Way Classification Performance

Our model achieved an average five-way classification accuracy that was well above chance level (51%). In practice, physicians usually have access to multiple different US images at different angles, as well as patient histories, and are therefore able to grade the US image by combining information from multiple views and timepoints. Although we are unable to compare our model's performance directly to a physician, achieving this level of accuracy with a single US image is very promising.

The model classified 94% (95% CI, 93–95%) of images either correctly or within one grade of the correct/provided label. Further investigation into the output of our model reveals that there are many borderline images where there is not an obvious choice for which class the image belongs to (e.g., **Figures 3A,C**). In cases such as these where two grades possible are, it must choose a single HN grade according to the SFU system, much like a physician (12, 13).

Considering that HN grading can be challenging, and that subjective assessments are used to differentiate between borderline cases (12, 13), we would argue that solely relying on whether the model's predictions matched the provided SFU labels is an incomplete assessment of our model's performance. Instead, the percentage of cases that are either "correct" of within one grade of the provided label (94%) is a more representative metric of our model's true performance. The nearly block-diagonal structure of the confusion matrix supports this (**Figure 2**) and indicates that the model is learning useful information for HN classification.

Binary Classification Performance

Discriminating between moderate HN grades is known to be challenging (12, 13), and therefore we wanted to investigate our model's performance on this same task. When comparing mild (0, I, II) and severe (III, IV) HN images, our model achieved an average accuracy of 78%, which is well above chance level. When the model discriminated between moderate grades (II and III), which is less reliable for physicians (12, 13), performance only dropped to 71%. There is no direct comparison to be made against physician accuracy, however, considering the known difficulties in distinguishing between moderate HN grades (12, 13), these results are encouraging.

Interpretability

We visualized regions of the HN US images that the CNN found important for five-way classification in a sample of images using layer-wise relevance propagation (21) from the DeepExplain toolbox (22). Layer-wise relevance propagation allows us to determine which features in the image contribute most strongly to the CNNs output (**Figure 3B**). Cyan pixels indicate that the model heavily relied on those features to classify the image. Visualizing can be used to validate whether our model is learning appropriate features that correspond with the SFU grading system and interpret its inner workings. Interpretability is crucial as we develop deep learning based clinical adjuncts since physicians will need to be able to understand why a model made a decision, rather than just blindly following the algorithm.

Of the examples we tested, we can see that our model is learning features that correspond appropriately with the SFU system (e.g., renal parenchyma, calyces), however, in some cases it is also relying on regions outside of the kidney. This can likely be attributed to image noise, and therefore removing the noise with segmentation (i.e., finding regions of interest in the image) would ensure that the model is only relying on appropriate regions for classification. However,

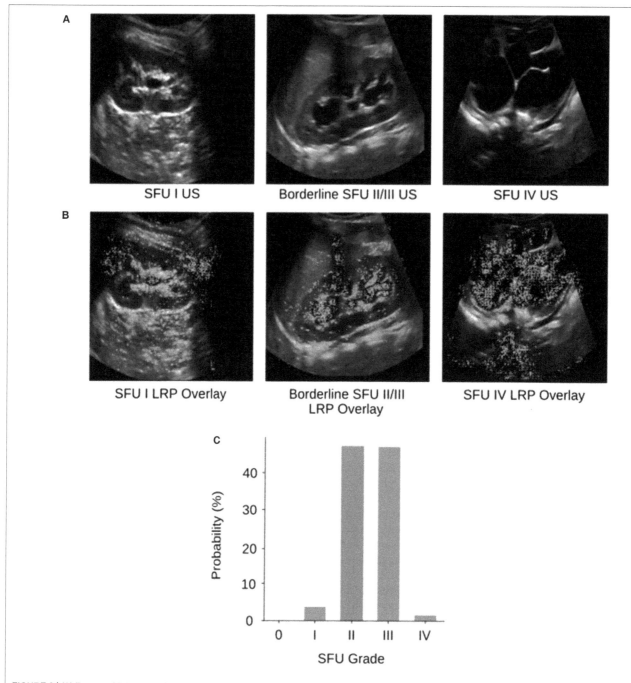

FIGURE 3 | (A) Example SFU I, borderline SFU II/III, and SFU IV US images from the database. **(B)** The corresponding layerwise relevance propagations of each of the example images. Layer-wise relevance propagations give a sparse representation of pixel importance. Propagations were visualized as heat maps and overlaid on top of the gray-scale input US images. The cyan colored pixels indicate regions that the CNN heavily relied upon for classification. **(C)** The corresponding softmax output probability distribution of the borderline SFU II/III US image. The image was labeled as SFU grade III by physicians; however, the CNN predicted SFU grade II which was incorrect. We can see based on the probability distribution that the model "thought" SFU grade II and III were almost equally likely but had to select one grade as its prediction. This behavior is analogous to that of physicians and can be partially explained by the poor inter-rater reliability and subjectivity of the SFU system (i.e., intrinsic limitations of that classification).

the model may be finding relevant features outside of those from the SFU classification system that are clinically relevant but not normally considered, and so this finding warrants further investigation.

Implications for Clinical Practice

Machine learning and deep learning models have been successfully applied in the context of HN to predict the need for surgical intervention (1), and the necessity of diuretic nuclear renography (2). More broadly, machine learning and deep learning have been used in the field of pediatric urology to classify between different kidney diseases (23), and between diseased and normal kidneys (24). In addition, deep learning has recently been used to perform automatic kidney segmentation in ultrasound imaging (25). Due to the different problems being evaluated in each of the studies, a direct comparison in performance cannot be made. It is important to highlight that along with investigating different questions, and therefore having differing levels of chance performance (i.e., 50 vs. 20% in the current study), these studies also differ from the current study in that many of these papers are asking objective questions (e.g., Was surgery required?) and are therefore able to utilize objective labels in their models. As discussed previously, the lack of objective ground truth in the current study presents challenges in interpreting the true performance of our model, and likely contributes to our model's lower accuracy metric as compared to other papers.

Considering the issue of subjectivity, our model's current level of performance in classifying HN is promising and in line with previous research from our group (14). Our findings suggest that applying these algorithms into clinical practice through decision aids and teaching aids has potential. It is important to clarify that we anticipate that deep learning models like the one presented here will 1 day be used to support physicians rather than replace them, as human-level reliability and generalizability remains a major challenge for medical applications (26). We outline below two new ways that we expect deep learning models can be applied to benefit clinical practice in the future.

Decision Aids

In clinical practice, decision aids are used to assess the structure of interest, and then provide its estimate of disease probability. Physicians are then free to use this estimate as they wish. To our knowledge, patient management is always left up to the physician, and the aids act more like a second opinion. Studies have shown that the combined synergistic effects of the decision aid and physician knowledge greatly improved the diagnostic accuracy (27). In the context of HN, we expect that the second opinion from the decision aid would be particularly useful for borderline cases, since currently consensus decisions are required to resolve these cases.

Teaching Aids

Deep learning models can also be used to develop teaching aids for trainees to teach and provide them with feedback on how to grade HN US images. These teaching features can be created by exploiting the rich information that these algorithms contain. For example, a deep learning-based teaching aid could provide trainees with informative feedback based on the inner workings of the algorithm to tell trainees whether their diagnosis was correct. Furthermore, the teaching aid could highlight parts of the image with a heat-map using visualization methods, such as layer-wise relevance propagation, to indicate which regions were of clinical importance, and to what degree. A teaching aid would alleviate at least some of the need for direct physician feedback and would allow trainees to work through examples at their own pace to maximize learning.

Limitations and Future Work

Considering that the current dataset was small by deep learning standards, slightly imbalanced, and only contained one image per patient visit, our model still achieved moderate to good accuracy across the different classification problems. This suggests that a richer and larger dataset could lead to even better performance and an eventual deep learning based clinical adjunct for HN. Future work should also investigate HN classification at the patient level and consider the time series in the data. HN patients are followed across time, and the trends in their HN severity provide physicians with important information that is incorporated into their clinical decision making. We would expect that providing a deep learning model with time series data would benefit model performance as well. Additionally, a model could convey its level of uncertainty in its diagnosis, flagging to the physician that this image merited a closer examination or additional measurements.

We applied relatively little preprocessing to our images, therefore future studies should investigate whether segmentation, a commonly recommended preprocessing technique, reduces model noise and improves performance (25). Within the current classification model, layer-wise relevance propagation revealed that regions outside of the kidney were contributing to model output. Further investigation on the impact of segmentation whereby the model is constrained to extract features from the kidney that correspond with the SFU grading system should elucidate whether these findings are attributable to image noise or useful features.

CONCLUSIONS

The purpose of the current study was to explore whether deep learning can effectively classify HN US images and separate them into 5 main categories. Overall, our model performs well above chance level across all classifications, categorizing images either correctly, or within one grade of the provided label. The model was also capable of discriminating well between mild and severe grades of HN, which has important clinical implications. The results of the current study suggest that CNNs can be applied to grade HN US images effectively, and that further investigation into using deep learning to grade HN US images is warranted. With further model refinement, and by addressing the limitations of our current data set, we expect that our model can be used to develop effective clinical adjuncts to improve clinical practice.

AUTHOR CONTRIBUTIONS

LS was responsible for data analysis and writing the first draft of the manuscript. LB provided clinical oversight for the project, and was responsible for acquisition and curation of the dataset used for model training. All authors were responsible for the design of the study, interpretation of the data, and writing the final manuscript.

REFERENCES

1. Lorenzo AJ, Rickard M, Braga LH, Guo Y, Oliveria JP. Predictive analytics and modeling employing machine learning technology: the next step in data sharing, analysis and individualized counseling explored with a large, prospective prenatal hydronephrosis database. *Urology.* (2018) 123:204–9. doi: 10.1016/j.urology.2018.05.041
2. Cerrolaza JJ, Peters CA, Martin AD, Myers E, Safdar N, Linguraru MG. Quantitative ultrasound for measuring obstructive severity in children with hydronephrosis. *J Urol.* (2016) 195:1093–9. doi: 10.1016/j.juro.2015.10.173
3. Krizhevsky A, Sutskever I, Hinton GE. ImageNet classification with deep convolutional neural networks. In: Pereira F, Burges CJC, Bottou L, Weinberger KQ, editors. *Advances in Neural Information Processing Systems 25.* Lake Tahoe, NV: Curran Associates Inc. (2012). p. 1097–105.
4. Le Cun Y, Bottou L, Bengio Y, Haffner P. Gradient-based learning applied to document recognition. *Proc IEEE.* (1998) 86:2278–324. doi: 10.1109/5.726791
5. Woodward M, Frank D. Postnatal management of antenatal hydronephrosis. *BJU Int.* (2002) 89:149–56. doi: 10.1046/j.1464-4096.2001.woodward.2578.x
6. Montini G, Tullus K, Hewitt I. Febrile urinary tract infections in children. *N Engl J Med.* (2011) 365:239–50. doi: 10.1056/NEJMra1007755
7. Yang Y, Hou Y, Niu ZB, Wang CL. Long-term follow-up and management of prenatally detected, isolated hydronephrosis. *J Pediatr Surg.* (2010) 45:1701–6. doi: 10.1016/j.jpedsurg.2010.03.030
8. Braga LH, McGrath M, Farrokhyar F, Jegatheeswaran K, Lorenzo AJ. Associations of initial society for fetal urology grades and urinary tract dilatation risk groups with clinical outcomes in patients with isolated prenatal hydronephrosis. *J Urol.* (2017) 197:831–7. doi: 10.1016/j.juro.2016.08.099
9. González R, Schimke CM. The prenatal diagnosis of hydronephrosis, when and why to operate? *Arch Esp Urol.* (1998) 51:575–9.
10. Hanna MK. Antenatal hydronephrosis and ureteropelvic junction obstruction: the case for early intervention. *Urology.* (2000) 55:612–5. doi: 10.1016/S0090-4295(00)00460-X
11. Nguyen HT, Benson CB, Bromley B, Campbell JB, Chow J, Coleman B, et al. Multidisciplinary consensus on the classification of prenatal and postnatal urinary tract dilation (UTD classification system). *J Pediatr Urol.* (2014) 10:982–98. doi: 10.1016/j.jpurol.2014.10.002
12. Rickard M, Easterbrook B, Kim S, Farrokhyar F, Stein N, Arora S, et al. Six of one, half a dozen of the other: a measure of multidisciplinary inter/intra-rater reliability of the society for fetal urology and urinary tract dilation grading systems for hydronephrosis. *J Pediatr Urol.* (2017) 13:80.e1–5. doi: 10.1016/j.jpurol.2016.09.005
13. Keays MA, Guerra LA, Mihill J, Raju G, Al-Asheeri N, Geier P, et al. Reliability assessment of society for fetal urology ultrasound grading system for hydronephrosis. *J Urol.* (2008) 180:1680–3. doi: 10.1016/j.juro.2008.03.107
14. Dhindsa K, Smail LC, McGrath M, Braga LH, Becker S, Sonnadara RR. Grading prenatal hydronephrosis from ultrasound imaging using deep convolutional neural networks. In: *15th Conference on Computer and Robot Vision.* Toronto, ON: IEEExplore (2018). p. 80–7. Available online at: https://bibbase.org/network/publication/dhindsa-smail-mcgrath-braga-becker-sonnadara-gradingprenatalhydronephrosisfromultrasoundimagingusingdeepconvolutionalneuralnetworks-2018 (accessed July 12, 2018).
15. Nguyen HT, Herndon CDA, Cooper C, Gatti J, Kirsch A, Kokorowski P, et al. The society for fetal urology consensus statement on the evaluation and management of antenatal hydronephrosis. *J Pediatr Urol.* (2010) 6:212–31. doi: 10.1016/j.jpurol.2010.02.205
16. Nieminen A, Heinonen P, Neuvo Y. A new class of detail-preserving filters for image processing. *IEEE Trans Pattern Anal Mach Intell.* (1987) 9:74–90. doi: 10.1109/TPAMI.1987.4767873
17. Simard PY, Steinkraus D, Platt JC. Best practices in convolutional neural networks applied to visual document analysis. In: *Seventh International Conference on Document Analysis and Recognition, 2003* (Edinburgh) (2003). p. 958–62. doi: 10.1109/ICDAR.2003.1227801
18. Le Cun Y, Bengio Y, Hinton G. Deep learning. *Nature.* (2015) 521:436–44. doi: 10.1038/nature14539
19. Chollet F. *Keras* (2015). Available online at: http://keras.io (accessed September 20, 2018).
20. Abadi M, Agarwal A, Barham P, Brevdo E, Chen Z, Citro C, et al. *TensorFlow: Large-Scale Machine Learning on Heterogeneous Distributed Systems* (2016). Available online at: http://arxiv.org/abs/1603.04467 (accessed March 14, 2019).
21. Bach S, Binder A, Montavon G, Klauschen F, Müller KR, Samek W. On pixel-wise explanations for non-linear classifier decisions by layer-wise relevance propagation. *PLoS ONE.* (2015) 10:e0130140. doi: 10.1371/journal.pone.0130140
22. Ancona M, Ceolini E, Öztireli C, Gross M. *Towards Better Understanding of Gradient-Based Attribution Methods for Deep Neural Networks* (2017). Available online at: http://arxiv.org/abs/1711.06104 (accessed September 20, 2018).
23. Yin S, Peng Q, Li H, Zhang Z, You X, Liu H, et al. Multi-instance deep learning with graph convolutional neural networks for diagnosis of kidney diseases using ultrasound imaging. In: Greenspan H, Tanno R, Erdt M, Arbel T, Baumgartner C, Dalca A, et al., editors. *Uncertainty for Safe Utilization of Machine Learning in Medical Imaging and Clinical Image-Based Procedures.* Cham: Springer International Publishing (2019). p. 146–54.
24. Zheng Q, Furth SL, Tasian GE, Fan Y. Computer-aided diagnosis of congenital abnormalities of the kidney and urinary tract in children based on ultrasound imaging data by integrating texture image features and deep transfer learning image features. *J Pediatr Urol.* (2019) 15:75.e1–7. doi: 10.1016/j.jpurol.2018.10.020
25. Sivanesan U, Braga LH, Sonnadara RR, Dhindsa K. *Unsupervised Medical Image Segmentation with Adversarial Networks: From Edge Diagrams to Segmentation Maps* (2019). Available online at: http://arxiv.org/abs/1911.05140 (accessed December 03, 2019).
26. Dhindsa K, Bhandari M, Sonnadara RR. What's holding up the big data revolution in healthcare? *BMJ.* (2018) 363:k5357. doi: 10.1136/bmj.k5357
27. Doi K. Computer-aided diagnosis in medical imaging: historical review, current status and future potential. *Comput Med Imaging Graph.* (2007) 31:198–211. doi: 10.1016/j.compmedimag.2007.02.002

4

Symptomatology and Clinic of Hydronephrosis Associated with Uretero Pelvic Junction Anomalies

Ilmay Bilge*

Division of Pediatric Nephrology, Department of Pediatrics, School of Medicine, Koc University, Istanbul, Turkey

Correspondence:
Ilmay Bilge
ibilge@ku.edu.tr

The most common cause of hydronephrosis in the pediatric age group is ureteropelvic junction-type hydronephrosis (UPJHN). Since the advent of widespread maternal ultrasound screening, clinical presentation of hydronephrosis associated with UPJ anomalies has changed dramatically. Today most cases are diagnosed in the prenatal period, and neonates present without signs or symptoms. For those who are not detected at birth, UPJHN eventually presents throughout childhood and even adulthood with various symptoms. Clinical picture of UPJHN highly depends on the presence and severity of obstruction, and whether it affects single or both kidneys. Abdominal or flank pain, abdominal mass, hematuria, kidney stones, urinary tract infections (UTI), and gastrointestinal discomfort are the main symptoms of UPJHN in childhood. Other less common findings in such patients are growth retardation, anemia, and hypertension. UTI is a relatively rare condition in UPJHN cases, but it may occur as pyelonephritis. Vesicoureteric reflux should be kept in mind as a concomitant pathology in pediatric UPJHN that develop febrile UTI. Although many UPJHN cases are known to improve over time, close clinical observation is critical in order to avoid irreversible kidney damage. The most appropriate approach is to follow-up the patients considering the presence of symptoms, the severity of hydronephrosis and the decrease in kidney function and, if necessary, to decide on early surgical intervention.

Keywords: ureteropelvic junction, hydronephrosis, urinary tract infection, pain, children

INTRODUCTION

Widespread use of prenatal ultrasonography (US) gave clinicians the opportunity to diagnose urinary tract abnormalities much earlier and more frequently than the past (1). The approximate varying incidence of 1 per 750–2,000, ureteropelvic junction type hydronephrosis (UPJHN) is the most common cause of childhood hydronephrosis (2). It occurs in 13% of children with prenatally detected renal pelvis dilatation, and is more common on the left side, more common in boys (2:1- male to female), and is rarely seen bilaterally (2–4).

An obstruction at ureteropelvic junction level which is defined as restriction of urine outflow from pelvis renalis to the ureter may result in progressive deterioration or hinder normal renal development (5–8). Over 50% of all cases considered to have kidney abnormalities in the prenatal period are hydronephrosis, but unfortunately there are currently no reliable prenatal diagnostic test that can distinguish obstructive hydronephrosis from non-obstructive (8–10). The differentiation between urinary tract obstruction and dilatation is the most important problem in the management of these patients (6, 11, 12). Since the clinical course are quite diverse, and generalization is rather difficult, the most appropriate approach of UPJHN seen in children would be to evaluate on a patient basis (4, 13–16).

In this review, the purpose is to provide general information about the clinical presentation and symptomatology of hydronephrosis associated with uretero pelvic junction anomalies, as well as discussing the clinical findings through some case examples.

CLINICAL PRESENTATION

Over the last decades, clinical presentation of patients with UPJHN has shifted from the "symptomatic" patients to the "asymptomatic" neonates who present with prenatal diagnosis (1–4, 15, 16). UPJHN cases without a prenatal diagnosis present with various symptoms such as febrile urinary tract infection (UTI), abdominal masses, pain, pyuria, hematuria, and some gastrointestinal symptoms in the post-natal period or later years. Failure to thrive, anemia, hypertension, and urinary extravasation are much more rare symptoms of UPJHN in childhood (14–16).

Clinical picture of hydronephrosis associated with uretero pelvic junction anomalies highly depends on the presence and severity of obstruction, and whether it affects single or both kidneys. However, most infants with severe hydronephrosis are otherwise asymptomatic and rarely require intervention during follow-up (6, 8, 12). Therefore, parallel to the change in its clinical presentation, the first enthusiasm for early intervention of hydronephrosis associated with UPJ anomalies has turned into a more conservative approach in recent years (11, 15, 17–19). Although there are numerous publications regarding conservative management of UPJ hydronephrosis, and the current trend is to follow the infants through clinical and US findings, the general practice shows a wide variety even today (20–26).

The most accurate answers to the questions of which treatment is better for symptomatic infants, which kidney will benefit from surgery and which patients should be followed up expectantly are still not clear. There are two issues that do not have much discussion during follow-up period of UPJHN patients. First; close monitoring is mandatory for high-grade hydronephrosis managed conservatively; secondly, severe hydronephrosis suggesting an obstruction in solitary kidney is an indisputable condition that requires urgent intervention. An urgent intervention may also be required in patients presenting with urosepsis or acute renal failure (13, 15, 26, 27). In general, the surgical decision in UPJOHN cases is made based on US findings. Therefore, accurate determination of hydronephrosis severity is very important for infants associated with UPJHN. In severe cases of hydronephrosis (SFU 4) with renal parenchymal thinning, clinicians should make a surgical decision without delay, as kidney function may also be impaired in a short time. Based on EAU and ESPU 2019 Guidelines on pediatric urology, surgical indications for UPJHN are impaired renal function (<40%), significant renal functional decrease (>10%) in control scans, poor drainage after furosemide injection, increased AP diameter, and SFU-III/IV (8, 26). Although there are problems

with some of these indications, absolute surgical indications in the follow-up of UPJHN cases can be considered as renal parenchymal thinning (<3 mm), contralateral kidney balancing hypertrophy and decreased kidney function. Differential renal uptake on diuretic renography <30% in unilateral cases and <35% in bilateral cases is usually required a surgical intervention. Surgical treatment can also be recommended in children whose SFU3 hydronephrosis continues for 3 years and develops compensated hypertrophy in the contralateral kidney (27). If the main goal during conservative monitoring is to protect the child from the risk of permanent kidney damage, waiting for ultrasonographic or functional deterioration is a cornerstone that must be distinguished very carefully in each case. It should be noted that at this cornerstone, the presence of symptoms such as recurrent UTI, hematuria, kidney stones or pain will speed up the decision of surgical intervention (21, 26, 27).

As mentioned above, the clinical picture of UPJHN should be evaluated in two different categories, considering that most cases are asymptomatic and diagnosed on routine prenatal US screening; (a) asymptomatic infants who are usually managed conservatively (b) children who present at an older ages with urinary symptoms or as a result of incidental findings during the analysis of unrelated problems.

INFANTS WITH PRENATAL DIAGNOSIS

Symptomatology in a newborn with antenatally diagnosed UPJHN is usually the absence of symptoms. However, the most frequent symptom of UPJHN in neonates and infants was a palpable flank mass in the past. Most of the abdominal masses encountered in the neonatal period are related to hydronephrotic kidneys. Therefore, a palpable abdominal mass may be the first finding to be considered in a physical examination in a newborn with UPJHN.

Since UPJHN is often associated with other congenital anomalies, including imperforated anus, contralateral multicystic kidney, congenital heart disease, VATER syndrome, and esophageal atresia, in a newborn with established prenatal diagnosis, a thorough examination of all systems should be performed (8). Occasionally, UPJHN can also be diagnosed during extended diagnostics of other congenital abnormalities. On the other hand, in all children with a diagnosis of urinary tract infection (UTI) within the early neonatal period, urinary tract obstruction, UPJHN should also be considered.

Urinary Tract Infection

Children with UPJHN and impaired urinary drainage are considered to be prone to severe UTIs (28, 29). Although UTI is an uncommon presentation in UPJHN cases with an incidence of 1.3–12%, it may be quite severe requiring urgent intervention and drainage (4, 30–35). Previous reports suggest that the risk of UTI increases with the degree of hydronephrosis, and patients with high-grade hydronephrosis have significantly higher UTI rates than those with mild hydronephrosis (13.8 vs. 4.1%) (36–39). Although the studies are not standardized in terms of the use of prophylactic antibiotics, the method of detecting infection or the selection of patients for VCUG, it has been clearly demonstrated that patients with mild or moderate hydronephrosis are at much lower risk of significant UTI than patients with severe hydronephrosis.

When a child with UPJHN applies with a febrile UTI, the possibility of associated VUR is an important issue to consider. Based on the fact that some studies show one-third of cases having a VUR (8, 40, 41); VCUG is often favored by European guidelines for all children with UPJO (42, 43). Before deciding to apply VCUG, an invasive procedure with radiation exposure in UPJHN patients, it should be taken into account that in many cases that are often asymptomatic, VUR may improve over time and the concept of benefit-harm to the patient (44–46).

Madden et al. (47) performed VCUG in more than 80% of their patients with UPJHN and in no case detected VUR. In the same study, it was reported that patients who did not undergo VCUG remained asymptomatic and no imaging was required except for follow-up ultrasounds (47). Given the low rate of UTI reported, it may be considered that antibiotic prophylaxis has a limited role in the management of such patients (13, 47–49), and VCUG screening is considered to be optional (50). However, more aggressive evaluation and intervention, including antibiotic prophylaxis and VCUG are often indicated in those with worsening or high-grade hydronephrosis (47, 51–53). It should be noted that the presence of ureter dilatation is also important to suspect VUR even in severe hydronephrosis cases.

Another issue that can be considered for the prevention UTI in boys with UPJHN may be circumcision. Ellison et al. (54) reported that the risk of UTI in boys with UPJHN decreased significantly when circumcised. Although there may be no direct relationship since the stasis is in renal pelvis away from the external urethral meatus, in clinical practice, circumcision may be recommended for infant boys who have UTI history.

CHILDREN WITHOUT PRENATAL DIAGNOSIS

Unlike asymptomatic presentation early in life, older children with UPJHN are often diagnosed due to their specific or non-specific symptoms. A carefully gathered clinical history played a very important role in the diagnosis of patients with UPJHN. These symptoms are usually febrile UTIs, a palpable mass, or unexplained abdominal or flank pain. In addition, UPJHN can be detected during evaluation of stone disease and sudden onset hypertension (8). Another small group ordered for a completely unrelated issue during imaging is diagnosed by chance.

Pain

In children with UPJHN/UPJO, pain is primarily the result of dilation, stretching and spasm of the urinary tract, when the urine flow exceeds the capacity to drain properly. The causes of pain are generally muscle spasm, increased proximal peristalsis, local inflammation, irritation and edema at the site of obstruction. It develops through chemoreptor activation and stretching of the submucosal free nerve endings. The severity of pain depends on the individual's pain threshold and perception, and on the speed and degree of changes in hydrostatic pressure within the

proximal ureter and renal pelvis. Chronic severe obstruction usually does not cause pain.

Although it is generally thought to have gastrointestinal symptoms, It should be noted that attacks of unexplained recurrent vomiting or abdominal discomfort may be associated with UPJ obstruction in infants (55). Sudden onset of severe abdominal pain, nausea, and vomiting, often in the late evening, is typical in older children with UPJO. This colicky-type pain usually begins in the upper lateral midback over the costovertebral angle and occasionally subcostally. It radiates inferiorly and anteriorly toward the groin. At their initial presentation, this symptomatology is far more common than febrile urinary tract infections or hematuria (8, 56). Pain along with increased diuresis should also raise the level of suspicion for an obstructive process. This usually occurs in children who receive a diuretic challenge during a furosemide renal scan.

It is important to recognize that patients with extrinsic anatomic abnormalities (e.g., lower pole crossing vessels) can present with colicky flank pain, which is sometimes associated with vomiting, and may present misleadingly unremarkable test results during their asymptomatic periods (56, 57). There is no history of hydronephrosis in the neonatal period In 75–100% of children with crossing vessels (57–59). The incidence of colickly pain in pure extrinsic UPJHN has been reported as 71.8–100%, increasing with age (57–59). The average age of patients with a crossing vessel is between 7 and 11 years and is statistically higher than in patients with pure intrinsic obstruction (58–61). An ultrasonography performed in the symptomatic period can prevent delay in diagnosis of extrinsic UPJHN due to crossing vessel.

Urinary Stone Disease

Hydronephrosis is considered as a risk factor for stone formation in children. Although the etiology of stone formation does not depend solely on the pelvicaliceal anatomy, impaired urinary drainage, decreased or abnormal peristalsis, increased urine transit times and larger pelvicaliceal volumes play a subtle role during the beginning of the nucleation process in UPJHN patients with nephro/urolithiasis (62) (**Figure 1**).

Hypertension

Published pediatric reports of hypertension obviously caused by hydronephrosis are few, and the numbers of patients included in these reports are very low (63–68). On clinical basis, the number of cases diagnosed with UPJHN/UPJO by referring to the results or symptoms of high blood pressure in the child age group is very few. While the development of clinically significant hypertension or proteinuria is very rare in patients with unilateral hydronephrosis, the same is not the case for bilateral disease (8, 63). Depending on the onset, level, and degree of obstruction as well as the presence of renal parenchymal damage or dysplasia, hypertension may develop during the follow-up.

It has been demonstrated that the function of the hydronephrotic kidney is rather well-preserved in young children, therefore it appears that the intrarenal mechanism leading to hypertension is also reversible (6, 11). The clinical importance of such finding is that surgical management may

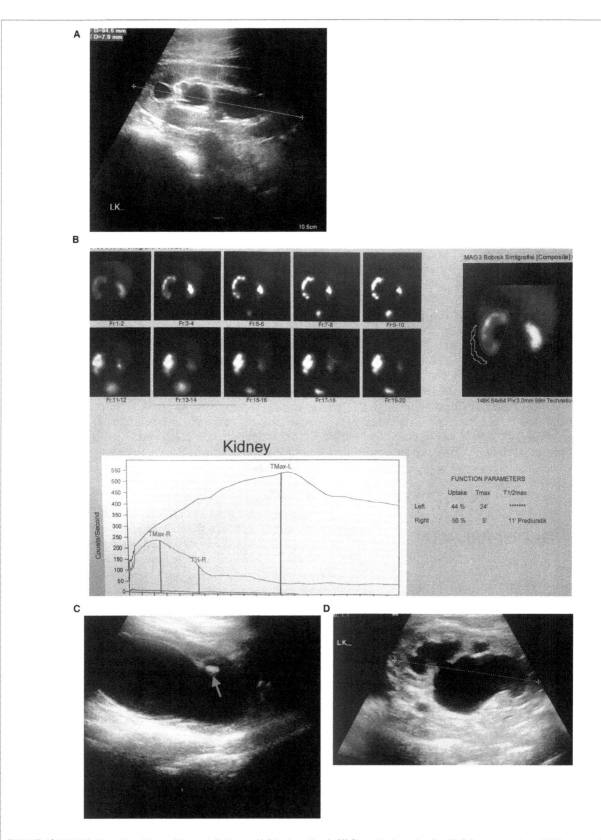

FIGURE 1 | UPJHN in 3 months-old boy with prenatally detected left hydronephrosis **(A)** Severe hydronephrosis with 2.4 mm paranchymal thickness and 22 mm in AP diameter of pelvis renalis **(B)** Left obstructive hydronephrosis with 44% of differential function on MAG 3 scintigraphy **(C)** Mobile hyperechogenic particules in renal pelvis and calyces, hyperechogenicity in the lower calyces which are suggested urinary stone formation **(D)** Mild hydronephrosis with 8 mm paranchymal thickness and 16 mm in AP diameter of pelvis renalis in 9 years after left pyeloplasty.

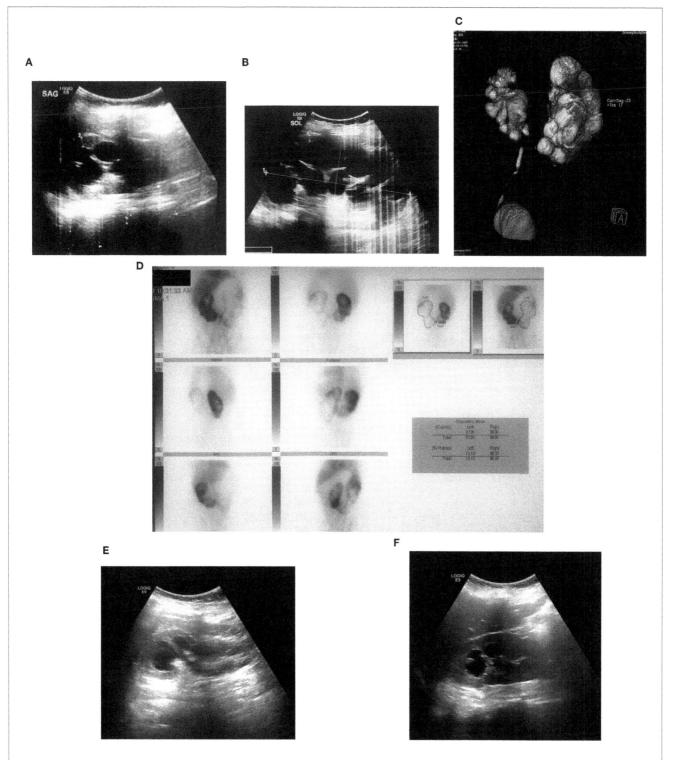

FIGURE 2 | Bilateral UPJHN in 12 years-old boy with prenatally detected bilateral hydronephrosis with no follow-up who presented with severe hypertension and high serum creatinine (1.6 mg/dl) **(A,B)** pre-operative US images showing right and left severe hydronephrosis **(C)** Severe renal paranchymal loss on left kidney with 13% of differential function on DMSA scintigraphy **(D)** bilateral obstructive UPJ type hydronephrosis shown by MR urography **(E,F)** post-operative (bilaterally pyeloplasty) US image showing a resolution of left and right hydronephrosis, which was followed by resolution serum creatinine (0.67 mg/dl) and hypertension.

prevent the development of chronic hypertension and associated comorbidities in patients with severe hydronephrosis (68–70). The pediatric urologist and nephrologist may have to pay more attention to the risk of development of high blood pressure in patients with severe hydronephrosis (**Figure 2**).

CONCLUSION

Current management approach for most children with UPJHN is often considered conservative follow-up because hydronephrosis associated with UPJ anomalies can safely improve over the time. However, it is clear that delayed decision making in the case of obstructive hydronephrosis, which requires surgical intervention, leads to impaired kidney function and long-term morbidity.

It should always be kept in mind that clinical and symptomatological findings, as well as radiological tests, should be carefully evaluated so that the conservative follow-up strategy does not put a single patient at risk for possibly irreversible kidney damage.

Although conservative management algorithms and surgical indications are still an ongoing problem and there is no consensus among different disciplines, it is very important to maintain a long follow-up in both conservatively managed and surgical cases, taking into account negative prognostic factors.

AUTHOR CONTRIBUTIONS

The author confirms being the sole contributor of this work and has approved it for publication.

REFERENCES

1. Thomas DFM. Prenatal diagnosis: what do we know of long term outcomes? *J Pediatr Urol.* (2010) 6:204–11. doi: 10.1016/j.jpurol.2010.01.013
2. Woodward M, Frank D. Postnatal management of antenatal hydronephrosis. *BJU Int.* (2002) 89:149–56. doi: 10.1046/j.1464-4096.2001.woodward.2578.x
3. Nguyen HT, Benson CB, Bromley B, Campbell JB, Chow J, Coleman B, et al. Multidisciplinary consensus on the classification of prenatal an postnatal urinary tract dilation (UTD classification system). *J Pediatr Urol.* (2014) 10:982–99. doi: 10.1016/j.jpurol.2014.10.002
4. Passerotti CC, Kalish LA, Chow J, Passerotti AM, Recabal P, Cendron M, et al. The predictive value of the first postnatal ultrasound in children with antenatal hydronephrosis. *J Pediatr Urol.* (2011) 7:128–36. doi: 10.1016/j.jpurol.2010.09.007
5. Whitaker RH. Some observations and theories on the wide ureter and hydronephrosis. *Br J Urol.* (1975) 47:377–85. doi: 10.1111/j.1464-410X.1975.tb03990.x
6. Koff SA. Requirements for accurately diagnosing chronic partial upper urinary tract obstruction in children with hydronephrosis. *Pediatr Radiol.* (2008) 38 (Suppl. 1):S41–8. doi: 10.1007/s00247-007-0590-2
7. Chevalier RL, Chung KH, Smith CD, Ficenec M, Gomez RA. Renal apoptosis and clusterin following ureteral obstruction: the role of maturation. *J Urol.* (1996) 156:1474–9. doi: 10.1097/00005392-199610000-00075
8. Lorenzo AJ, Csaicsich D, Aufricht C, Khoury AE. *Obstructive Genitourinary Disorders.* Elsevier BV (2008). doi: 10.1016/B978-0-323-04883-5.50043-X
9. Elder JS. Antenatal hydronephrosis. Fetal and neonatal management. *Pediatr Clin North Am.* (1997) 44:1299–321. doi: 10.1016/S0031-3955(05)70558-7
10. Reddy PP, Mandell J. Prenatal diagnosis. Therapeutic implications. *Urol Clin North Am.* (1998) 25:171–80. doi: 10.1016/S0094-0143(05)70005-7
11. Ulman I, Jayanthi V, and Koff SA. The longterm follow-up of newborns with severe unilateral hydronephrosis managed nonoperatively. *J Urol.* (2000) 164 (3 pt 2):1101–5. doi: 10.1097/00005392-200009020-00046
12. Ransley PG, Dhillon HK, Gordon I, Duffy PG, Dillon MJ, Barrat TM. The postnatal management of hydronephrosis diagnosed by prenatal ultrasound. *J Urol.* (1990) 144:584–7. doi: 10.1016/S0022-5347(17)39528-9
13. Nguyen HT, Herndon CD, Cooper C,Gatti J, Kirsch A, Kokorowski P, et al. The Society for fetal urology consensus statement on the evaluation and management of antenatal hydronephrosis. *J Pediatr Urol.* (2010) 6:212–31. doi: 10.1016/j.jpurol.2010.02.205
14. Keays MA, Guerra LA, Mihill J, Raju G, Al-Asheeri NA, Pike J, et al. Reliability assessment of society for fetal urology ultrasound grading system for hydronephrosis. *J Urol.* (2008) 180:1680–2; discussion 1682–3. doi: 10.1016/j.juro.2008.03.107
15. Herndon A. Antenatal hydronephrosis: differential diagnosis, evaluation, and treatment options. *ScientificWorld J.* (2006) 6:2345–65. doi: 10.1100/tsw.2006.366
16. Onen A. Treatment and outcome of prenatally detected newborn hydronephrosis. *J Pediatr Urol.* (2007) 3:469–76. doi: 10.1016/j.jpurol.2007.05.002
17. King L. Fetal hydronephrosis: what is the urologist to do? *Urology.* (1993) 42:229–31. doi: 10.1016/0090-4295(93)90609-E
18. Koff SA. Postnatal management of antenatal hydronephrosis using an observational approach. *Urology.* (2000) 55:609–11. doi: 10.1016/S0090-4295(00)00459-3
19. Perez L, Friedman R, King L. The case for relief of ureteropelvic junction in neonates and young children at time of diagnosis. *Urology.* (1991) 38:195–201. doi: 10.1016/S0090-4295(91)80343-6
20. Weitz M, Schmidt M, Laube G. Primary non surgical management of unilateral ureteropelvic junction obstruction in children: a systematic review. *Pediatr Nephrol.* (2017) 32:2203–13. doi: 10.1007/s00467-016-3566-3
21. Braga LH, Ruzhynsky V, Pemberton J, Farrokhyar F, Demeira J, Lorenzo AJ. Evaluating practice patterns in postnatal management of antenatal hydronehrosis: a national survey of Canadian pediatric urologists and nephrologists. *Urology.* (2014) 83:909–14. doi: 10.1016/j.urology.2013.10.054
22. Williams B, Tareen B, Resnick MI. Pathophysiology and treatment of ureteropelvic junction obstruction. *Curr Urol Rep.* (2007) 8:111–7. doi: 10.1007/s11934-007-0059-8
23. Ingraham SE, McHugh KM. Current perspectives on congenital obstructive nephropathy. *Pediatr Nephrol.* (2011) 26:1453–61. doi: 10.1007/s00467-011-1799-8
24. Chertin B, Rolle U, Farkas A, Puri P. Does delaying pyeloplasty affect renal function in children with prenatal diagnosis of pelvi-ureteric junction obstruction? *BJU Int.* (2002) 90:72–5. doi: 10.1046/j.1464-410X.2002.02829.x
25. Onen A, Jayanthi VR, Koff SA. Long-term follow-up of prenatally detected severe bilateral newborn hydronephrosis initially managed non operatively. *J Urol.* (2002) 168:1118–20. doi: 10.1016/S0022-5347(05)64604-6
26. Radmayr C, Bogaert G, Dogan HS, Kocvara R, Nijman JM, Stein R, et al. *EAU Guidelines on Pediatric Urology.* European Society for Paediatric Urology and European Association of Urology (2020). p. 59–61. Arnhem: EAU Guidelines Office. Available online at: http://uroweb.org/guidelines/compilations-of-all-guidelines/
27. Onen A. Grading of hydronephrosis: an ongoing challenge. *Front. Pediatr.* (2020). doi: 10.3389/fped.2020.00458

28. Riccabona M, Sorantin E, Hausegger K. Imaging guided interventional procedures in pediatric urradiology- a case based overview. *Eur J Radiol.* (2002) 43:167–79. doi: 10.1016/S0720-048X(02)00110-9

29. Khan A, Jhaveri R, Seed PC, Arshad M. Update on associated risk factors, diagnosis, and management of recurrent urinary tract infections in children. *J Pediatric Infect Dis Soc.* (2019) 8:152–9. doi: 10.1093/jpids/piy065

30. Yang Y, Hou Y, Niu ZB, Wang CL. Long-term follow-up and management of prenatally detected, isolated hydronephrosis. *J Pediatr Surg.* (2010) 45:1701–6. doi: 10.1016/j.jpedsurg.2010.03.030

31. Sidhu G, Beyene J, Rosenblum ND. Outcome of isolated antenatal hydronephrosis: a systematic review and meta-analysis. *Pediatr Nephrol.* (2006) 21:218–24. doi: 10.1007/s00467-005-2100-9

32. Lee RS, Cendron M, Kinnamon DD, Nguyen HT. Antenatal hydronephrosis as a predictor of postnatal outcome: a meta-analysis. *Pediatrics.* (2006) 118:586–93. doi: 10.1542/peds.2006-0120

33. Tombesi MM, Alconcher LF. Short-term outcome of mild isolated antenatal hydronephrosis conservatively managed. *J Pediatr Urol.* (2012) 8:129–33. doi: 10.1016/j.jpurol.2011.06.009

34. Estrada CR, Peters CA, Retik AB, Nguyen HT. Vesicoureteral reflux and urinary tract infection in children with a history of prenatal hydronephrosis-should voiding cystourethrography be performed in cases of postnatally persistent grade II hydronephrosis? *J Urol.* (2009) 181:801–6; discussion 806–7. doi: 10.1016/j.juro.2008.10.057

35. Coelho GM, Bouzada MC, Lemos GS, Pereira AK, Lima BP, Oliveira EA. Risk factors for urinary tract infection in children with prenatal renal pelvic dilatation. *J Urol.* (2008) 179:284–9. doi: 10.1016/j.juro.2007.08.159

36. Timberlake MD, Herndorn A. Mild to moderate postnatal hydronephrosis-grading systems and management. *Nat Rev Urol.* (2013) 10:649–56. doi: 10.1038/nrurol.2013.172

37. Coelho GM, Bouzada MC, Pereira AK, Figueiedo BF, Leite MR, Oliveira DS, et al. Outcome of isolated antenatal hydronephrosis: a prospective cohort study. *Pediatr Nephrol.* (2007) 22:1727–34. doi: 10.1007/s00467-007-0539-6

38. Szymanski KM, Al-Said AN, Pippi Salle JL, Capolicchio JP. Do infants with mild prenatal hydronephrosis benefit from screening for vesicouretral reflux? *J Urol.* (2012) 188:576–81. doi: 10.1016/j.juro.2012.04.017

39. Stein R, Dogan HS, Hoebeke P, Kočvara R, Nijman RJ, Radmayr C, et al. European association of urology; european society for pediatric urology. *Eur Urol.* (2015) 67:546–58. doi: 10.1016/j.eururo.2014.11.007

40. Woo HH, Farnsworth RH. Vesico-ureteric reflux and surgically treated pelvi-ureteric junction obstruction in infants under the age of 12 months. *Aust N Z J Surg.* (1996) 66:824–5. doi: 10.1111/j.1445-2197.1996.tb00758.x

41. Perrelli L, Calisti A, Pintus C, D'Errico G. Management of pelviureteric junction obstruction in the first six months of life. *Z Kinderchir.* (1985) 40:158–62. doi: 10.1055/s-2008-1059736

42. Beetz R, Bokenkamp A, Brandis M, Hoyer P, John U, Kemper MJ, et al. Diagnosis of congenital dilatation of the urinary tract. Consensus Group of the Pediatric Nephrology Working Society in cooperation with the pediatric urology working Group of the German Society of urology and with the pediatric urology working Society in the Germany Society of pediatric surgery. *Urologe A.* (2001) 40:495–507; quiz 508–499. doi: 10.1007/s001200170015

43. Silay MS, Undre S, Nambiar AK, Dogan HS, Kocvara R, Nijman RJM, et al. Role of antibiotic prophylaxis in antenatal hydronephrosis: a systematic review from the European Association of Urology/European Society for Paediatric Urology Guidelines Panel. *J Pediatr Urol.* (2017) 13:306–15. doi: 10.1016/j.jpurol.2017.02.023

44. Weitz M, Schmidt M. To screen or not to screen for vesicoureteral reflux in children with ureteropelvic junction obstruction: a systematic review. *Eur J Pediatr.* (2017) 176:1–9. doi: 10.1007/s00431-016-2818-3

45. Williams G, Fletcher JT, Alexander SI, Craig JC. Vesicoureteral Reflux. *J Am Soc Nephrology.* (2008) 19:847–62. doi: 10.1681/ASN.2007020245

46. Stratton KL, Pope JC, Adams MC, Brock JW III, Thomas JC. Implications of ionizing radiation in the pediatric urology patient. *J Urol.* (2010) 183:2137–42. doi: 10.1016/j.juro.2010.02.2384

47. Madden JM, Wiener JS, Routh JC, Ross SS. Resolution rate of isolated low-grade hydronephrosis diagnosed within the first year of life. *J Pediatr Urol.* (2014) 10:639–44. doi: 10.1016/j.jpurol.2014.07.004

48. Lee JH, Choi HS, Kim JK, Won HS, Kim KS, Moon DH, et al. Nonrefluxing neonatal hydronephrosis and the risk of urinary tract infection. *J Urol.* (2008) 179:1524–8. doi: 10.1016/j.juro.2007.11.090

49. Skoog SJ, Peters CA, Arant BS Jr, Copp HL, Elder JS, Hudson RG, et al. Pediatric vesicoureteral reflux guidelines panel summary report: clinical practice guidelines for screening siblings of children with vesicoureteral reflux and neonates/infants with prenatal hydronephrosis. *J Urol.* (2010) 184:1145–51. doi: 10.1016/j.juro.2010.05.066

50. Nicolau N, Renkama KY, Bongers EM, Giles RH, Knoers NV. Genetic, environmental and epigenetic factors involved in CAKUT. *Nat Rev Nephrol.* (2015) 11:720–31. doi: 10.1038/nrneph.2015.140

51. Shaikh N, Ewing AL, Bhatnagar S, Hoberman A. Risk of renal scarring in children with a first urinary tract infection: a systematic review. *Pediatrics.* (2010) 126:1084–91. doi: 10.1542/peds.2010-0685

52. Zanetta VC, Rosman BM, Bromley B, Shipp TD, Chow JS, Campbell JB, et al. Variations in management of mild prenatal hydronephrosis among maternal-fetal medicine obstetricians, and pediatric urologists and radiologists. *J Urol.* (2012) 188:1935–9. doi: 10.1016/j.juro.2012.07.011

53. Docimo SG, Silver RI. Renal ultrasonography in newborns with prrenatally detected hydronephrosis: why wait? *J Urol.* (1997) 157:1387–9. doi: 10.1016/S0022-5347(01)64996-6

54. Ellison JS, Geolani W, Fu BC, Holt SK, Gore JL, Merguerian PA Neonatal circumcision and urinary tract infections in infants with hydronephrosis. *Pediatrics.* (2018) 142:1–7. doi: 10.1542/peds.2017-3703

55. Mergener K, Weinerth JL, Baillie J. Dietl's crisis: a syndrome of episoodic abdominal pain of urologic origin that may present to gastroenterologist. *Am J Gastroenterol.* (1997) 92:2289–91.

56. Cain MP, Rink RC, Thomas AC, Austin PF, Kaefer M, Casale AJ. Symptomatic ureteropelvic junction obstruction in children in the era of prenatal sonography- is there a higher incidence of crossing vessels? *Urology.* (2001) 57:338–41. doi: 10.1016/S0090-4295(00)00995-X

57. Polok M, Toczewski K, Borselle D, Apoznanski W, Jedrzejuk D, Patkowski D. Hydronephrosis in children caused by lower pole crossing vessels—how to choose the proper method of treatment? *Front Pediatr.* (2019) 7:1–4. doi: 10.3389/fped.2019.00083

58. Esposito C, Bleve C, Escolino M, Caione P, GerocarniNappo S, Farina A, et al. Laparoscopic transposition of lower pole crossing vessels (vascular hitch) in children with pelviureteric junction obstruction. *Transl Pediatr.* (2016) 5:256–61. doi: 10.21037/tp.2016.09.08

59. Weiss D, Kadakia S, Kurzweil R, Srinivasan A, Darge K, Shukla A. Detection of crossing vessels in pediatric ureteropelvic junction obstruction: clinical patterns and imaging findings. *J Pediatr Urol.* (2015) 11:173.e1–5. doi: 10.1016/j.jpurol.2015.04.017

60. Chiarenza F, Bleve C, Fasoli L, Battaglino F, Bucci V, Novek S, et al. Ureteropelvic junction obstruction in children by polar vessels. Is laparoscopic vascular hitching procedure a good solution? Single center experience on 35 consecutive patients. *J Pediatr Surg.* (2016) 51:310–4. doi: 10.1016/j.jpedsurg.2015.10.005

61. Schneider A, Ferreira CG, Delay C, Lacreuse I, Moog R, Becmeur F. Lower pole vessels in children with pelviureteric junction obstruction: laparoscopic vascular hitch or dismembered pyeloplasty? *J Pediatr Urol.* (2013) 9:419–23. doi: 10.1016/j.jpurol.2012.07.005

62. Khan SR, Pearle MS, Robertson WG, Gambaro G, Canales BK, Doizi S, et al. Kidney Stones. *Nat Rev Dis Primers.* (2016) 2:16008. doi: 10.1038/nrdp.2016.8

63. Farnham SB, Adams MC, Brock JW, Pope JC. Pediatric urologogical causes of hypertension. *J Urol.* (2005) 173:697–704. doi: 10.1097/01.ju.0000153713.46735.98

64. Abramson M, Jackson B. Hypertension and unilateral hydronephrosis. *J Urol.* (1984) 132:746–8. doi: 10.1016/S0022-5347(17)49855-7

65. Wanner C, Luscher TF, Schollmeyer P, Vetter W. Unilateral hydronephrosis and hypertension: cause or coincidence? *Nephron.* (1987) 45:236–41. doi: 10.1159/000184125

66. Carlström M, Wåhlin N, Sällström J, Skøtt O, Brown R, Persson AE. Hydronephrosis causes salt-sensitive hypertension in rats. *J Hypertens.* (2006) 24:1437–43. doi: 10.1097/01.hjh.0000234126.78766.00

67. Mizuiri S, Amagasaki Y, Hosaka H, Fukasawa K, Nakayama K, Nakamura N, et al. Hypertension in unilateral atrophic kidney secondary to ureteropelvic junction obstruction. *Nephron.* (1992) 61:217–9. doi: 10.1159/000186876

68. Chalisey A, Karim M. Hypertension and hydronephrosis: rapid resolution of high blood pressure following relief of bilateral ureteric obstruction. *J Gen Intern Med.* (2013) 28:478–81. doi: 10.1007/s11606-012-2183-5

69. Al-Mashhadi A, Häggman M, Läckgren G, Ladjevardi S, Nevéus T, Stenberg A, et al. Changes of arterial pressure following relief of obstruction in adults with hydronephrosis. *Ups J Med Sci.* (2018) 123:216–24. doi: 10.1080/03009734.2018.1521890

70. de Waard D, Dik P, Lilien MR, Kok ET, de Jong TP. Hypertension is an indication for surgery in children with ureteropelvic junction obstruction. *J Urol.* (2008) 179:1976–8; discussion 1978–9. doi: 10.1016/j.juro.2008.01.058

5

Managing Ureteropelvic Junction Obstruction in the Young Infant

5

Niccolo Maria Passoni and Craig Andrew Peters*

University of Texas Southwestern Medical Center, Dallas, TX, United States

Correspondence:
Craig Andrew Peters
craig.peters@utsouthwestern.edu

In the last decade, management of congenital UPJ obstruction has become progressively observational despite the lack of precise predictors of outcome. While it is clear that many children will have resolution of their hydronephrosis and healthy kidneys, it is equally clear that there are those in whom renal functional development is at risk. Surgical intervention for the young infant, under 6 months, has become relatively infrequent, yet can be necessary and poses unique challenges. This review will address the clinical evaluation of UPJO in the very young infant and approaches to determining in whom surgical intervention may be preferable, as well as surgical considerations for the small infant. There are some clinical scenarios where the need for intervention is readily apparent, such as the solitary kidney or in child with infection. In others, a careful evaluation and discussion with the family must be undertaken to identify the most appropriate course of care. Further, while minimally invasive pyeloplasty has become commonly performed, it is often withheld from those under 6 months. This review will discuss the key elements of that practice and offer a perspective of where minimally invasive pyeloplasty is of value in the small infant. The modern pediatric urologist must be aware of the various possible clinical situations that may be present with UPJO and feel comfortable in their decision-making and surgical care. Simply delaying an intervention until a child is bigger may not always be the best approach.

Keywords: robotic assisted pyeloplasty, infant–age, prenatal hydronephrosis, diuretic nephrogram, ureteropelvic junction (UPJ) obstruction

INTRODUCTION

Hydronephrosis is the most commonly diagnosed genito-urinary abnormality on prenatal ultrasounds (1). In the past, corrective surgery was offered to every child who presented with uretero-pelvic junction obstruction (UPJO). Indeed, prior to diffusion of fetal ultrasound, patients with this condition were identified due to their signs and symptoms (2). Children were commonly diagnosed between the ages of 6 and 15 years, with only 14% of them being younger than 1 year of age (3).

However, prenatal imaging has increased the rate of diagnosis of asymptomatic cases that may not have otherwise not been detected until later in life. A multitude of studies has questioned the earlier operative paradigm by demonstrating a high rate of spontaneous resolution. Unfortunately, this culminated in a conundrum which today still has no clear solution: which asymptomatic infant with hydronephrosis will lose precious renal function if left untreated?

Finally, diagnosis of a UPJO that warrants surgical correction in an infant poses technical challenges in the modern era of minimally invasive surgery.

In this chapter the threats posed by chronic obstruction to the kidney as well as the natural history of prenatally diagnosed UPJO will be discussed. Surveillance algorithms aimed at identifying early candidates for surgery will be described prior to introducing novel markers and imaging methodologies to improve risk stratification. In the end, traditional and minimally invasive approaches will be compared with a particular attention to tips and tricks for the infant patient.

THE EFFECTS OF OBSTRUCTION ON THE KIDNEY

Hydronephrosis is an abnormal dilation of the collecting system. However, not all hydronephrosis is associated with clinically significant obstruction that will lead to renal function deterioration (4). Unfortunately, long-term complications of renal damage may not be evident until the patient reaches adulthood. Even if a child has normal renal function, these patients are four times more likely to develop ESRD (5) and can require renal replacement therapy in young adulthood (6). Nephrogenesis terminates at 36 weeks of gestation, without any more nephrons formed after birth. Premature babies will have a lower number of nephrons compared to children born at term (7). Therefore, any insult that leads to renal injury will not be followed by replacement of damaged nephrons but by adaptive changes of the remaining nephrons (8). While this mechanism maintains glomerular filtration rate at first, in the long term it appears to lead to renal damage in both the obstructed and the contralateral kidney, as shown in murine models (9).

Furthermore, obstruction that originates *in utero* can lead to more deleterious effects by altering the pathways of renal development (10, 11).

Initial series of biopsies obtained at time of surgical repair showed that up to 21% of children with a differential renal uptake (DRU) on diuretic renography >40% at time of surgery had histological changes, while only 34% of patients with a DRU <40% had normal findings (12). Interestingly, when grouping children by presentation, they demonstrated that only 19% of children diagnosed due to symptoms harbored moderate or severe histological changes, compared to 50% of children diagnosed either prenatally or due to a palpable mass (up to 80%). A larger more recent study found that 67% of biopsies from 61 children had glomerular sclerosis (13). Interestingly, the number of affected glomeruli did not significantly correlate with either degree of hydronephrosis nor DRU. In addition, tubulointerstitial changes were found in only 26% of patients, and significant fibrosis was more common in patients older than 1 year of age, suggesting a potentially progressive process with chronic obstruction. Alteration of the renal parenchyma secondary to obstruction has been documented in human fetuses as well. An autopsy study conducted on fetuses with evidence of UPJO on prenatal ultrasound showed that obstructed kidneys have a reduction in glomerular number and cortical thickness as well as an increase

in fibrosis when compared to specimens from age-matched fetuses with normal kidneys (14). The authors found that fibrosis and reduced glomerular numbers correlated strongly with hyperechogenicity on prenatal ultrasound, which is consistent with clinical observations.

In reality, damage from obstruction is likely secondary to partial obstruction that develops later in pregnancy once nephrogenesis is almost complete, otherwise it would lead to cystic dysplasia or renal agenesis (15).

Just as not all hydronephrosis will persist, as will be discussed in the next section, not all obstructed systems harbor the same damage potential. Therefore, the clinician must be able to synthesize the clinical history and diagnostic data to identify the child more at risk of losing renal function.

NATURAL HISTORY OF PRENATALLY DETECTED HYDRONEPHROSIS

While at first it was believed that most UPJ obstructions with severe dilation detected prenatally required intervention, several studies have shown a relatively high rate of spontaneous resolution. This has led to a shift in management, centered on the serial monitoring of renal dilation and function to hopefully identify the children that will eventually require surgery as early as possible without irreversible loss of renal functional potential.

Several statistics are useful when counseling families of newborns with hydronephrosis secondary to UPJO.

First, that rates of resolution and/or improvement even for severe dilation, as in grade 3 and 4 as defined by the Society for Fetal Urology (SFU) are reasonably good. Indeed, complete resolution rates in observed children range from 33 to 70% (16–23). In the literature, lower rates of resolution are associated with more severe hydronephrosis. Furthermore, another important parameter is improvement in hydronephrosis. Indeed, a change in SFU Grade from 3–4 to 1–2 is considered significant and likely reflects a kidney without significant risk of functional deterioration.

Second, not all children with moderate and severe hydronephrosis have poor DRU as measured on diuretic renography. Data from studies shows that between 10 and 39% of children with SFU grade 3 or 4 have a reduced DRU at diagnosis, defined as <40%. These children are usually offered early pyeloplasty. However, if observation is performed for kidneys with a DRU <40%, renal function remains stable in ~80% of them at 1 year (17, 24). It remains undefined how many may experience later deterioration without intervention.

DIAGNOSIS AND INITIAL EVALUATION

The challenges in managing infants with prenatally detected UPJO are secondary to a lack of diagnostic tools that can identify obstruction that will lead to deterioration of renal function or prevent normal renal functional development. To further complicate matters, the current gold standard evaluation of renal function is diuretic renography; however, we are not sure if a kidney with "normal" DRU on nephrography can be considered completely normal since it likely has received some insults from *in-utero* obstruction (13). Also, diuretic renography does not provide any information regarding the multiple other important functions of the kidney, including tubular homeostatic and endocrine functions. Therefore, urologists need to rely on a combination of ultrasound and diuretic renography findings to individualize management.

Once a baby with prenatal hydronephrosis is delivered, a postnatal ultrasound is obtained to assess persistence of hydronephrosis. Usually it is obtained between 48 and 72 h after birth, due to transient neonatal dehydration. However, it is recommended to obtain this study earlier in specific cases, such as bilateral hydronephrosis, solitary kidney or a history of oligohydramnios. It is also important to record size of the kidney, thickness and echogenicity of the renal parenchyma, as well as appearance of the bladder and post void residuals. Important information can be obtained from the initial ultrasound. Severe hydronephrosis is associated with diffuse and uniform dilation of the calyces with flattening of the renal papillae (**Figure 1**). In severe cases, the hydronephrosis leads to thinning of the renal parenchyma. Asymmetric dilation should raise suspicion of a duplicated system. It is important to remember that a severely dilated renal pelvis with mild-to-moderate dilation of the intra-renal collecting system is usually a hallmark of milder obstruction and pelvic dilation should not be used to draw therapeutic conclusions by itself. Isolated dilation of the extra-renal pelvis is usually considered a benign finding (25). One study showed that while infants extra-renal pelvis dilation have slightly higher rates of UTI, it resolves in 98% of patients on follow-up (26). Furthermore, dilation of the intra-renal pelvis has by far as more significant prognostic values, as highlighted by the adoption of anterio-posterior renal pelvis diameter by the UTD classification (27). Finally, the presence of a dilated ureter can indicate either the presence of vesicoureteral reflux or a more distal obstruction.

A voiding cystourethrogram is usually obtained to rule out lower urinary tract obstruction or vesicoureteral reflux, especially for cases with bilateral hydronephrosis, unilateral hydronephrosis in solitary kidneys or oligohydramnios. However, for a child with unilateral renal dilation without ipsilateral ureteral involvement, a voiding cystourethrogram to rule out reflux might not be needed. Indeed, a recent review showed that among children with UPJO the pooled prevalence of vesicoureteral reflux is 8.2%, 3-fold higher than in children without UPJO (28). Lee et al. demonstrated a higher rate of vesicoureteral reflux among patients with higher grades of hydronephrosis. With the goal or reducing unnecessary radiation exposure and testing, they developed a risk-based approach based on ultrasound findings such as presence of duplication, hydroureteronephrosis and renal dysplasia (29). Performing a VCUG only in children with all three aforementioned ultrasound criteria would reduce the number of tests ordered by 40% while maintaining the same miss rate of reflux as if ordering a VCUG

only if severe hydronephrosis were present. However, it remains controversial as to how valuable the VCUG and identification of reflux might be in this population.

DIURETIC NEPHROGRAPHY

Once severe hydronephrosis is confirmed, diuretic renography is ordered to assess the degree of obstruction as well as the level of renal function. Technetium-99m (99mTc) mercaptoacetyltriglycine (MAG3) is the preferred radionuclide due to its short half-life and its excretion via both glomerular filtration and active tubular secretion, allowing for assessment of poorly functioning kidneys. In general, the amount of tracer uptake in the first 2 min after injection correlates with the glomerular filtration rate.

Several elements can be controlled in order to obtained the most informative study (3). The patient should be adequately hydrated prior to the procedure. Second, the bladder should be emptied with a catheter since a full bladder can impair upper tract drainage, as well-increasing gonadal radiation exposure. Finally, the diuretic has been described as being administered 15 min prior to radionuclide injection, at the same time, or 20–30 min after. The most common approach includes administration of the diuretic once the entire dilated collected system is filled with radionuclide in order to better assess washout. The diuretic that is commonly used is furosemide, at a dose of 1 mg/kg for infants.

Diuretic renography provides several useful parameters. First, it estimates differential renal function. It has been shown that unilateral variation within 5% is considered physiological (30), while a loss >5% should be considered as loss of renal function (31). Second, washout curves can be interpreted to assess the degree of obstruction. However, the traditional T1/2 cut-offs used for obstruction should not be used as rigid checkpoints for therapeutic algorithms.

The astute clinician should remember that UPJO can be a dynamic process and should consider changes in degree of hydronephrosis, DRU as well as washout curves when formulating a treatment strategy. The washout curve can show prompt drainage (**Figure 1**) or obstruction if a flat, plateauing shape is seen (**Figure 2**). However, a biphasic curve can show dynamic obstruction. This curve normally shows prompt drainage that eventually plateaus or even raises, suggesting varying degrees of obstruction (**Figure 3**). Finally, delayed cortical transit time, which is defined as the absence of radionuclide in the sub-cortical renal parenchyma within 3–8 min of injection has been associated with outcomes after pyeloplasty. Song et al. demonstrated that children with delayed cortical transit time had greater improvement of their DRU after surgery compared to those with normal values (32). Furthermore, a delayed transit time has been shown to be a prognostic factor identifying which children will progress to surgery while on observation (33, 34). Interestingly, in a porcine model, delayed cortical transit time has been linked to histological changes such as glomerulosclerosis, decreased number of glomeruli, tubular atrophy, and increased fibrosis (35). However, the correlation between hydronephrosis and diuretic renography findings is

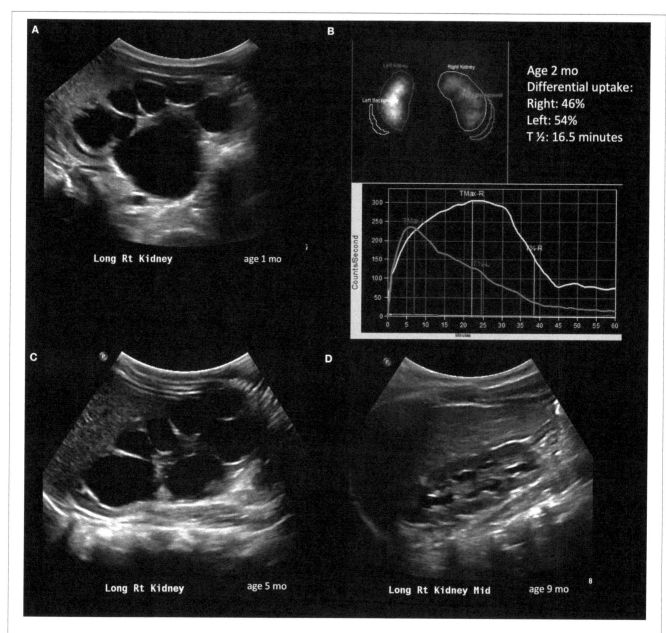

FIGURE 1 | Radiological history of an infant with resolution of severe hydronephrosis. **(A)** Postnatal ultrasound confirming prenatally diagnosed hydronephrosis; the image shows SFU grade 4 hydronephrosis with thinned isoechoic parenchyma. **(B)** Diuretic renogram performed at 2 months of age, showing symmetric uptake; despite the right kidney exhibits a delayed washout curve, it is still considered adequate. **(C)** Repeat ultrasound at 5 months showing persistent SFU grade 4 hydronephrosis. **(D)** Follow-up ultrasound at 9 months showing significant spontaneous improvement of hydronephrosis; the child will still however need follow-up imaging to ensure persistent improvement.

poor (36). Among 13% of children with improving or stable hydronephrosis, DRU worsened more than 5%.

BIOMARKERS

For a long time there has been a focus on urine biomarkers to screen for children with UPJO who will ultimately develop renal damage, yet none are in regular clinical practice to date. Kostic et al. sampled urine and blood from newborns with either lower or upper urinary obstruction and compared values of biomarkers with healthy infants matched by gender and gestational age (37). They identified NGAL (Neutrophil Gelatinase-Associated Lipocalin), RBP (Retinol Binding Protein), TGF-ß1 (Transcription Growth Factor-ß1), and KIM-1 (Kidney Injury Molecule-1) as promising markers, compared to serum creatinine and cystatin, for identifying which patients with unilateral hydronephrosis will progress and require surgery. All their values decreased after surgery.

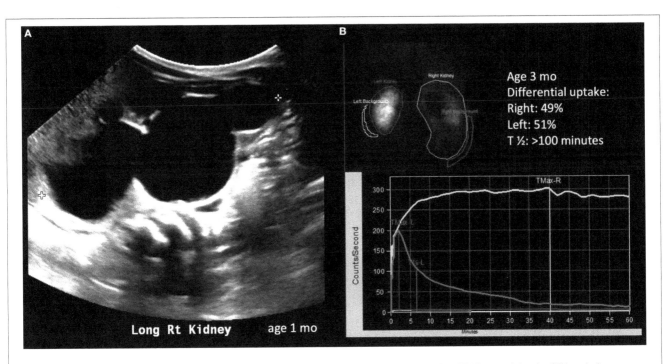

FIGURE 2 | Radiological history of an infant with severe hydronephrosis secondary to significant UPJ obstruction. **(A)** Ultrasound showing SFU grade 4 hydronephrosis on postnatal imaging. **(B)** Diuretic renogram showing symmetrical uptake; unlike the case described in **Figure 1**, the drainage curve of the right kidney does not show any drainage, even after diuretic administration.

These proteins are markers of ischemic and tubule-interstitial pathology, and herald renal damage prior to radiological findings.

The benefits of using urine is that it is readily available, can be collected longitudinally and in a non-invasive manner. However, voided urine contains a mix of urine from both kidneys, and markers from an obstructed system can easily be diluted. Froelich et al. performed urine proteomics analysis by sampling urine from both the obstructed kidney at time of surgery and the bladder (38). They identified 76 proteins that were present both in renal and bladder samples, showing that obstruction produces changes in the urine proteome that are also secondary to compensatory changes in the non-obstructed kidney. A significant number of these proteins were part of the oxidative stress pathway, underling its important role in the pathogenesis of UPJO. Future areas of development for novel biomarkers are magnetic resonance imaging and proteomics and metabolomics (39). While the latter can provide quantitative information on glomerular numbers and volume, the former still requires generation of age-specific normative-data.

Further multi-disciplinary and multi-institutional studies are needed however to identify a marker that can reliably identify obstructed renal units that are at risk of deterioration.

CLINICAL RISK FACTORS OF RENAL DETERIORATION

A copious literature exists investigating what factors are able to predict renal deterioration and thus identify candidate who would benefit from early surgery. This is based on the belief that operating on a child whose DRU has not deteriorated yet will lead to better long-term results. However, there are reports showing that lost function during observation will be recovered after surgical correction (18) and will last into puberty (40). Furthermore, early detection of surgical candidates can potentially reduce costs of follow-up imaging as well as stress for the families. The prediction usually relies on parameters obtained from ultrasound and nuclear medicine imaging. With regard to renal function, infants with a >10% difference in DRU between then hydronephrotic kidney and contralateral healthy one at initial evaluation has been found to experience renal deterioration 3 times more often and to be two times more likely to develop symptoms (41). As mentioned earlier, delayed cortical transit time has been found to be a predictor of deterioration, once having adjusted for other factors such as DRU, T1/2 and hydronephrosis (32, 42). Anterior-posterior diameter (APD) on initial ultrasound has been found to be an independent predictor of resolution of hydronephrosis (43). An APD of 24 mm an initial evaluation has been shown to have high specificity and sensitivity to predict need of surgery, secondary to either a drop of 10% or greater in DRU or worsening hydronephrosis with an obstructed nephrogram (44).

The idea of creating a variable that includes information from both degree of hydronephrosis severity and renal parenchyma thinning was first introduced by Shapiro and coworkers with hydronephrosis index (45). This was obtained by subtracting the area of the calyces and renal pelvis from the total area of the

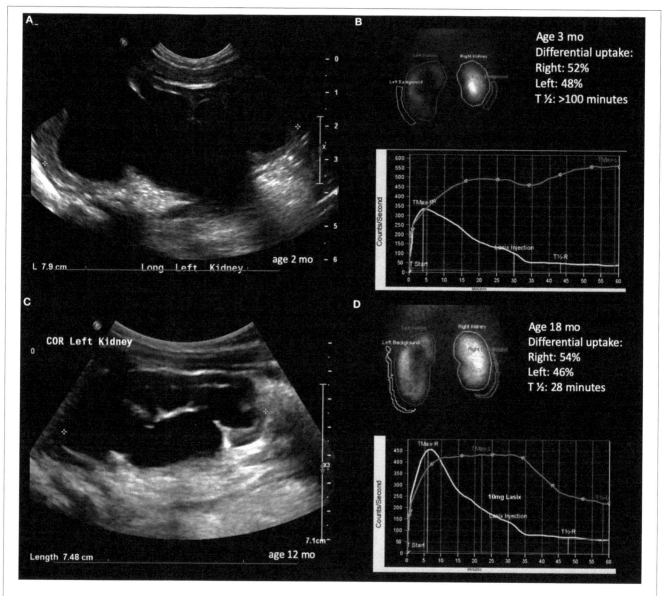

FIGURE 3 | Radiological history of an infant with severe hydronephrosis secondary to UPJ obstruction and biphasic diuretic curve. **(A)** Ultrasound confirming SFU grade 4 hydronephrosis at 2 months of age. **(B)** Diuretic renogram showing symmetrical uptake with biphasic washout curve. **(C)** Ultrasound at 12 months of age showing slightly improving but still SFU grade 4 hydronephrosis. **(D)** Improved washout curve on diuretic renogram, but still with delayed emptying.

kidney and then dividing it by the total area. The hydronephrosis index was shown to be easily reproducible and associated with resolution or worsening of hydronephrosis. Later, Cerrolaza et al. (46), by applying machine learning to ultrasound images and diuretic renogram curves, described how quantitative analysis of renal ultrasound images can predict diuretic renography curves and help reduce the number of nuclear medicine studies. More recently, Rickard et al. (47) showed that the renal parenchyma to hydronephrosis area ratio correlates well with DRU and T1/2, and demonstrated a very good performance in selecting children who will require surgery.

TREATMENT ALGORITHM

Absolute candidates for surgical treatment are symptomatic patients, however defining symptoms of UPJO in infants can be challenging, since most won't be able to complain about pain. Significant symptoms also include recurrent urinary tract infections despite antibiotic prophylaxis, hematuria, kidney stones, or mass effect from the severely dilated kidney. Another absolute indication for surgery is the child with clinical obstruction in a solitary kidney and evidence of reduced overall renal function. For all other patients, the algorithm (**Figure 4**) is a suggested clinically pragmatic approach.

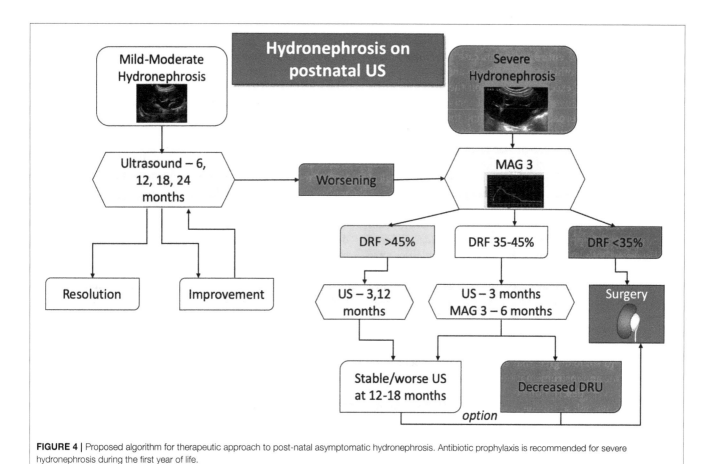

FIGURE 4 | Proposed algorithm for therapeutic approach to post-natal asymptomatic hydronephrosis. Antibiotic prophylaxis is recommended for severe hydronephrosis during the first year of life.

In essence, patients with mild or moderate hydronephrosis, defined as SFU grade 1 or 2, should be followed with serial ultrasounds to detect either improvement and resolution or progression. Children with confirmed severe hydronephrosis on post-natal imaging or those who progress to it should undergo a MAG3 study. The findings of the diuretic renography will dictate the follow up. If the DRU is more than 45%, ultrasound is repeated to assess for degree of dilation, whereas if the DRU is <35% surgery is usually recommended. If the hydronephrosis does not improve on repeated ultrasound images, despite a normal DRU, then surgery can be appropriately offered. For all other patients, US and MAG3 should be repeated, and in case of worsening hydronephrosis or DRU the surgery should be considered. It has been shown that if a patient demonstrates two consecutive drops in their DRU on two consecutive scans, then there is an 85% he or she will require surgery (48). As mentioned earlier, a delayed cortical transit time is also a strong indicator of future renal deterioration and should be incorporated into clinical algorithms without having to wait for actual loss of function.

If the DRU is <10%, some authors argue that a nephrectomy is indicated where there is development of symptoms such as infections or hypertension; otherwise non-intervention is warranted. There are reports of a significant improvement of function in kidneys with a pre-operative DRU <10%. Wagner et al. reported a return to function to a range of 27–53% at 1 year after pyeloplasty (49). Other authors instead recommend placement of a nephrostomy tube for 4 weeks to determine if there will be some recovery of renal function. In their series, up to 70% of kids treated with a urinary diversion recovered from <10% DRU to an average or 29% (50, 51). While this can occur, significant functional improvement has not been common in the senior author's experience, raising concern as to the validity of initial functional assessments, which can be problematic.

SURGICAL TREATMENT OF UPJO IN THE INFANT PATIENT

The challenges of surgical correction of UPJO in patients younger than 1 year of age mainly reside in the adaptation of minimally invasive techniques due to the patient's size. The open Anderson-Hynes dismembered pyeloplasty is considered the gold standard approach in this population. In the very small infant, the dorsal lumbotomy is preferred by the authors for several reasons. First, it avoids muscle splitting, reducing post-operative pain. Second, it allows for direct access to the posterior aspect of the renal pelvis and ureter. Finally, the incision is in a more discrete area, compared to a lateral approach. However, the open approach, unlike the laparoscopic or robotic ones, does not allow for access to the entire ureter, in case of a longer than expected stricture. Another potential disadvantage of the open approach is the use of excessive traction on the tissues in order to improve exposure toward the surgical incision. Indeed, the minimally invasive approach allows to bring the instruments to the tissues, instead of having to bring the tissues to the surgical site, avoiding unnecessary tension that could damage the ureter. Furthermore, unless for selective circumstances like a posterior renal pelvis, minimally-invasive pyeloplasty allows for surgical correction without the need to rotate the kidney.

Minimally invasive approaches have shown direct patient benefit in terms of reduced hospital stay, reduced need of pain medications and improved cosmetics results in older children (52). However, both laparoscopic and robotic pyeloplasties were originally received with skepticism in infant populations. The main concerns raised by critics were the smaller operative field offered by an infant pneumoperitoneum, the limited space for port placement, lack of appropriate-sized instruments for the robot and finally the fact that the robotic system would limit access to the patient by the anesthesia team. It was also argued, appropriately to some degree, that there was limited benefit for the costs in time and instrumentation.

The first ever description of a successful laparoscopic dismembered pyeloplasty in the pediatric literature was by the senior author in 1995, on a 7 years old child (53). Subsequently, Dr. Tan (54) reported on a series of 16 children, in which two had persistent post-operative obstruction, and both these patients were 3 months of age at time of surgery. Hence laparoscopic pyeloplasty was discouraged for patients younger than 6 months. Kutikov et al. subsequently published their outcomes of laparoscopic pyeloplasties in children young than 6 months of age, using 3 mm instruments, showing good results and challenging the conclusion that infants are not candidates for minimally invasive approaches (55). Several other series corroborated the feasibility, safety and good outcomes of laparoscopic management for UPJO in infants (56–61). However, all authors acknowledged the technical difficulty of such procedure and advocate for the need of an experienced surgeon and team in order to perform this surgery.

While conventional laparoscopic pyeloplasty has not gained popularity due to its longer learning curve and high technical demands (62), robotic surgery has become vastly more popular due to instruments that allow for 7 degrees of motion, thee-dimensional displays with magnification, tremor reduction and surgeon ergonomics (63). Furthermore, the learning curve for robotic pyeloplasty has been shown to be similar to that of open surgery (64).

In a study comparing robotic to laparoscopic pyeloplasty in children of all ages, Lee et al. were the first to report on the feasibility of the robotic approach in infants (52). The first published series of robotic pyeloplasties just in infants, Kutikov et al. reported resolution of hydronephrosis in seven of nine, while the remaining two patients had no evidence of obstruction on diuretic renography (65). Dangle and coworkers (66) were the first to compare 10 infants who underwent open pyeloplasty to 10 who underwent robotic surgery. They showed similar outcomes with improved aesthetic results and pain control. These authors also recommended using 8-mm instruments instead of the 5-mm ones, which due to their goose-neck joint design require a greater distance from the tissues to fully articulate, reducing the functional space. However, in the hands of an experienced surgeon, 5 mm instruments do not increase either total operative time nor console time when used in infants, compared to larger children (67). The largest-to-date series on robotic pyeloplasty in infants is a multi-center report that includes 62 surgeries in 60 patients, with a mean age of 7.3 months and a median weight of 8.1 kg (68). Resolution or improvement in hydronephrosis was documented in 91% of kidneys and only two patients required redo pyeloplasty, with no intra-operative and only 7 (11%) post-operative complications.

The robotic approach is however under critique for the perceived increase in medical costs, especially when compared to open surgery. Data show that even if robotic equipment increases costs, the shortened post-operative stay and the frequent usage of the system eventually lead to savings (69). In addition, a shorter hospital stay translates into an increased human capital gain for the parents (70). Further data have that robotic surgery is not more expensive than pure laparoscopic pyeloplasty (71). Robotic costs will continue to decrease as more surgeries are performed with this approach. Indeed, between 2003 and 2015, the utilization of robotic pyeloplasty increased by 29% annually. However, this growth was mainly in children and adolescents. While 40% of pyeloplasties in children and adolescents in 2015 were performed robotically, 85% of infant cases were still performed via an open approach (72). Infant patients accounted for 2% and 19% of all robotic and laparoscopic pyeloplasties performed (73), but these trends are likely to change as more surgeons are trained in minimally invasive approaches.

In the end, surgical experience and volume with either open or minimally invasive technique should be a significant factor in the approach chosen to treat UPJO. In the largest report of minimally-invasive pyeloplasties, including 575 pure laparoscopic and robotic cases, a prolonged operative time, but not patient age, was associated with higher complication rates (74). However, success rates were similar. While operative time can be increased by surgical difficulty, it is also a proxy of surgical experience, since progression on the learning curve is associated with shorter operative times (75). Nationwide data from 2008 to 2010 stressed the importance of hospital volume with regards to outcomes of pyeloplasties (76). At high volume centers, peri-operative outcomes of open or minimally-invasive pyeloplasties were similar, however children who underwent minimally-invasive surgery had a shorter hospital stay. Furthermore, the worse outcomes were seen in patients undergoing minimally invasive surgery at low volume centers. Luckily, the same data showed that minimally-invasive pyeloplasties in infants are more frequently performed in high-volume centers than low-volume ones (2.8 vs. 0.4%).

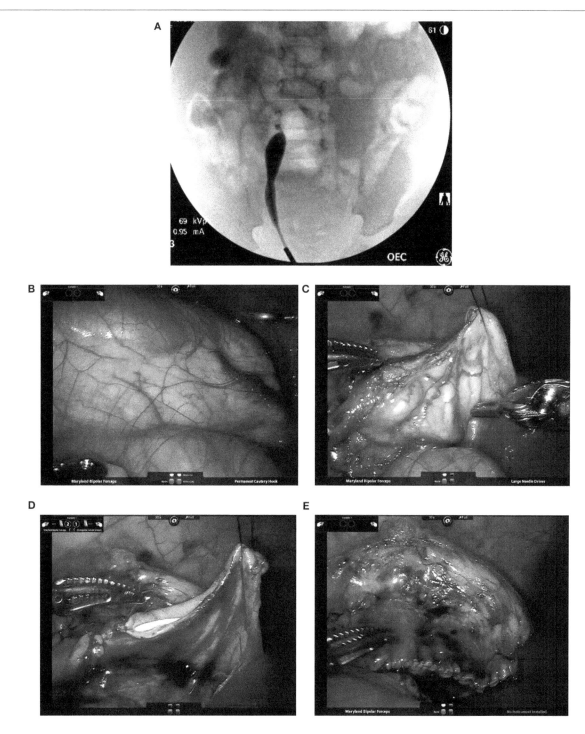

FIGURE 5 | Intra-operative pictures and findings of robotic-assisted laparoscopic pyeloplasty in an infant. **(A)** A retrograde pyelogram performed at the beginning of the case allows for localization of the stricture as well as assessment of its length. This allows for easier planning of reconstructive technique (e.g., dismembered pyeloplasty vs. the need of a flap for longer narrow segments). In addition, it allows for detection of possible distal strictures. A stent is placed at the end prior to the robotic portion of the case. **(B)** Identification of the right kidney with a dilated renal pelvis visible underneath the peritoneum. **(C)** Once the renal pelvis and proximal ureter are dissection, placement of trans-abdominal hitch stich facilitate exposure of the operative field while avoiding the potential use of excessive retraction force by robotic instruments. **(D)** Suturing over the ureteral stent that was placed in a retrograde fashion at time of retrograde pyelogram. **(E)** Complete repair. In the case used for the images, a fair amount of redundant renal pelvis was excised.

TECHNICAL CONSIDERATIONS FOR THE ROBOTIC APPROACH IN THE INFANT PATIENT

At the beginning of the procedure, the authors recommend performing a cystoscopy with retrograde pyelogram. This can rule out any potential distal obstruction as well as delineating the exact extension of the UPJ obstruction. This also allows for placement of a stent in a retrograde manner with an extraction string, eliminating the need for a second cystoscopy (**Figure 5**).

To facilitate port placement in infants we recommend decompression of the bladder with a catheter and the stomach with an orogastric tube as well as a rectal tube to help with colonic decompression. Placement of the ports in the midline can facilitate reduction of instrument clashing. This port configuration can be performed easily with either the daVinci Si or Xi systems. The surgeon should must be aware of the extension of intra-abdominal movements which are amplified externally with the robotic arms. The depth of the ports can also be reduced, placing the proximal thin line on port at the skin level. We strongly recommend using a box-stitch secured to the fascia to facilitate port placement and prevent port slippage. This will also help with port closure at the end of the procedure. The use of a hitch stitch to elevate the renal pelvis can facilitate anastomotic suturing. Finally, since there will be less gas to dissolve the heat from the electrocautery, it is better to reduce the settings to 15 or less. We have found that use of AirSeal® insufflation reduces the problems of fogging significantly.

OUTCOMES

Outcomes of minimally invasive pyeloplasty in the hands of experienced surgeons have been excellent. Reported success rates for laparoscopic surgery are 92–99% while for the robotic approach are 94–100%. The range of complications is wider, 6–30% for laparoscopic and 6–33% for robotic, depending on criterion for consideration as a surgical complication (63, 66, 68, 72, 76).

CONCLUSIONS

Prenatal detection of hydronephrosis secondary to UPJO has increased the numbers of asymptomatic cases from which the clinician must discern who will benefit from surgery and who is best observed. The majority of these children will have resolution of their hydronephrosis, however a non-trivial minority will not improve and may be best managed with surgical intervention to preserve renal functional potential. Early signs of worsening obstruction should be caught promptly in order to offer surgical correction, which can be performed safely with a minimally invasive approach in the hands of an experienced surgeon. Leaving significant obstruction untreated for a prolonged period of time can lead to long-term consequences that will manifest later in the life of the child.

AUTHOR CONTRIBUTIONS

CP and NP were involved in literature review. NP drafted the manuscript. CP provided critical review of the manuscript.

REFERENCES

1. Ficara A, Syngelaki A, Hammami A, Akolekar R, Nicolaides KH. Value of routine ultrasound examination at 35–37 weeks' gestation in diagnosis of fetal abnormalities. *Ultrasound Obstet Gynecol*. (2020) 55:75–80. doi: 10.1002/uog.20857

2. Johnston JH, Evans JP, Glassberg KI, Shapiro SR. Pelvic hydronephrosis in children: a review of 219 personal cases. *J Urol*. (1977) 117:97–101. doi: 10.1016/S0022-534758355-X

3. Bayne CE, Majd M, Rushton HG. Diuresis renography in the evaluation and management of pediatric hydronephrosis: what have we learned? *J Pediatr Urol*. (2019) 15:128–37. doi: 10.1016/j.jpurol.2019.01.011

4. Peters CA. Urinary tract obstruction in children. *J Urol*. (1995) 154:1874–83; discussion 83-4. doi: 10.1016/S0022-534766815-0

5. Calderon-Margalit R, Golan E, Twig G, Leiba A, Tzur D, Afek A, et al. History of childhood kidney disease and risk of adult end-stage renal disease. *N Engl J Med*. (2018) 378:428–38. doi: 10.1056/NEJMoa1700993

6. Wuhl E, van Stralen KJ, Verrina E, Bjerre A, Wanner C, Heaf JG, et al. Timing and outcome of renal replacement therapy in patients with congenital malformations of the kidney and urinary tract. *Clin J Am Soc Nephrol*. (2013) 8:67–74. doi: 10.2215/CJN.03310412

7. Rodriguez MM, Gomez AH, Abitbol CL, Chandar JJ, Duara S, Zilleruelo GE. Histomorphometric analysis of postnatal glomerulogenesis in extremely preterm infants. *Pediatr Dev Pathol*. (2004) 7:17–25. doi: 10.1007/s10024-003-3029-2

8. Chevalier RL. Congenital urinary tract obstruction: the long view. *Adv Chronic Kidney Dis*. (2015) 22:312–9. doi: 10.1053/j.ackd.2015.01.012

9. Chevalier RL, Thornhill BA, Chang AY. Unilateral ureteral obstruction in neonatal rats leads to renal insufficiency in adulthood. *Kidney Int*. (2000) 58:1987–95. doi: 10.1111/j.1523-1755.2000.00371.x

10. Peters CA, Carr MC, Lais A, Retik AB, Mandell J. The response of the fetal kidney to obstruction. *J Urol*. (1992) 148:503–9. doi: 10.1016/S0022-534736640-5

11. Peters CA. Animal models of fetal renal disease. *Prenat Diagn*. (2001) 21:917–23. doi: 10.1002/pd.211

12. Elder JS, Stansbrey R, Dahms BB, Selzman AA. Renal histological changes secondary to ureteropelvic junction obstruction. *J Urol*. (1995) 154:719–22. doi: 10.1016/S0022-534767143-X

13. Huang WY, Peters CA, Zurakowski D, Borer JG, Diamond DA, Bauer SB, et al. Renal biopsy in congenital ureteropelvic junction obstruction: evidence for parenchymal maldevelopment. *Kidney Int*. (2006) 69:137–43. doi: 10.1038/sj.ki.5000004

14. Suresh S, Jindal S, Duvuru P, Lata S, Sadiya N. Fetal obstructive uropathy: impact of renal histopathological changes on prenatal interventions. *Prenat Diagn*. (2011) 31:675–7. doi: 10.1002/pd.2798

15. Rosen S, Peters CA, Chevalier RL, Huang WY. The kidney in congenital ureteropelvic junction obstruction: a spectrum from normal to nephrectomy. *J Urol*. (2008) 179:1257–63. doi: 10.1016/j.juro.2007.11.048

16. Koff SA, Campbell K. Nonoperative management of unilateral neonatal hydronephrosis. *J Urol*. (1992) 148:525–31. doi: 10.1016/S0022-534736644-2

17. Koff SA, Campbell KD. The nonoperative management of unilateral neonatal hydronephrosis: natural history of poorly functioning kidneys. *J Urol*. (1994) 152:593–5. doi: 10.1016/S0022-534732658-7

18. Ulman I, Jayanthi VR, Koff SA. The long-term followup of newborns with severe unilateral hydronephrosis initially treated nonoperatively. *J Urol.* (2000) 164:1101–5. doi: 10.1016/S0022-534767262-X

19. Onen A, Jayanthi VR, Koff SA. Long-term followup of prenatally detected severe bilateral newborn hydronephrosis initially managed nonoperatively. *J Urol.* (2002) 168:1118–20. doi: 10.1016/S0022-534764604-6

20. Chertin B, Pollack A, Koulikov D, Rabinowitz R, Hain D, Hadas-Halpren I, et al. Conservative treatment of ureteropelvic junction obstruction in children with antenatal diagnosis of hydronephrosis: lessons learned after 16 years of follow-up. *Eur Urol.* (2006) 49:734–8. doi: 10.1016/j.eururo.2006.01.046

21. Yang Y, Hou Y, Niu ZB, Wang CL. Long-term follow-up and management of prenatally detected, isolated hydronephrosis. *J Pediatr Surg.* (2010) 45:1701–6. doi: 10.1016/j.jpedsurg.2010.03.030

22. Ross SS, Kardos S, Krill A, Bourland J, Sprague B, Majd M, et al. Observation of infants with SFU grades 3-4 hydronephrosis: worsening drainage with serial diuresis renography indicates surgical intervention and helps prevent loss of renal function. *J Pediatr Urol.* (2011) 7:266–71. doi: 10.1016/j.jpurol.2011.03.001

23. Arena S, Chimenz R, Antonelli E, Peri FM, Romeo P, Impellizzeri P, et al. A long-term follow-up in conservative management of unilateral ureteropelvic junction obstruction with poor drainage and good renal function. *Eur J Pediatr.* (2018) 177:1761–5. doi: 10.1007/s00431-018-3239-2

24. Thorup J, Jokela R, Cortes D, Nielsen OH. The results of 15 years of consistent strategy in treating antenatally suspected pelvi-ureteric junction obstruction. *BJU Int.* (2003) 91:850–2. doi: 10.1046/j.1464-410X.2003.04228.x

25. Lam BC, Wong SN, Yeung CY, Tang MH, Ghosh A. Outcome and management of babies with prenatal ultrasonographic renal abnormalities. *Am J Perinatol.* (1993) 10:263–8. doi: 10.1055/s-2007-994736

26. Katzir Z, Witzling M, Nikolov G, Gvirtz G, Arbel E, Kohelet D, et al. Neonates with extra-renal pelvis: the first 2 years. *Pediatr Nephrol.* (2005) 20:763–7. doi: 10.1007/s00467-005-1851-7

27. Nguyen HT, Benson CB, Bromley B, Campbell JB, Chow J, Coleman B, et al. Multidisciplinary consensus on the classification of prenatal and postnatal urinary tract dilation (UTD classification system). *J Pediatr Urol.* (2014) 10:982–98. doi: 10.1016/j.jpurol.2014.10.002

28. Weitz M, Schmidt M. To screen or not to screen for vesicoureteral reflux in children with ureteropelvic junction obstruction: a systematic review. *Eur J Pediatr.* (2017) 176:1–9. doi: 10.1007/s00431-016-2818-3

29. Lee NG, Rushton HG, Peters CA, Groves DS, Pohl HG. Evaluation of prenatal hydronephrosis: novel criteria for predicting vesicoureteral reflux on ultrasonography. *J Urol.* (2014) 192:914–8. doi: 10.1016/j.juro.2014.03.100

30. Klingensmith WC, 3rd, Briggs DE, Smith WI. Technetium-99m-MAG3 renal studies: normal range and reproducibility of physiologic parameters as a function of age and sex. *J Nucl Med.* (1994) 35:1612–7.

31. Taylor A, Manatunga A, Halkar R, Issa MM, Shenvi NV. A 7% decrease in the differential renal uptake of MAG3 implies a loss in renal function. *Urology.* (2010) 76:1512–6. doi: 10.1016/j.urology.2010.03.066

32. Song SH, Park S, Chae SY, Moon DH, Park S, Kim KS. Predictors of renal functional improvement after pyeloplasty in ureteropelvic junction obstruction: clinical value of visually assessed renal tissue tracer transit in (99m)Tc-mercaptoacetyltriglycine renography. *Urology.* (2017) 108:149–54. doi: 10.1016/j.urology.2017.05.044

33. Harper L, Bourquard D, Grosos C, Abbo O, Ferdynus C, Michel JL, et al. Cortical transit time as a predictive marker of the need for surgery in children with pelvi-ureteric junction stenosis: preliminary study. *J Pediatr Urol.* (2013) 9:1054–8. doi: 10.1016/j.jpurol.2013.03.002

34. Lee JN, Kang JK, Jeong SY, Lee SM, Cho MH, Ha YS, et al. Predictive value of cortical transit time on MAG3 for surgery in antenatally detected unilateral hydronephrosis caused by ureteropelvic junction stenosis. *J Pediatr Urol.* (2018) 14:55 e1–6. doi: 10.1016/j.jpurol.2017.08.009

35. Schlotmann A, Clorius JH, Rohrschneider WK, Clorius SN, Amelung F, Becker K. Diuretic renography in hydronephrosis: delayed tissue tracer transit accompanies both functional decline and tissue reorganization. *J Nucl Med.* (2008) 49:1196–203. doi: 10.2967/jnumed.107.049890

36. Jacobson DL, Flink CC, Johnson EK, Maizels M, Yerkes EB, Lindgren BW, et al. The correlation between serial ultrasound and diuretic renography in children with severe unilateral hydronephrosis. *J Urol.* (2018) 200:440–7. doi: 10.1016/j.juro.2018.03.126

37. Kostic D, Beozzo G, do Couto SB, Kato AHT, Lima L, Palmeira P, et al. The role of renal biomarkers to predict the need of surgery in congenital urinary tract obstruction in infants. *J Pediatr Urol.* (2019) 15:242 e1–9. doi: 10.1016/j.jpurol.2019.03.009

38. Froehlich JW, Kostel SA, Cho PS, Briscoe AC, Steen H, Vaezzadeh AR, et al. Urinary proteomics yield pathological insights for ureteropelvic junction obstruction. *Mol Cell Proteomics.* (2016) 15:2607–15. doi: 10.1074/mcp.M116.059386

39. Chevalier RL. Prognostic factors and biomarkers of congenital obstructive nephropathy. *Pediatr Nephrol.* (2016) 31:1411–20. doi: 10.1007/s00467-015-3291-3

40. Chertin B, Pollack A, Koulikov D, Rabinowitz R, Shen O, Hain D, et al. Does renal function remain stable after puberty in children with prenatal hydronephrosis and improved renal function after pyeloplasty? *J Urol.* (2009) 182(4 Suppl.):1845–8. doi: 10.1016/j.juro.2009.03.008

41. Assmus MA, Kiddoo DA, Hung RW, Metcalfe PD. Initially asymmetrical function on MAG3 renography increases incidence of adverse outcomes. *J Urol.* (2016) 195:1196–202. doi: 10.1016/j.juro.2015.11.011

42. Duong HP, Piepsz A, Collier F, Khelif K, Christophe C, Cassart M, et al. Predicting the clinical outcome of antenatally detected unilateral pelviureteric junction stenosis. *Urology.* (2013) 82:691–6. doi: 10.1016/j.urology.2013.03.041

43. Longpre M, Nguan A, Macneily AE, Afshar K. Prediction of the outcome of antenatally diagnosed hydronephrosis: a multivariable analysis. *J Pediatr Urol.* (2012) 8:135–9. doi: 10.1016/j.jpurol.2011.05.013

44. Arora S, Yadav P, Kumar M, Singh SK, Sureka SK, Mittal V, et al. Predictors for the need of surgery in antenatally detected hydronephrosis due to UPJ obstruction–a prospective multivariate analysis. *J Pediatr Urol.* (2015) 11:248 e1–5. doi: 10.1016/j.jpurol.2015.02.008

45. Shapiro SR, Wahl EF, Silberstein MJ, Steinhardt G. Hydronephrosis index: a new method to track patients with hydronephrosis quantitatively. *Urology.* (2008) 72:536–8. doi: 10.1016/j.urology.2008.02.007

46. Cerrolaza JJ, Peters CA, Martin AD, Myers E, Safdar N, Linguraru MG. Quantitative ultrasound for measuring obstructive severity in children with hydronephrosis. *J Urol.* (2016) 195:1093–9. doi: 10.1016/j.juro.2015.10.173

47. Rickard M, Lorenzo AJ, Braga LH, Munoz C. Parenchyma-to-hydronephrosis area ratio is a promising outcome measure to quantify upper tract changes in infants with high-grade prenatal hydronephrosis. *Urology.* (2017) 104:166–71. doi: 10.1016/j.urology.2017.01.015

48. Kaselas C, Papouis G, Grigoriadis G, Klokkaris A, Kaselas V. Pattern of renal function deterioration as a predictive factor of unilateral ureteropelvic junction obstruction treatment. *Eur Urol.* (2007) 51:551–5. doi: 10.1016/j.eururo.2006.05.053

49. Wagner M, Mayr J, Hacker FM. Improvement of renal split function in hydronephrosis with less than 10 % function. *Eur J Pediatr Surg.* (2008) 18:156–9. doi: 10.1055/s-2008-1038445

50. Gupta DK, Chandrasekharam VV, Srinivas M, Bajpai M. Percutaneous nephrostomy in children with ureteropelvic junction obstruction and poor renal function. *Urology.* (2001) 57:547–50. doi: 10.1016/S0090-429501046-3

51. Ismail A, Elkholy A, Zaghmout O, Alkadhi A, Elnaggar O, Khairat A, et al. Postnatal management of antenatally diagnosed ureteropelvic junction obstruction. *J Pediatr Urol.* (2006) 2:163–8. doi: 10.1016/j.jpurol.2005.07.005

52. Lee RS, Retik AB, Borer JG, Peters CA. Pediatric robot assisted laparoscopic dismembered pyeloplasty: comparison with a cohort of open surgery. *J Urol.* (2006) 175:683–7. doi: 10.1016/S0022-534700183-7

53. Peters CA, Schlussel RN, Retik AB. Pediatric laparoscopic dismembered pyeloplasty. *J Urol.* (1995) 153:1962–5. doi: 10.1016/S0022-534767378-6

54. Tan HL. Laparoscopic Anderson-Hynes dismembered pyeloplasty in children. *J Urol.* (1999) 162:1045–7. doi: 10.1016/S0022-534768060-1

55. Kutikov A, Resnick M, Casale P. Laparoscopic pyeloplasty in the infant younger than 6 months–is it technically possible? *J Urol.* (2006) 175:1477–9. doi: 10.1016/S0022-534700673-7

56. Piaggio LA, Franc-Guimond J, Noh PH, Wehry M, Figueroa TE, Barthold J, et al. Transperitoneal laparoscopic pyeloplasty for primary repair of ureteropelvic junction obstruction in infants and children: comparison with open surgery. *J Urol.* (2007) 178:1579–83. doi: 10.1016/j.juro.2007.03.159

57. Fuchs J, Luithle T, Warmann SW, Haber P, Blumenstock G, Szavay P. Laparoscopic surgery on upper urinary tract in children younger than 1

year: technical aspects and functional outcome. *J Urol.* (2009) 182:1561–8. doi: 10.1016/j.juro.2009.06.063

58. Szavay PO, Luithle T, Seitz G, Warmann SW, Haber P, Fuchs J. Functional outcome after laparoscopic dismembered pyeloplasty in children. *J Pediatr Urol.* (2010) 6:359–63. doi: 10.1016/j.jpurol.2009.10.015

59. Turner RM, 2nd, Fox JA, Tomaszewski JJ, Schneck FX, Docimo SG, Ost MC. Laparoscopic pyeloplasty for ureteropelvic junction obstruction in infants. *J Urol.* (2013) 189:1503–7. doi: 10.1016/j.juro.2012.10.067

60. Garcia-Aparicio L, Blazquez-Gomez E, Martin O, Manzanares A, Garcia-Smith N, Bejarano M, et al. Anderson-hynes pyeloplasty in patients less than 12 months old. Is the laparoscopic approach safe and feasible? *J Endourol.* (2014) 28:906–8. doi: 10.1089/end.2013.0704

61. Chandrasekharam VV. Laparoscopic pyeloplasty in infants: single-surgeon experience. *J Pediatr Urol.* (2015) 11:272 e1–5. doi: 10.1016/j.jpurol.2015.05.013

62. Casale P. Robotic pyeloplasty in the pediatric population. *Curr Opin Urol.* (2009) 19:97–101. doi: 10.1097/MOU.0b013e32831ac6e8

63. Barbosa JA, Kowal A, Onal B, Gouveia E, Walters M, Newcomer J, et al. Comparative evaluation of the resolution of hydronephrosis in children who underwent open and robotic-assisted laparoscopic pyeloplasty. *J Pediatr Urol.* (2013) 9:199–205. doi: 10.1016/j.jpurol.2012.02.002

64. Sorensen MD, Delostrinos C, Johnson MH, Grady RW, Lendvay TS. Comparison of the learning curve and outcomes of robotic assisted pediatric pyeloplasty. *J Urol.* (2011) 185(6 Suppl.):2517–22. doi: 10.1016/j.juro.2011.01.021

65. Kutikov A, Nguyen M, Guzzo T, Canter D, Casale P. Robot assisted pyeloplasty in the infant-lessons learned. *J Urol.* (2006) 176:2237–9. doi: 10.1016/j.juro.2006.07.059

66. Dangle PP, Kearns J, Anderson B, Gundeti MS. Outcomes of infants undergoing robot-assisted laparoscopic pyeloplasty compared to open repair. *J Urol.* (2013) 190:2221–6. doi: 10.1016/j.juro.2013.07.063

67. Baek M, Silay MS, Au JK, Huang GO, Elizondo RA, Puttmann KT, et al. Does the use of 5 mm instruments affect the outcomes of robot-assisted laparoscopic pyeloplasty in smaller working spaces? A comparative analysis of infants and older children. *J Pediatr Urol.* (2018) 14:537 e1–6. doi: 10.1016/j.jpurol.2018.06.010

68. Avery DI, Herbst KW, Lendvay TS, Noh PH, Dangle P, Gundeti MS, et al. Robot-assisted laparoscopic pyeloplasty: multi-institutional experience in infants. *J Pediatr Urol.* (2015) 11:139 e1–5. doi: 10.1016/j.jpurol.2014.11.025

69. Rowe CK, Pierce MW, Tecci KC, Houck CS, Mandell J, Retik AB, et al. A comparative direct cost analysis of pediatric urologic robot-assisted laparoscopic surgery versus open surgery: could robot-assisted surgery be less expensive? *J Endourol.* (2012) 26:871–7. doi: 10.1089/end.2011.0584

70. Behan JW, Kim SS, Dorey F, De Filippo RE, Chang AY, Hardy BE, et al. Human capital gains associated with robotic assisted laparoscopic pyeloplasty in children compared to open pyeloplasty. *J Urol.* (2011) 186(4 Suppl.):1663–7. doi: 10.1016/j.juro.2011.04.019

71. Casella DP, Fox JA, Schneck FX, Cannon GM, Ost MC. Cost analysis of pediatric robot-assisted and laparoscopic pyeloplasty. *J Urol.* (2013) 189:1083–6. doi: 10.1016/j.juro.2012.08.259

72. Varda BK, Wang Y, Chung BI, Lee RS, Kurtz MP, Nelson CP, et al. Has the robot caught up? National trends in utilization, perioperative outcomes, and cost for open, laparoscopic, and robotic pediatric pyeloplasty in the United States from 2003 to 2015. *J Pediatr Urol.* (2018) 14:336 e1–8. doi: 10.1016/j.jpurol.2017.12.010

73. Varda BK, Johnson EK, Clark C, Chung BI, Nelson CP, Chang SL. National trends of perioperative outcomes and costs for open, laparoscopic and robotic pediatric pyeloplasty. *J Urol.* (2014) 191:1090–5. doi: 10.1016/j.juro.2013.10.077

74. Silay MS, Spinoit AF, Undre S, Fiala V, Tandogdu Z, Garmanova T, et al. Global minimally invasive pyeloplasty study in children: results from the pediatric urology expert group of the european association of urology young academic urologists working party. *J Pediatr Urol.* (2016) 12:229 e1–7. doi: 10.1016/j.jpurol.2016.04.007

75. Tasian GE, Wiebe DJ, Casale P. Learning curve of robotic assisted pyeloplasty for pediatric urology fellows. *J Urol.* (2013) 190(4 Suppl.):1622–6. doi: 10.1016/j.juro.2013.02.009

76. Sukumar S, Djahangirian O, Sood A, Sammon JD, Varda B, Janosek-Albright K, et al. Minimally invasive vs. open pyeloplasty in children: the differential effect of procedure volume on operative outcomes. *Urology.* (2014) 84:180–4. doi: 10.1016/j.urology.2014.02.002

6

Comparing Robot-Assisted Laparoscopic Pyeloplasty vs. Laparoscopic Pyeloplasty in Infants Aged 12 Months or Less

Yuenshan Sammi Wong, Kristine Kit Yi Pang and Yuk Him Tam*

Division of Paediatric Surgery and Paediatric Urology, Department of Surgery, Prince of Wales Hospital, The Chinese University of Hong Kong, Shatin, Hong Kong

*Correspondence:
Yuk Him Tam
pyhtam@surgery.cuhk.edu.hk

Objective: To investigate the outcomes of minimally invasive approach to infants with ureteropelvic junction (UPJ) obstruction by comparing the two surgical modalities of robot-assisted laparoscopic pyeloplasty (RALP) and laparoscopic pyeloplasty (LP).

Methods: We conducted a retrospective review of all consecutive infants aged $\leq$12 months who underwent either LP or RALP in a single institution over the period of 2008–Jul 2020. We included primary pyeloplasty cases that were performed by or under the supervision of the same surgeon.

Results: Forty-six infants (LP = 22; RALP = 24) were included with medians of age and body weight at 6 months (2–12months) and 8.0 kg (5.4–10 kg), respectively. There was no difference between the two groups in the patients' demographics and pre-operative characteristics. All infants underwent LP or RALP successfully without conversion to open surgery. None had intraoperative complications. Operative time (OT) was 242 min (SD = 59) in LP, compared with 225 min (SD = 39) of RALP ($p = 0.25$). Linear regression analysis showed a significant trend of decrease in OT with increasing case experience of RALP($p = 0.005$). No difference was noted in the post-operative analgesic requirement. RALP was associated with a shorter hospital length of stay than LP (3 vs. 3.8 days; $p = 0.009$). 4/22(18%) LP and 3/24(13%) RALP developed post-operative complications ($p = 0.59$), mostly minor and stent-related. The success rates were 20/22 (91%) in LP and 23/24 (96%) in RALP ($p = 0.49$).

Conclusions: Pyeloplasty by minimally invasive approach is safe and effective in the infant population. RALP may have superiority over LP in infants with its faster recovery and a more manageable learning curve to acquire the skills.

Keywords: ureteropelvic junction obstruction, infant, standard laparoscopy, pyeloplasty in infants, robot assisted laparoscopy

INTRODUCTION

Previous studies of meta-analysis have shown that both laparoscopic pyeloplasty (LP) and robot-assisted laparoscopic pyeloplasty (RALP) are viable options to treat ureteropelvic junction (UPJ) obstruction in children with the benefits of shorter hospital stay and decreased morbidity while maintaining a success rate comparable to open pyeloplasty (OP) (1–3).

The contemporary evidence of performing pyeloplasty by minimally invasive approach in the infant population, however, are less robust than in older children as there are few comparative studies ever published (4–6).

The expanding interest in minimally invasive pyeloplasty in children is mainly brought by the momentum of the robotic technology. National trends study in the United States between 2003 and 2015 showed that LP decreased annually by a rate of 12% while RALP grew by 29% annually (7). By 2015, RALP accounted for 40% of total cases and comprised 84% of cases among adolescents (7). A big contrast, however, was noted in the infant population in which 85% of cases were OP while RALP and LP accounted for 10 and 5%, respectively in 2015 (7). Adoption of minimally invasive approach in infants has been slow due to the perceived technical challenges associated with the anatomical and physiological constraints of infants and the high success rate by OP (5, 6, 8). Infants were excluded in some of the comparative studies (9, 10).

Our institution has adopted the minimally invasive approach for correction of UPJ obstruction across the entire pediatric age groups for two decades (11). LP had been our standard until Jan 2014 when it was replaced by RALP. In this study we aimed to compare the outcomes of the two minimally invasive modalities in infants. We hypothesized that RALP has superiority over LP in infants.

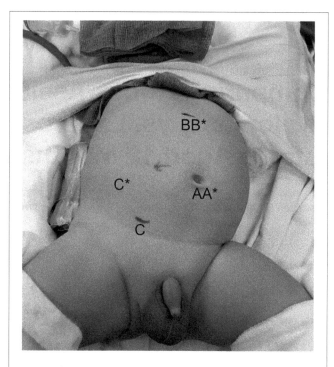

FIGURE 1 | Positions of the ports in a 3-month-old infant who underwent right-sided RALP. A, B, and C, positions of the ports in RALP; A*, B*, and C*, positions of the ports if the procedure were LP.

MATERIALS AND METHODS

After getting the approval of the clinical research ethics committee of our institution, we retrospectively reviewed the medical records of all consecutive infants aged 12 months or less who underwent either LP or RALP for UPJ obstruction in our institution over the period of 2008–July 2020. We included those primary pyeloplasties which were performed by or under the supervision of the senior author of this study using standardized surgical techniques, and similar pre- and post-operative management protocols. Re-operative pyeloplasty was excluded. All the LP cases were recruited before Jan 2014, and since then all the infant pyeloplasties had been performed by the robotic approach.

Before surgery, all patients had ultrasound (US) and MAG3 scan which showed Society of Fetal Urology (SFU) grade 3 or 4 hydronephrosis, and obstructed drainage with diuretic t-half > 20 min of the affected kidney. Indications for surgery included progressive worsening of hydronephrosis in serial US, drop in split renal function $<45\%$ in the initial or repeat MAG3, giant hydronephrosis with mass effect requiring percutaneous nephrostomy (PCN) decompression in neonatal period, and urosepsis.

All patients had double-J stent inserted at the time of pyeloplasty and was removed in 3–4 weeks. Routine post-operative evaluation included both US and MAG3 scan in 2–3 months after double-J stent removal. US was then repeated in 6 months and then yearly if the initial post-operative investigations suggested successful pyeloplasty. Success of surgery was defined by absence of repeat intervention plus 1 or more of the

following radiological criteria: (i) resolution of hydronephrosis with anteroposterior diameter (APD) of renal pelvis <10 mm in US, (ii) improved drainage in MAG3 scan with diuretic t-half < 20 min, (iii) reduction in hydronephrosis with stable split renal function in MAG3 scan.

We collected data on patients' demographics, clinical characteristics at baseline, post-operative radiological findings, operative details, complications, analgesic requirement, length of hospital stay (LOS), and follow-up period. Operative time (OT) was defined by the time interval from the first skin incision to completion of wound closure. Post-operative complications were graded according to the Clavien classification (12).

We have previously described our technique of LP and RALP (13). Transperitoneal approach was used in both LP and RALP. The surgical steps of the two approaches were almost identical. Only three ports were used in both approaches with a single transabdominal hitching suture to lift and stabilize the renal pelvis. No accessory port was used in RALP. We used 3-mm instruments in LP and 8-mm instruments in RALP. The initial cases of RALP were performed by the da Vinci S model (Intuitive Surgical, Sunnyvale, CA) which was subsequently replaced by the Xi model. In RALP, we placed a purse-string suture to tighten the musculofascial defect around the camera port at the umbilicus and the suture was further tied onto the short rubber latex tube placed around the port. The two working ports were placed at sub-xiphoid and suprainguinal region just lateral to the inferior epigastric vessels under the laparoscopic view (**Figure 1**). A double-J stent was routinely inserted by antegrade method

TABLE 1 | Summary of the baseline characteristics of the two groups.

	LP; $n = 22$	RALP; $n = 24$	p-values
Median age in months at the time of surgery (range)	6 (3–12)	5.5 (2–12)	0.97
Median body weight in kg at the time of surgery (range)	8.5 (5.4–10)	7.9 (5.7–10)	0.56
Gender: male/female	17/5	20/4	0.61
Laterality: left/right	16/6	13/11	0.19
Antenatal diagnosis	22/22	24/24	NA
Temporary PCN before surgery	3/22	6/24	0.33
Pre-operative imaging:			
APD in US	31 ± 12 mm	32 ± 12 mm	0.89
SRF in MAG3	44.8 ± 6.5%	45.6 ± 9.5%	0.74

LP, laparoscopic pyeloplasty; RALP, robot-assisted laparoscopic pyeloplasty; US, ultrasound; APD, anteroposterior diameter; SRF, split renal function; PCN, percutaneous nephrostomy; NA, not applicable.

over guidewire introduced transabdominally. Cystoscopy would be used if difficulty was encountered in passing the double-J stent into bladder by antegrade method. Intraoperative fluroscopy was used in every case to confirm the position of the distal end of double-J stent.

Comparative analysis was performed between the two groups. Primary outcome was success of surgery. Secondary outcomes were other perioperative parameters. Categorical data were compared using chi-square or Fisher exact test. Continuous data were expressed as median with range or mean with standard deviation (SD). Continuous data were compared by Student t test or Mann-Whitney test as appropriate. Linear regression was used to investigate the trend of OT against increasing case experience. A p-value of < 0.05 was considered to be significant.

RESULTS

A total of 46 infants (LP = 22; RALP = 24) were included in this study. The medians of age and body weight were 6 months (2–12 months) and 8.0 kg (5.4–10 kg), respectively. There was no difference between the two groups in the patients' demographics and clinical characteristics at baseline (**Table 1**). No OP was performed for infants during the study period.

All infants underwent LP or RALP successfully without conversion to open surgery or requirement of additional ports. None of the patients had intraoperative complications such as vascular or bowel injury, and none required blood transfusion. The estimated blood loss recorded was minimal with 5 ml or less.

Table 2 summarized the perioperative parameters and post-pyeloplasty outcomes. OT was 242 min (SD = 59) in LP, compared with 225 min (SD = 39) of RALP ($p = 0.25$). Linear regression analysis showed a significant trend of decrease in OT with increasing case experience of RALP ($p = 0.005$) (**Figure 2**).

No difference was noted in the post-operative analgesic requirement. RALP was associated with a shorter LOS of 3

TABLE 2 | Summary of the perioperative parameters and surgical success of the two groups.

	LP; $n = 22$	RALP; $n = 24$	p-values
OT in minutes	242 ± 59	225 ± 3 9	0.25
Intraoperative cystoscopy	2/22	2/24	0.93
Aberrant crossing vessels	0/22	3/24	0.09
Participation of surgeon-in-training	7/22	12/24	0.21
Conversion to open or placement of additional ports	Nil	Nil	NA
Intraoperative complications or blood transfusion	Nil	Nil	NA
Mean number of doses of oral acetominophen per patient	3.8 ± 2.5	4.3 ± 3.2	0.55
Mean number of doses of intramuscular narcotics per patient	0.15 ± 0.50	0.04 ± 0.20	0.31
LOS in days	3.8 ± 1.3	3.0 ± 0.3	0.009
Post-operative complications (%)	4/22 (18)	3/24 (13)	0.59
Clavien Grade I – II	Prolonged ileus = 1 Stent-related UTI = 3	Stent-related UTI =2	
Clavien Grade IIIb		Proximal migration of Double-J stent = 1	
Operative success (%)	20/22 (91)	23/24 (96)	0.49
Mean follow-up in months	40 ± 16	23 ± 12	<0.001

LP, laparoscopic pyeloplasty; RALP, robot-assisted laparoscopic pyeloplasty; OT, operative time; LOS, length of stay; UTI, urinary tract infection; NA, not applicable.

days (SD = 0.3) compared with 3.8 days (SD = 1.3) of LP ($p = 0.009$). 4/22(18%) LP and 3/24(13%) RALP developed post-operative complications ($p = 0.59$). All but one of the complications were minor of Clavien grade I-II (prolonged ileus = 1; stent-related urinary tract infection = 5). The only Clavien grade III complication happened in the RALP group due to proximal migration of the double-J stent which was removed cystoscopically by a Fr 4 Amplatz Gooseneck snare catheter.

The success rates were 20/22(91%) in LP and 23/24(96%) in RALP ($p = 0.49$). The two failures in LP underwent redo-LP as they occurred before the introduction of RALP in our institution, and the single failure in RALP was treated by redo-RALP. All three redo-pyeloplasties were successful.

DISCUSSION

The existing data of minimally invasive pyeloplasty in infants are derived from case series (14, 15), comparative studies with OP (16, 17), and comparative studies with older children (18, 19). To the best of our knowledge, the present study is the first single-institution study to compare LP vs. RALP in infants. Others

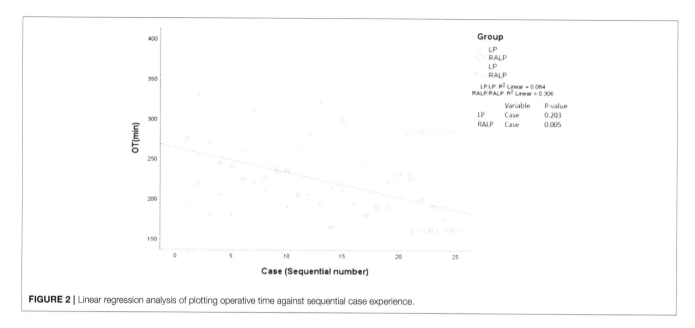

FIGURE 2 | Linear regression analysis of plotting operative time against sequential case experience.

have reported their findings by comparing two cohorts of infants who underwent LP and RALP in two different institutions (20). Our study design of recruiting patients managed by the same surgeon may reduce the confounding effects caused by variations in surgical techniques, post-operative protocols, and in-patient practices which happened in multi-institutional studies (15, 20).

Our finding of 91% success rate of LP is similar to 92% reported by previous studies (14, 20) in infants. Concern has been raised whether the failure rate of LP could be higher in infants than in older children (21). A recent systematic review found an average success rate of 96.9% for LP in children (4). The authors, however, reported that there were very few studies targeted at infants (4). Failures of LP in infants may have been underreported, and the world-wide declining interest in LP has hampered further studies in infants for whom few surgeons perform LP (7).

The largest published series of RALP in infants was from a multi-institutional study which recruited 60 patients and reported 91% success rate (15). Two recent single-institution studies reported 93.8 and 94.1% success rates of RALP in 16 and 34 infants, respectively (18, 19). In both studies the authors did not note any difference in success rates between infants and older children (18, 19).

The latest meta-analysis performed by Taktak et al. included eight more studies comparing RALP vs. LP in pediatric populations (22) than the previous meta-analysis by Cundy et al. (1). The authors found a significantly higher success rate and shorter LOS in RALP than LP in children (22). Our findings of 96% success rate in RALP did not reach significant difference when compared with the 91% of LP. Further studies are warranted to investigate whether the potential superiority of pediatric RALP over LP in treatment success can be expanded to the infant population.

A bi-institutional study reported a significantly shorter LOS of RALP than LP in infants (1 vs. 7 days) (20). The authors, however, explained the finding by the difference in the healthcare systems

and hospitalization polices of the two institutions where LP and RALP were separately performed (20). We found a statistically significant but small difference in LOS in favor of RALP(3 vs. 3.8 days). Our finding, however, needs to be interpreted with caution. The clinical significance of a difference in LOS of <1 day is questionable. Given the small number in either group, any outliers might have significant effect in the statistical analysis. Although all our study subjects were under the care of the same surgeon over the entire study period, we cannot exclude the possibility of a slight change in discharge criteria over time which might have disadvantaged the LP group in LOS. Nevertheless, it is our subjective experience that the robotic technology enhances the precision in tissue approximation and suturing, and thus has the potential to promote a faster recovery by allowing better tissue healing with less subclinical urine leakage.

It is debatable whether 5- or 8-mm instruments should be used in infant RALP. Use of 5-mm instruments allows a smaller incision at the cost of requiring a longer intracorporeal length for articulation due to its pulley system, which is the concern raised by some surgeons (8, 15). Proponents of 5-mm instruments, however, have reported the safety and similarly high success rates in infant and non-infant pediatric populations (18, 19). We have had no experience in using 5-mm instruments which are not supported by the current da Vinci Xi platform. Our findings of the post-operative analgesic requirement do not suggest any significant negative effects associated with the use of 8-mm ports in RALP when compared with LP using 5- and 3-mm ports. Nevertheless, we fully echo with others the need of the development of miniaturized robotic instruments specific for infants and small children (23).

Our OT of 225 min in infant RALP is much longer than the 115 and 144 min reported by master surgeons working at high-volume centers (16, 18), but similar to the 232 min reported by a multi-institutional study involving teaching hospitals with fellowship or residency training programs (15). Given our small case volume, we are still at a distance from achieving mastery in infant RALP. Our OT also included the time spent on undocking and redocking for fluoroscopy, and some cases involved training of surgeons who had not attained competency in pediatric RALP. We did not detect any difference in OT between the two groups of LP and RALP. However, the additional time spent on docking in RALP might suggest a faster procedure in RALP than LP, particularly during the intracorporeal suturing which the robotic platform alleviates much of the technical difficulty. The linear regression analysis demonstrated a significant trend of decrease in OT with increasing experience in RALP, and a trend of OT in favor of RALP after the first 10 cases. Given the two groups were comparable in other study variables, our finding suggests a faster learning curve of RALP than LP in infants.

Despite our long history of performing pediatric pyeloplasty by minimally invasive approach, our institution had only one surgeon left who was competent to perform LP in 2013. Since the adoption of RALP in 2014, there are currently three surgeons in our institution who are competent to perform pediatric RALP. We agree with others that the robotic technology offers the advantage of creating a more manageable learning curve for minimally invasive pyeloplasty, thus making it more accessible particularly to the infant population in which application of LP is even more challenging than older children (4).

We followed the technical tricks in infant RALP as described before with some modifications. Air leakage at the port site is more of a concern in infants than older children given the thin abdominal wall and its laxity in infants. We prevent air leakage by placing a purse-string suture to tighten the musculofascial defect around the camera port at the umbilicus and the suture was further tied onto the short rubber latex tube placed around the port to prevent it from accidentally slipping out. We did not anchor the two working ports to skin by sutures, and we made the incisions precisely such that the wounds were not any bigger than the trocars. Creating an adequate working space both intracorporeally and extracorporeally is critical to success in performing RALP in infants. Our ports positioning allows adequate distance to prevent trocar collision while avoiding the risk of bladder injury if the ports are all placed in midline as preferred by some surgeons (8, 15, 18). Elevation of the ports against the abdominal wall, and keeping a minimal depth of working ports inside the peritoneal cavity are both pivotal in maximizing the intracorporeal working space for small infants. It should be emphasized that excessive force in traction or grasping tissues may go unnoticed due to lack of tactile feedback of the robotic instruments, and extra caution must be exercised in infants whose tissues are more fragile than older children.

We acknowledged the limitations of our study including the retrospective nature, small case numbers over a long review period, lack of breakdown of OT, difference in follow-up periods, and lack of details of participation of surgeon-in-training.

Patients were assigned the surgical approach chronologically without any randomization, and all the RALP cases were recruited after we had stopped performing LP. The prior acquisition of skills in LP may have given advantage in subsequent RALP. Our study findings did not allow estimation of the number of cases required to complete the learning phase of either technique. The generalizability of our data from a single institution is questionable, although some of the potential bias may be reduced by the standardized surgical techniques and management protocols. It was beyond the scope of the present study to investigate and compare the costs of the two procedures. The public healthcare service in our society is heavily subsidized by government such that it was almost free of charge for our patients' families whether the procedure was LP or RALP. There are no data in the billing system or from the finance department of our institution that we can retrieve to investigate the costs incurred from each surgical procedure. There is no question that it is a huge investment in purchasing a robotic platform, and the costs for maintenance and the disposable instruments are substantial. Previous single-institution studies have reported no difference in cost when RALP was compared with OP in infants (17), and when RALP was compared with LP in pediatric patients (24). At a national level, pediatric RALP was found to be associated with a higher cost than OP, and the relatively small number of pediatric pyeloplasty even in high-volume children's hospitals remained to be a limiting factor for reducing the cost of RALP (7). The robotic platform in our institution is shared among pediatric and adult patients. The high-volume adult robotic surgeries might give us an advantage in cost-effectiveness of performing pediatric RALP.

Given the paucity of data comparing the two minimally invasive modalities in infants, we believe our findings would contribute to the existing literature with addition evidence despite all the study limitations. Both LP and RALP are safe and effective modalities via a minimally invasive approach for correction of UPJ obstruction in infants. RALP appears to have superiority over LP in infants with its faster recovery, and a more manageable learning curve for skills acquisition. Our findings support the application of RALP across the entire pediatric population including infants.

AUTHOR CONTRIBUTIONS

YW: study design, data collection and analysis, literature review, and draft manuscript. KP: data collection and analysis and literature review. YT: study design, literature review, and revised manuscript. All authors contributed to the article and approved the submitted version.

REFERENCES

1. Cundy TP, Harling L, Hughes-Hallett A, Mayer EK, Najmaldin AS, Athanasiou T, et al. Meta-analysis of robot-assisted vs conventional laparoscopic and open pyeloplasty in children. *BJU Int.* (2014) 114:582–94. doi: 10.1111/bju.12683

2. Mei H, Pu J, Yang C, Zhang H, Zheng L, Tong Q. Laparoscopic versus open pyeloplasty for ureteropelvic junction obstruction in children: a systematic review and meta-analysis. *J Endourol.* (2011) 25:727–36. doi: 10.1089/end.2010.0544

3. Huang Y, Wu Y, Shan W, Zeng L, Huang L. An updated meta-analysis of

laparoscopic versus open pyeloplasty for ureteropelvic junction obstruction in children. *Int J Clin Exp Med.* (2015) 8:4922–31.

4. Andolfi C, Adamic B, Oommen J, Gundeti MS. Robot-assisted laparoscopic pyeloplasty in infants and children: is it superior to conventional laparoscopy? *World J Urol.* (2020) 38:1827–33. doi: 10.1007/s00345-019-02943-z

5. Villanueva J, Killian M, Chaudhry R. Robotic urologic surgery in the infant: a review. *Curr Urol Rep.* (2019) 20:35. doi: 10.1007/s11934-019-0902-8

6. Passoni NM, Peters CA. Managing ureteropelvic junction obstruction in the young infant. *Front Pediatr.* (2020) 8:242. doi: 10.3389/fped.2020.00242

7. Varda BK, Wang Y, Chung BI, Lee RS, Kurtz MP, Nelson CP, et al. Has the robot caught up? National trends in utilization, perioperative outcomes, and cost for open, laparoscopic, and robotic pediatric pyeloplasty in the United States from 2003 to 2015. *J Pediatr Urol.* (2018) 14:336.e1–8. doi: 10.1016/j.jpurol.2017.12.010

8. Boysen WR, Gundeti MS. Robot-assisted laparoscopic pyeloplasty in the pediatric population: a review of tenchique, outcomes, complications, and special considerations in infants. *Pediatr Surg Int.* (2017) 33:925–35. doi: 10.1007/s00383-017-4082-7

9. Esposito C, Masieri L, Castagnetti M, Sforza S, Farina A, Cerulo M, et al. Robot-assisted vs laparoscopic pyeloplasty in children with uretero-pelvic junction obstruction (UPJO): technical considerations and results. *J Pediatr Urol.* (2019) 15:667.e1–8. doi: 10.1016/j.jpurol.2019.09.018

10. Gatti JM, Amstutz SP, Bowlin PR, Stephany HA, Murphy JP. Laparoscopic vs open pyeloplasty in children: results of a randomized, prospective, controlled trial. *J Urol.* (2017) 197:792–7. doi: 10.1016/j.juro.2016.10.056

11. Yeung CK, Tam YH, Sihoe JD, Lee KH, Liu KW. Retroperitoneoscopic dismembered pyeloplasty for pelvi-ureteric junction obstruction in infants and children. *BJU Int.* (2001) 87:509–13. doi: 10.1046/j.1464-410X.2001.00129.x

12. Dindo D, Demartines N, Clavien PA. Classification of surgical complications: a new proposal with evaluation in a cohort of 6336 patients and results of a survey. *Ann Surg.* (2004) 240:205–13. doi: 10.1097/01.sla.0000133083.54934.ae

13. Tam YH, Pang KKY, Wong YS, Chan KW, Lee KH. From laparoscopic pyeloplasty to robot-assisted laparoscopic pyeloplasty in primary and reoperative repairs for ureteropelvic junction obstruction in children. *J Laparoendosc Adv Surg Tech A.* (2018) 28:1012–8. doi: 10.1089/lap.2017.0561

14. Turner RM,II, Fox JA, Tomaszewski JJ, Schneck FX, Docimo SG, Ost MC. Laparoscopic pyeloplasty for ureteropelvic junction obstruction in infants. *J Urol.* (2013) 189:1503–7. doi: 10.1016/j.juro.2012.10.067

15. Avery DI, Herbst KW, Lendvay TS, Noh PH, Dangle P, Gundeti MS, et al. Robot-assisted laparoscopic pyeloplasty: multi-institutional experience in infants. *J Pediatr Urol.* (2015) 11:139.e1–5. doi: 10.1016/j.jpurol.2014.11.025

16. Bansal D, Cost NG, DeFoor WR, Jr, Reddy PP, Minevich EA, Vanderbrink BA, et al. Infant robotic pyeloplasty: comparison with an open cohort. *J Pediatr Urol.* (2014) 10:380–5. doi: 10.1016/j.jpurol.2013.10.016

17. Dangle PP, Kearns J, Anderson B, Gundeti MS. Outcomes of infants undergoing robot-assisted laparoscopic pyeloplasty compared to open repair. *J Urol.* (2013) 190:2221–6. doi: 10.1016/j.juro.2013.07.063

18. Baek M, Silay MS, Au JK, Huang GO, Elizondo RA, Puttmann KT, et al. Does the use of 5 mm instruments affect the outcomes of robot-assisted laparoscopic pyeloplasty in smaller working spaces? A comparative analysis of infants and older children. *J Pediatr Urol.* (2018) 14:537.e1–6. doi: 10.1016/j.jpurol.2018.06.010

19. Kawal T, Srinivasan AK, Shrivastava D, Chu DI, Van Batavia J, Weiss D, et al. Pediatric robotic-assisted laparoscopic pyeloplasty: does age matter? *J Pediatr Urol.* (2018) 14:540.e1–6. doi: 10.1016/j.jpurol.2018.04.023

20. Neheman A, Kord E, Zisman A, Darawsha AE, Noh PH. Comparison of robotic pyeloplasty and standard laparoscopic pyeloplasty in infants: a bi-institutional study. *J Laparoendosc Adv Surg Tech A.* (2018) 28:467–70. doi: 10.1089/lap.2017.0262

21. Farhat WA. Editorial comment on "Laparoscopic pyeloplasty for ureteropelvic junction obstruction in infants". *J Urol.* (2013) 189:1506–7. doi: 10.1016/j.juro.2012.10.134

22. Taktak S, Llewellyn O, Aboelsoud M, Hajibandeh S, Hajibandeh S. Robot-assisted laparoscopic pyeloplasty versus laparoscopic pyeloplasty for pelvi-ureteric junction obstruction in the paediatric population: a systematic review and meta-analysis. *Ther Adv Urol.* (2019) 11:1756287219835704. doi: 10.1177/1756287219835704

23. Kawal T, Sahadev R, Srinivasan A, Chu D, Weiss D, Long C, et al. Robotic surgery in infants and children: an argument for smaller and fewer incisions. *World J Urol.* (2020) 38:1835–40. doi: 10.1007/s00345-019-02765-z

24. Casella DP, Fox JA, Schneck FX, Cannon GM, Ost MC. Cost analysis of pediatric robot-assisted and laparoscopic pyeloplasty. *J Urol.* (2013) 189:1083–6. doi: 10.1016/j.juro.2012.08.259

7

Comparison of Drainage Methods after Pyeloplasty in Children: A 14-Year Study

Xiangpan Kong [1,2], Zhenpeng Li [1,2], Mujie Li [1,2], Xing Liu [1,2] and Dawei He [1,2]*

[1] Department of Urology, Children's Hospital of Chongqing Medical University, Chongqing, China, [2] Ministry of Education Key Laboratory of Child Development and Disorders, International Science and Technology Cooperation Base of Child Development and Critical Disorders, National Clinical Research Center for Child Health and Disorders, Chongqing Key Laboratory of Pediatrics, Chongqing Key Laboratory of Children Urogenital Development and Tissue Engineering, Chongqing, China

Correspondence:
Dawei He
hedawei@hospital.cqmu.edu.cn

Objective: To summarize our experiences with drainage methods after laparoscopic pyeloplasty with a 14-year study.

Methods: We reviewed the data of the 838 children operated on for hydronephrosis due to congenital ureteropelvic junction obstruction (UPJO) between July 2007 and July 2020. Patients' demographics, perioperative details, postoperative drainage stents [including double-J stent, percutaneous trans-anastomotic (PU) stent, and trans-uretero-cystic external urethral stent (TEUS)], complications, hospital stay, and long-term follow-up outcomes were analyzed. Long-term follow-up was performed by outpatient visits and telephone follow-up. Moreover, we reviewed the details of nine cases of recurrence after laparoscopic pyeloplasty.

Results: Comparison of preoperative general data among the three groups indicated that there was no statistical difference in age, gender, and surgical side of the three groups. Statistical differences were found in the incidence of postoperative complications from the three postoperative drainage method groups, especially the incidence of reoperations ($p < 0.01$): there were six cases (3.19%) of recurrences in the TEUS group, two cases (0.36%) in the DJ group, and one case (0.93%) in the PU group. In the six recurrent cases from the TEUS group, four cases (44.4%) were found to have stenosis, and two cases (22.2%) have iatrogenic valvular formation.

Conclusion: Not all three types of drainage methods are suitable for drainage after pyeloplasty. Based on our findings, TEUS is not recommended.

Keywords: pyeloplasty, hydronephrosis, ureteropelvic junction obstruction, drainage methods, outcomes

INTRODUCTION

Congenital ureteropelvic junction obstruction (UPJO) is one of the most commonly encountered abnormalities that are responsible for persistent hydronephrosis in children (1). The classic option of treatment for UPJO is pyeloplasty. Since the first descriptions of laparoscopic pyeloplasty (LP) in 1993 by Schlussel (2) and in 1995 by Peters (3), LP has become the gold standard in the treatment of UPJO, with its safety and minimal invasiveness. Usually, surgeons will choose to use a drainage stent after pyeloplasty; however, which drainage method is the best choice is still quite controversial (4, 5).

After LP, the choice of stent type has always been the focus of debate. For now, double-J (DJ) stent and percutaneous trans-anastomotic (PU) are widely used due to their reliable efficacy, but their disadvantages are also obvious, such as displacement and secondary anesthesia in the DJ stent (5–8) and urine leakage, kinks, and obstruction in the PU stent (5, 9, 10). Therefore, the ideal drainage method should be effective while being minimally invasive and safe. We used the trans-uretero-cystic external urethral stent (TEUS) approach to solve the problems caused by the DJ stent and PU stent; in the previous research (11), we proved it to be safe and effective by comparing it with the DJ stent, but there is a lack of verification of long-term follow-up results in the study.

After a long-term postoperative follow-up work, we found some abnormal results (postoperative recurrence rates were higher in children treated with TEUS than other drainage methods), which made us question the safety of this new drainage method. Therefore, we conducted this study to answer the question, summarize the relevant experience and findings, and share them with other scholars.

MATERIALS AND METHODS

Patients and Data

We retrospectively reviewed 838 patients with congenital UPJO without other urinary system deformities between July 2007 and June 2020 in the Children's Hospital of Chongqing Medical University. All patients underwent standard LP according to Anderson–Hynes technique (12); surgeries were performed by three senior surgeons with extensive experience in pediatric urology surgery. Patients' demographics, data of preoperative and postoperative exams, perioperative details, complications, hospital stay, and regular postoperatively follow-up results were collected (the occurrence of long-term complications).

Surgical Method and Follow Up

Stenting is selected by the surgeon according to the preoperative or intraoperative situation. The TEUS stent was placed by a cystoscope preoperatively; a Fr3 or Fr4 stent was inserted in a retrograde fashion into the ureter via cystoscopy, with a Foley catheter placed in the bladder. The other stents were used intraoperatively (**Figure 1**). Seven to 10 days after surgery, the PU stent and TEUS stent were removed, while the DJ stent was removed about 1–4 weeks after surgery.

Follow-up included outpatient follow-up at 3 and 6 months and once a year after surgery. Patients who were followed up for <1 year or were lost to follow-up were excluded.

Abbreviations: UPJO, ureteropelvic junction obstruction; LP, laparoscopic pyeloplasty; DJ, double-J; PU, percutaneous trans-anastomotic; TEUS, trans-uretero-cystic external urethral stent.

Statistical Analysis

Postoperative complications were analyzed by the Clavien–Dindo system (13). Analyses were performed using SPSS®, version 25.0 (IBM Corp., Armonk, NY, USA). Qualitative or categorical variables were expressed as numbers and compared using the χ^2 or Fisher's exact test, as appropriate. Data were compared between groups using Students' t-test or chi-square test. Data that did not comply with a normal distribution were expressed as median range and compared between groups using the Mann–Whitney test. All statistical tests were two-sided and performed with a significance level set at $p < 0.05$.

Ethics Approval

We obtained ethical approval for this study from the local institutional research ethics board. Written informed consent for participation was signed by the guardian of the child when hospitalized.

RESULTS

This study included a total of 838 children who underwent LP. The demographics data (gender, age, and surgical side) of the three groups were not statistically significant ($p > 0.05$). From the comparison of the operative duration, intraoperative blood loss, and hospitalization duration of patients in the three groups, statistically significant differences were found between groups. The operative duration was significantly different between the DJ group and the other two groups ($p < 0.05$). Bleeding volume in the PU group was significantly different from that of the other two groups ($p < 0.05$). Hospitalization duration was statistically different among the three groups. Among them, compared with the other two groups, the DJ group had the shortest hospitalization duration and the shortest operation duration; the PU group had the most blood loss; and the TEUS group had the longest operation duration (**Table 1**).

We calculated the time of the stent removal and postoperative complications in the three groups. The time of the stent removal of the three groups was 28.5 ± 12.2, 7.4 ± 1.8, and 10.9 ± 8.2 days, which was significantly different between groups. Meanwhile, the overall complication rate in the three groups was significantly different too. They are 24 (4.42%) cases, 23 (12.23%), and nine (8.41%) cases; especially, the incidence of reoperation in Group B (six cases) was significantly higher than in other groups (**Table 2**).

At last, we collected clinical data from the nine children (six boys and three girls) who underwent reoperation; all developed severe hydronephrosis before the first surgery. After the first operation, five children had a recent complication (two cases of urinary tract infection (UTI), two cases of anastomotic obstruction, and one case of persistent hematuria). In the choice of postoperative drainage stent, we used TEUS in six children, the DJ stent in two children, and the PU stent in one child. During the reoperation, surprisingly, four cases showed that the ureteropelvic junction still had scar stenosis, and two cases showed iatrogenic valve; it is worth noting that TEUS was used in all these six children. In the remaining three reoperation cases, two cases were found to have surrounding tissues adhering to the stent, ureteropelvic junction did not have obvious stenosis, and

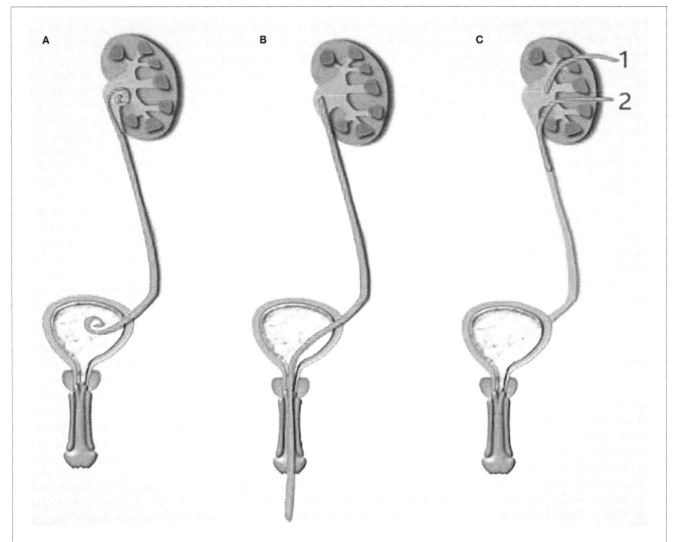

FIGURE 1 | Schematic diagram of three types of postoperative drainage stents. **(A)** DJ stent. **(B)** TEUS. **(C)** PU stent: 1, drainage stent; 2, stent. DJ, double-J stent; TEUS, trans-uretero-cystic external urethral stent; PU, percutaneous trans-anastomotic.

these patients had UTI after the first surgery. The last case had angulation distortion.

DISCUSSION

More than 30 years ago, open pyeloplasty (OP) was the gold standard for the treatment of UPJO. The first LP was reported in 1993 (2), which is safe, reliable, and minimally invasive. LP has gradually become the standard method for the treatment of UPJO in children. However, due to the peculiarities of children, which type of drainage method is the best choice has been controversial after pyeloplasty.

Should a stent be used after LP, and if a stent is used, which stent is the most ideal?

At present, there are two kinds of stent tubes widely used: the DJ stent and PU stent. Recently, Sarhan et al. (5) reported a multicenter study of the efficacy of drainage methods in 175

children between the two groups, which showed no significant difference in the incidence of postoperative complications or long-term outcomes. DJ stent insertion provides a shorter hospital stay, but a second operating room visit and anesthesia for removal are unavoidable. Similarly, in the study of Irene et al. (8), they also compared the costs incurred by the two drainage methods, and they believed that the DJ and PU stents were equivalent in terms of overall complications and success rate. Moreover, PU stents can avoid the need for additional general anesthesia and reduce overall hospital costs. Therefore, the advantages of the DJ stent are that is minimally invasive, safe, and reliable, but it requires reoperation to remove the stent. The PU stent has the advantages of convenient stent removal and precise curative effect and the disadvantages of more trauma.

Since some catheter-related complications are inevitable with all types of drainage methods, what is the efficacy of stent-less pyeloplasty? Bayne et al. (14) proved that the incidence

TABLE 1 | Patients' demographics and data of operation.

	DJ group	TEUS group	PU group	*p*-Value
Number, *n*	543	188	107	-
Male, gender, *n* (%)	445 (82.0)	147 (78.2)	79 (73.8)	0.285
Age, months, median (IQR)	57 (14–91)	30 (11–83)	48 (13–83)	0.064
Side, left, n (%)	427 (78.6)	146 (77.7)	77 (72.0)	0.285
• Operative duration, min • Median (IQR)	100 (79–130)	120 (95–155)	115 (90–140)	0.000*
• Bleeding volume, ml • Median (IQR)	10 (5–10)	10 (5–10)	10 (5–15)	0.000*
• Hospitalization duration, days • Median (IQR)	12 (10–15)	15 (14–18)	18 (16–20)	0.000*

DJ, double-J stent; TEUS, trans-uretero-cystic external urethral stent; PU, percutaneous trans-anastomotic; IQR, interquartile range.
*Significant.

TABLE 2 | The three drainage stents' removal time and complications.

	DJ group (*n* = 543)	TEUS group (*n* = 188)	PU group (*n* = 107)	*p*-Value
Stent removal time, day (mean ± SD)	28.5 ± 12.2	7.4 ± 1.8	10.9 ± 8.2	0.000*
Complications, *n* (%)	24	23	9	0.001*
UTI (CDG II)	12 (50)	6 (26.1)	3 (33.3)	0.715
Urine leakage (CDG II)	10 (41.7)	6 (26.1)	4 (44.4)	0.299
Stent drop (CDG II)	0 (0)	3 (13.0)	1 (11.1)	-
Omental hernia (CDG II)	0 (0)	1 (4.35)	0 (0)	-
Paralytic intestinal obstruction (CDG IIIb)	0 (0)	1 (4.35)	0 (0)	-
Recurrence (CDG IIIb)	2 (8.3)	6 (26.1)	1 (11.1)	0.007*

DJ, double-J stent; TEUS, trans-uretero-cystic external urethral stent; PU, percutaneous trans-anastomotic; UTI, urinary tract infection; CDG, clavien-dindo grading.
*Significant.

of postoperative urinary leakage was significantly higher in the stent-free group than in the stent-less group in their study. And in another meta-analysis reported by Liu (9) to evaluate the efficacy and safety of the DJ stent, PU stent, and stent-less pyeloplasty in pediatric pyeloplasty, the network meta-analysis (NMA) results showed that there were no significant differences between the three groups in surgical duration, surgical success rate, length of hospital stay, improvement in renal function, overall complications, and recurrence rates. Compared with the stent-less group, the incidence of postoperative pain was higher for the DJ stent and PU stent. The urine leakage rate of the DJ stent was lower than that of the PU stent and stent-less pyeloplasty. No significant differences were observed in other types of complications such as UTI, stent displacement, and postoperative recurrence. This is consistent with other similar studies (15, 16), so the cost of stent-less pyeloplasty is an unavoidable high incidence of urinary leakage. Unfortunately, almost all postoperative urine leakage needs to be treated by intubation; it means that reoperation is conducted within a short period of time after the first surgery, which is unacceptable for children and their parents, and it may cause doctor–patient conflict and bring great challenges to clinical work.

Combined with the above discussions, we find that stent-less pyeloplasty is the most minimally invasive, but it has a high incidence of urinary leakage. Combined with the results of the other studies (5, 6, 10, 15–17), we found that the advantages of the DJ stent are that it is safe, reliable, effective, and more minimally invasive, while the removal time of the PU stent is shorter, which can reduce the occurrence of catheter-related complications. And the disadvantages are obvious too, such as issues with anesthesia during DJ stent removal and the high risk of urine leakage associated with the PU stent. In order to solve these problems, we tried a new drainage stent, TEUS. This drainage stent through the natural cavity solves not only the problem of DJ stent removal difficulty but also the problem of PU stent urine leakage around the catheter. Is this drainage method safe and effective? In an early short-term retrospective study, we compared the efficacy of the TEUS stent and DJ stent, and we found that in addition to the operation duration of the TEUS group, which was longer than that of the DJ group ($p < 0.05$), there was no difference in intraoperative blood loss, length of hospital stay, and incidence of complications [10 cases (22.2%) and eight cases (20%) of catheter-related complications in the DJ group and TEUS group, respectively ($p > 0.05$)] ($p > 0.05$). However, this study on the safety of TEUS lacked long-term follow-up results.

With the increased time of follow-up, we compared the removal time of stents and incidence/types of postoperative complications of 884 patients in the LP group who respectively used the DJ stent, TEUS, and PU stent for drainage. One unexpected finding was the extent to which the removal time of stents and overall complication rate of the three groups were statistically different, and the average catheter duration of the three groups was as follows: DJ group (28.5 days), TEUS group (7.4 days), and PU group (10.9 days). The incidence of postoperative complications in the three groups was as follows: 24 cases (4.42%) in the DJ group, 23 cases (12.23%) in the TEUS group, and nine cases (8.41%) in the PU group; especially, the incidence of reoperation in the TEUS group (six cases, 26.1%) was significantly higher than that in the other groups (two cases, 8.3%; one case, 1.1%). The finding that the incidence of postoperative complications was significantly different among the three groups was seriously inconsistent with the previous conclusion. Then what causes the postoperative recurrence rate of the TEUS group to be significantly higher than that of the other groups?

Current studies suggest that stenting and drainage after pyeloplasty are necessary to facilitate anastomotic healing and reduce urinary leakage (18). Both the DJ and PU stents have this function, but the TEUS stent had no supporting effect due to its special structure. In addition, TEUS is placed prior to pyeloplasty, which means that the renal pelvis will be emptied before pyeloplasty begins, and it may affect the judgment of the length of the stenosis, which may lead to residual stenosis. Moreover, the TEUS was inserted before surgery, which interferes with the surgical field during surgery, which is also not conducive to complete resection and suture of the stenosis and may eventually lead to residual stenosis and inaccurate suture. These hypotheses were also confirmed by pathological findings during reoperation (four cases with residual stenosis and two cases with close adhesion to surrounding tissues). And to further test this hypothesis, we are now conducting further experimental studies. Now, we do not recommend the use of TEUS stents, and we suggest that other scholars should not ignore our findings when trying new stents.

Compared with other reported literature (5, 8, 13–16), the advantages of our study lie in the long follow-up time and importantly in the number of patients. To our knowledge, this is the first long-term follow-up of TEUS and study of the results. The limitations of this study are that the data were retrospectively analyzed, the study group was not randomized, and the study was a single-center observation.

In summary, not all three types of drainage methods are suitable for pyeloplasty. We suggest that the use of the TEUS stent should be performed carefully, and we suggest that other scholars should not ignore our findings when trying new stents.

AUTHOR CONTRIBUTIONS

XL and DH contributed to conception and design. DH contributed to administrative support. XK, ZL, and ML contributed to collection and assembly of data. XK contributed to manuscript writing. All authors contributed to manuscript revision, read, and approved the submitted version.

ACKNOWLEDGMENTS

We would like to thank the parents and children who enrolled in the study. And we thank Dr. Wang Quan (Department of Cardiothoracic Surgery) for his valuable advice on the manuscript revision.

REFERENCES

1. Jiang D, Tang B, Xu M, Lin H, Jin L, He L, et al. Functional and morphological outcomes of pyeloplasty at different ages in prenatally diagnosed society of fetal urology grades 3-4 ureteropelvic junction obstruction: is it safe to wait? *Urology.* (2017) 101:45–9. doi: 10.1016/j.urology.2016.10.004
2. Schuessler WW, Grune MT, Tecuanhuey LV, Preminger GM. Laparoscopic dismembered pyeloplasty. *J Urol.* (1993) 150:1795–9. doi: 10.1016/S0022-5347(17)35898-6
3. Peters CA, Schlussel RN, Retik AB. Pediatric laparoscopic dismembered pyeloplasty. *J Urol.* (1995) 153:1962–5. doi: 10.1016/S0022-5347(01)67378-6
4. Ludwikowski BM, Botländer M, González R. The BULT method for pediatric mini laparoscopic pyeloplasty in infants: technique and results. *Front Pediatr.* (2016) 4:54. doi: 10.3389/fped.2016.00054
5. Sarhan O, Al Awwad A, Al Otay A, Al Faddagh A, El Helaly A, Al Ghanbar M, et al. Comparison between internal double J and external pyeloureteral stents in open pediatric pyeloplasty: a multicenter study. *J Pediatr Urol.* (2021) 17:511.e1. doi: 10.1016/j.jpurol.2021.03.027
6. Ates KM, Vaizer RP, Newton DC, Hao S, Mahoney K, Morganstern BA. Rare case: ureteropelvic junction complication presenting with bilateral labial abscesses and urosepsis requiring nephrectomy. *Urol Case Rep.* (2021) 37:101705. doi: 10.1016/j.eucr.2021.101705

7. Abedi AR, Dargahi M, Hosseini SJ. Misplacement of DJ stent into inferior vena cava in a patient with retroperitoneal fibrosis, a case report. *Urol Case Rep.* (2021) 38:101650. doi: 10.1016/j.eucr.2021.101650
8. Paraboschi I, Jannello L, Mantica G, Roberts L, Olubajo S, Paul A, et al. Outcomes and costs analysis of externalized pyeloureteral versus internal double-j ureteral stents after paediatric laparoscopic Anderson-Hynes pyeloplasty. *J Pediatr Urol.* (2021) 17:232.e1-e7. doi: 10.1016/j.jpurol.2020.12.006
9. Liu X, Huang C, Guo Y, Yue Y, Hong J. Comparison of DJ stented, external stented and stent-less procedures for pediatric pyeloplasty: a network meta-analysis. *Int J Surg.* (2019) 68:126–33. doi: 10.1016/j.ijsu.2019.07.001
10. Chu DI, Shrivastava D, Van Batavia JP, Bowen DK, Tong CC, Long CJ, et al. Outcomes of externalized pyeloureteral versus internal ureteral stent in pediatric robotic-assisted laparoscopic pyeloplasty. *J Pediatr Urol.* (2018) 14:450.e1–450.e6. doi: 10.1016/j.jpurol.2018.04.012
11. Dong JJ, Wen S, Liu X, Lin T, Liu F, Wei GH. Trans-uretero-cystic external urethral stent for urinary diversion in pediatric laparoscopic pyeloplasty: a novel approach. *Medicine.* (2020) 99:e22135. doi: 10.1097/MD.0000000000022135
12. Anderson JC, Hynes W. Retrocaval ureter; a case diagnosed pre-operatively and treated successfully by a plastic operation. *Br J Urol.* (1949) 21:209–14. doi: 10.1111/j.1464-410X.1949.tb10773.x

13. Clavien PA, Barkun J, de Oliveira ML, Vauthey JN, Dindo D, Schulick RD, et al. The Clavien–Dindo classification of surgical complications: five-year experience. *Ann Surg.* (2009) 250:187–96. doi: 10.1097/SLA.0b013e3181b 13ca2

14. Bayne AP, Lee KA, Nelson ED, Cisek LJ, Gonzales ET Jr, Roth DR. The impact of surgical approach and urinary diversion on patient outcomes in pediatric pyeloplasty. *J Urol.* (2011) 186(4 Suppl):1693– 98. doi: 10.1016/j.juro.2011.03.103

15. Lombardo Alyssa., Toni Tiffany., Andolfi Ciro., Gundeti Mohan S. Comparative outcomes of double-J and cutaneous pyeloureteral stents in pediatric robot-assisted laparoscopic pyeloplasty. *J Endourol.* (2021) 35:1616– 22. doi: 10.1089/end.2020.1115

16. Zhu H, Wang J, Deng Y, Huang L, Zhu X, Dong J, et al. Use of double-J ureteric stents post-laparoscopic pyeloplasty to treat ureteropelvic junction obstruction in hydronephrosis for pediatric patients: a single-center experience. *J Int Med Res.* (2020) 48:300060520918781. doi: 10.1177/0300060520918781

17. Braga LH, Lorenzo AJ, Farhat WA, Bägli DJ, Khoury AE, Pippi Salle JL. Outcome analysis and cost comparison between externalized pyeloureteral and standard stents in 470 consecutive open pyeloplasties. *J Urol.* (2008) 180(4 Suppl):1693–8. doi: 10.1016/j.juro.2008.05.084

18. Elmalik K, Chowdhury MM, Capps SN. Ureteric stents in pyeloplasty: a help or a hindrance? *J Pediatr Urol.* (2008) 4:275–9. doi: 10.1016/j.jpurol.2008.01.205

8

Searching for the Least Invasive Management of Pelvi-Ureteric Junction Obstruction in Children

Marco Castagnetti[1], Massimo Iafrate[1], Ciro Esposito[2] and Ramnath Subramaniam[3,4]*

[1] Section of Paediatric Urology, Department of Surgical, Oncological, and Gastrointestinal Sciences, University Hospital of Padova, Padua, Italy, [2] Department of Paediatrics, Federico II University of Naples, Naples, Italy, [3] Department of Paediatric Urology, Leeds Teaching Hospitals NHS Trust, University of Leeds, Leeds, United Kingdom, [4] Department of Paediatric Urology, University of Ghent, Ghent, Belgium

Correspondence:
Ramnath Subramaniam
r.subramaniam@leeds.ac.uk

Introduction: To review the published evidence on the minimally invasive pyeloplasty techniques available currently with particular emphasis on the comparative data about the various minimally invasive alternatives to treat pelvi-ureteric junction obstruction and gauge if one should be favored under certain circumstances.

Materials and Methods: Non-systematic review of literature on open and minimally invasive pyeloplasty including various kinds of laparoscopic procedures, the robotic-assisted laparoscopic pyeloplasty, and endourological procedures.

Results: Any particular minimally invasive pyeloplasty procedure seems feasible in experienced hands, irrespective of age including infants. Comparative data suggest that the robotic-assisted procedure has gained wider acceptance mainly because it is ergonomically more suited to surgeon well-being and facilitates advanced skills with dexterity thanks to 7 degrees of freedom. However, costs remain the major drawback of robotic surgery. In young children and infants, instead, open surgery can be performed via a relatively small incision and quicker time frame.

Conclusions: The best approach for pyeloplasty is still a matter of debate. The robotic approach has gained increasing acceptance over the last years with major advantages of the surgeon well-being and ergonomics and the ease of suturing. Evidence, however, may favor the use of open surgery in infancy.

Keywords: pyeloplasty, pelvi-ureteric junction, obstructive uropathy, hydronephrosis, minimally-invasive surgery, robotic surgery

INTRODUCTION

Open pyeloplasty has been for ages considered the gold standard treatment of pyelo-ureteric junction (PUJ) obstruction, and the standards of open pyeloplasty were set back in 1998 by Gerard Monfort (1). Using optical magnification and fine suture materials, it has been shown that the procedure can be performed as a day case surgery, without any indwelling stent, with >95% success rate. Long-term durability of open pyeloplasty has also been well-documented (2).

Despite the good outcomes of open pyeloplasty, the search for less invasive treatment modalities alternative to open pyeloplasty has continued. The potential advantages of a minimally invasive approach for the dissection have never been questioned; the main hurdle lies with the accomplishment of the pyelo-ureteral anastomosis that can require advanced suturing skills and can be time-consuming even in experienced hands, a fact particularly true with laparoscopic techniques (3). Consistently, in a systematic review and meta-analysis of open vs. minimally invasive pyeloplasty (MIP) performed in 2014, Autorino et al. observed that although MIP procedures can achieve complication and success rates comparable to open surgery, the operating time still largely favors open pyeloplasty (4). More importantly, multiple reports coming for different institutions prove that open pyeloplasty is safe and duplicable in the widespread use, and duplicability of the MIP procedure is more controversial as the skills necessary to perform the procedure can be hard to achieve and maintain (5). The most complex scenario is clearly that of a pyeloplasty performed in an infant (6), which is not an uncommon scenario with prenatal diagnosis, the most common presentation of PUJ obstruction, and most of these patients who require surgery do so in infancy (7).

The aim of the present review was to summarize the available evidence on the MIP techniques currently available with particular emphasis on the comparative data about the various MIP alternatives to gauge if one should be favored under certain circumstances.

MIP TECHNIQUES

MIP is an umbrella term that encompasses several techniques including laparoscopic surgery and robotic-assisted laparoscopic pyeloplasty (RALP) and can be performed using a trans-peritoneal or a retro-peritoneal route. The standard robotic instruments are 8 mm with cable-driven hinges, and although 5-mm instruments with metal hinges are available, the range of movements is difficult to realize especially in limited space. Traditional laparoscopic approach can be achieved with a 5-mm camera and 3-mm instruments, also referred to as "Mini-laparoscopy." Other recognized approaches include single-site surgery or one-trocar-assisted pyeloplasty (OTAP).

Single-site surgery also known as LESS (laparo-endoscopic single site) surgery is performed introducing all the instruments necessary to perform the procedure via a single umbilical incision, with or without a specific device (8). In the OTAP, instead, the dissection is performed laparoscopically using a retroperitoneal approach, whereas the PUJ is delivered outside the abdomen to perform the pyeloplasty externally like in open surgery (9). This procedure potentially combines the putative advantages of both a minimally invasive dissection and an easier open pyeloplasty keeping the incision small at the same time. The major limitation of the OTAP is patient size, as delivery of the PUJ can possibly be difficult in older patients.

In terms of the procedure, dismembered Anderson–Hynes pyeloplasty is the standard technique of choice. In MIP, this

TABLE 1 | Single institution series on minimally invasive treatment of pelvi-ureteric junction obstruction.

Series	Technique	N of Pts	Conversion rate	Failure rate
Chandarasekaram (17)	Laparoscopy	111	0	1%
Blanc et al. (18)	Retroperitoneoscopy	104	3%	2%
Lima et al. (9)	OTAP	155	8%	1%
Minnillo et al. (19)	RALP	155	0	3%
Parente et al. (14)	Baloon dilatation	50	0	10%

procedure requires advanced skills of suturing, which some surgeons find tedious and not comfortable ergonomically (10, 11). In order to circumvent the problems related to the suturing skills necessary to perform the procedure minimally invasively, in recent years, interest has increased with alternatives, such as the vascular hitch for PUJ obstructions due to extrinsic compression by a crossing vessel (12), or non-dismembered pyeloplasty for intrinsic PUJ obstructions (13). RALP is definitely the superior approach facilitating advanced suturing skills in MIP although cost is the main prohibitive factor preventing widespread acceptance as alluded to later on in this article.

Endourological techniques can also be considered minimally invasive modalities to treat PUJ obstruction. These include a range of procedures, such as the balloon dilatation of the PUJ and the endopyelotomy (14, 15) with availability of cutting balloons combining dilatation and endopyelotomy (16). Any endourological procedures can be performed using a retrograde or antegrade approach.

SINGLE-INSTITUTION RESULTS

For any of the mentioned minimally invasive treatment modalities, single-surgeon or single-institution series exist documenting feasibility and effectiveness (**Table 1**). The procedure can be carried out successfully at any age including infancy, although it is clearly more demanding in small patients given the small available operating space (20). Only endourological techniques are probably an exception; even in the most experienced hands, reported failure rate is 2- to 3-fold higher than the other techniques (**Table 1**). Consistently, a systematic review published in 2015 shows that this treatment modality has not gained wide acceptance (only 128 cases reported) and the complication rate (14.8%) is much higher and the median success rate (71%) is much lower than those reported for MIP (15). Nevertheless, for all the MIP techniques, duplicability and cost-effectiveness remain to be proven and we still need comparative data to assess which technique is more effective and under which circumstances.

COMPARATIVE DATA ON MIP PROCEDURES

An analysis of the published literature regarding RALP shows that despite the constantly increasing number of publications over years, the level of evidence for available studies remains limited to case reports, case series, and retrospective comparative studies (21). This issue, however, is unfortunately true for any MIP procedure (21).

In terms of comparative data, we have studies comparing laparoscopy pyeloplasty vs. endourological management, laparoscopic vs. retroperitoneoscopic pyeloplasty, and laparoscopic vs. robot-assisted pyeloplasty.

In the single series comparing retrograde balloon dilatation and laparoscopic pyeloplasty, balloon dilatation had a significantly shorter operating time and hospital stay, and significantly lower analgesic requirement and costs (22). The study confirms, however, that the real issue with the endourological techniques is the success rate, particularly in the long term. Balloon dilatation seems not to be a durable procedure. Both procedures indeed had comparable success rate at 3 months, 94.7% for balloon dilatation vs. 97.1% of laparoscopic pyeloplasty, but the success rate of balloon dilatation progressively dropped to 71% at 2 years follow-up, becoming significantly lower than laparoscopic pyeloplasty, the success rate for which instead remained pretty steady over time (22).

The comparison of laparoscopic vs. retroperitoneoscopic pyeloplasty has been the objective of one of the few randomized clinical trials available in pediatric urology. Badawy et al. compared 19 patients randomized to each MIP approach (23). Success rate was comparable, whereas the retroperitoneal approach had shorter operative time by an average 40 min with earlier resumption of oral feeding and, as a consequence, shorter hospital stay. These data are in contrast with those of what is probably the largest single surgeon series of pyeloplasty available in the literature by Liu et al. (8). This series includes 1,750 pyeloplasties, 451 retroperitoneoscopic, 311 laparoscopic, 322 LESS, and 805 trans-umbilical multiport. The two approaches had comparable complication and success rate in both these reports, with the retroperitoneoscopic approach having quicker resumption of oral feeding and shorter hospital stay. However, in the latter series (8), the complication rate was higher and operative time was significantly longer for retroperitoneoscopy than any other MIP procedure in contrast to the report by Badawy et al. (23). These results are consistent with a meta-analysis of one randomized clinical trial and eight clinical trials (776 participants) in adults (24). In summary, these data suggest that the trans-peritoneal approach may be easier to perform while the creation of a retroperitoneal working chamber might increase the complexity of the procedure, making it longer and increasing the risk of conversion. Potential disadvantages of trans-peritoneal route include a longer post-operative ileus, the risk of intraperitoneal urine leakage post-operatively and adhesions formation in the long term.

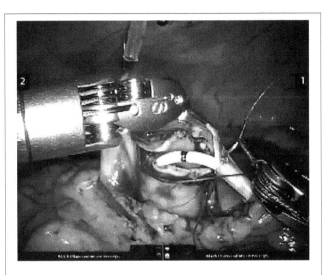

FIGURE 1 | Intraoperative picture showing the potential for articulation of the robotic instruments, which greatly simplifies suturing.

The comparison between laparoscopic and RALP is the one that has attracted more attention in the recent past. Since 2009, four systematic reviews and meta-analyses have been published on this topic (4, 25–27). The most recent one includes 14 studies: 1 prospective trial, 1 case–control, and 12 retrospective series (27). Once again, the general level of evidence is low, but the quality of studies was quite good with a low risk of bias in 10 out of 14. The meta-analysis showed that the operating time was equivalent, whereas all the other outcome parameters including hospital stay, complication rate, success rate, and re-intervention rate favored or tended to favor the robotic-assisted procedure.

This is consistent with the putative advantages of the robotic approach, including comfortable position for the surgeon, 3D view, and steady instruments with 7 degrees of freedom that make suturing much easier (**Figure 1**). It sounds reasonable that operating in a more comfortable way allows better results. It is well-documented that long-lasting laparoscopic procedures might cause chronic musculo-skeletal discomfort to the surgeon (11).

Consistently with this observation, Varda et al., analyzing the trend in utilization of open, laparoscopic, and robotic pyeloplasty in the United States from 2003 to 2015, reported since 2004, when the Da Vinci system became available, that the number of MIP procedures has progressively increased, mainly due to an increase in the number of robotic-assisted procedures, whereas the number of laparoscopic procedure has progressively decreased (28). Although not considered in the meta-analyses, another potential advantage of the robotic approach over conventional laparoscopy is that its learning curve is less steep (29), and since the use of robotic surgery further limits the volume of cases undergoing laparoscopic surgery, it is likely that the increased use of robotic surgery will permanently limit the use of conventional laparoscopic pyeloplasty in children, in the centers where the robot is available.

ROBOTIC-ASSISTED LAPAROSCOPIC PYELOPLASTY

The two major drawbacks of robotic-assisted pyeloplasty include costs and the size of the instruments.

Varda et al. estimated costs of open, laparoscopic, and robotic pyeloplasty and noted that the latter has a significantly higher cost mainly due to the cost of the consumables (28). This model, however, does not take into account the cost of the robot itself. Using a mathematical model, Behan et al. estimated that, in a center performing 100 RALP per year, the cost of the robot would not be neutralized even after 10 years (30).

Costs can be reduced using appropriate strategies. The first step is to reduce the console time and operating room turnover. Seideman et al. estimated that with a 2-days in-stay, RP could be cost-effective (when compared with LP) if it was carried out in under 120 min (31). Console time normally decreases with increasing experience and progression in the learning curve. It should be noted, however, that trainee involvement with the robot may make it difficult to lower console time as fellows and residents turnover regularly (32). Having a team specialized and dedicated just to robotic cases, instead, can reduce turnover time, particularly docking and undocking time (32, 33).

Increased and regular utilization of the robot by multiple services, i.e., increasing the volume of robotic procedures, is another important cost-saving strategy (32, 33).

Finally, increasing competition within the industry could translate into the end of the current monopoly, which could then translate to steadily reduce the cost of the robotic equipment, making robotics a more cost-effective and affordable technique (33).

The other issue is the size of the robotic instruments. The most modern standard instruments are 8 mm in size and also the arms of the robot are cumbersome. Smaller, 5-mm instruments do exist (34), but they have a pulley system that limits articulation and precludes certain movements. For this reason, many surgeons recommend the routine use of 8-mm instruments for all pediatric cases irrespective of age (35).

Consistently, splitting the results reported by Varda et al. by the age of the patients undergoing pyeloplasty, it is apparent that the use of the RALP mainly increased in the adolescent age group (13–18 years), whereas its use was very limited in infants (28).

PYELOPLASTY IN INFANTS

In the era of antenatal diagnosis of hydronephrosis, the infantile group represents an important age group for surgery. In this group of patients, RALP is feasible, but its role seems limited and has not gained wide acceptance. One issue is the size of the instruments mentioned above. In this, the use of 3-mm instruments, the so called mini-laparoscopy, can be advantageous (36) (**Figure 2**). Nevertheless, the accomplishment of a pyeloplasty in the limited space of an infant abdomen can be extremely demanding. Moreover, in younger patients, MIP does not seem to offer the same advantages in terms of shorter hospital stay and lower narcotic requirements observed instead in pre-adolescent and adolescent patients (37).

The second and perhaps the most relevant issue in this age group is the concern about the potential neurotoxicity of the drugs for the general anesthesia in early childhood (38, 39). For this reason, many authors and scientific societies recommend in this age group, if surgery cannot be postponed, at least

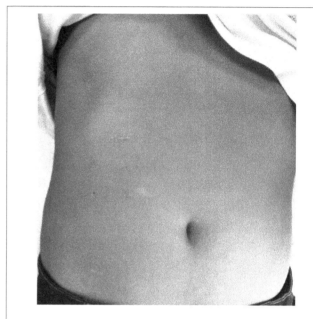

FIGURE 2 | Scar appearance after laparoscopic pyeloplasty.

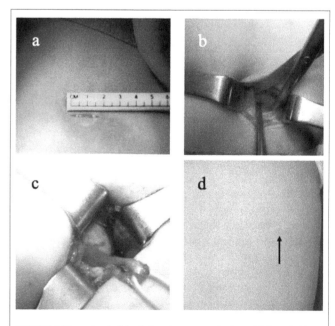

FIGURE 3 | Example of minimally invasive open pyeloplasty. **(a)** 2-cm incision; **(b)** muscle-sparing approach; **(c)** delivery of the pelvi-ureteric junction via the incision; **(d)** barely visible scar 6 months after the procedure.

the quickest procedure should be preferred. Published evidence overall thus far, as regards operative time, favors open pyeloplasty over MIP procedures (4).

In this respect, it is relevant that the procedure can be performed via such a small approach in infants to be called "minimally invasive open pyeloplasty" (40–42). Chako et al. reported that in patients <5 years, the procedure can be performed via an incision <3 cm in about 100 min on average combining a quick procedure with good cosmetic outcome (42) (**Figure 3**). However, some potential limitations of this approach should be considered. A small incision limits exposure of the anatomical structures, which can be an issue in case of unexpected anatomical variants. For this reason, advocates of this approach have underscored the importance of determining the exact incision site by intraoperative renal ultrasonography (40), and/or performing a retrograde pyelogram at the beginning of the surgery to define exactly the PUJ anatomy (41). Otherwise, a minimally invasive approach might prove somewhat more flexible while dealing with unexpected variants. Nevertheless, performing a pyeloplasty in an abnormal kidney and in an infant abdomen remains a formidable endeavor.

COSMETIC RESULTS OF OPEN VS. MIP

Cosmetic results are a relevant aspect in the decision-making. Gatte et al. performing a randomized, prospective, controlled trial comparing laparoscopic vs. open pyeloplasty concluded that both approaches are comparable and equally effective methods for repair of PUJ obstruction. Although operative time seems statistically shorter in the open group and length of stay seems shorter in the laparoscopic group, the choice should be based on family preference for incision aesthetics and surgeon comfort with either approach, rather than more classically objective outcome measures (43). In this respect, Wang et al. confirmed that larger initial incisions tend to grow more; therefore, at the same follow-up interval, laparoscopic incisions are smaller than those of open procedures (44). Barbossa et al. studied family preferences based on the assessment of pictures and diagrams of the scars of open pyeloplasty and RALP (45). They reported that families prefer the RALP scars both based on pictures and diagrams. Nevertheless, this held true only provided that there was no apparent medical benefit associated with one of the two procedures. Moreover, the approach did not seem to be a statistically significant factor in patients being pleased or not with the scar appearance in the study by Wang et al. (44).

CONCLUSIONS

Any MIP procedure seems feasible in experienced hands, even in infants. The best approach for pyeloplasty is still a matter of debate. The robotic approach seems to have gained increasing acceptance over the last years with major advantages being ergonomics and the ease of suturing. Costs and the size of the instruments remain major drawbacks for the application of the robotic approach in children. Evidence may favor the use of open surgery in infancy.

AUTHOR CONTRIBUTIONS

MC and RS drafted the manuscript, reviewed the literature, and also supplied one figure each. MI and CE suggested the articles for review and gave advice during the process of writing the manuscript. CE also supplied one figure.

REFERENCES

1. Guys JM, Borella F, Monfort G. Ureteropelvic junction obstructions: prenatal diagnosis and neonatal surgery in 47 cases. *J Pediatr Surg.* (1988) 23:156–8. doi: 10.1016/S0022-3468(88)80148-9
2. O'Reilly PH, Brooman PJ, Mak S, Jones M, Pickup C, Atkinson C, et al. The long-term results of Anderson-Hynes pyeloplasty. *BJU Int.* (2001) 87:287–9. doi: 10.1046/j.1464-410x.2001.00108.x
3. Esposito C, Masieri L, Castagnetti M, Sforza S, Farina A, Cerulo M, et al. Robot-assisted vs laparoscopic pyeloplasty in children with uretero-pelvic junction obstruction (UPJO): technical considerations and results. *J Pediatr Urol.* (2019) 15:667.e1–8. doi: 10.1016/j.jpurol.2019.09.018
4. Autorino R, Eden C, El-Ghoneimi A, Guazzoni G, Buffi N, Peters CA, et al. Robot-assisted and laparoscopic repair of ureteropelvic junction obstruction: a systematic review and meta-analysis. *Eur Urol.* (2014) 65:430–52. doi: 10.1016/j.eururo.2013.06.053
5. Silay MS, Spinoit AF, Undre S, Fiala V, Tandogdu Z, Garmanova T, et al. Global minimally invasive pyeloplasty study in children: results from the pediatric urology expert group of the european association of urology young academic urologists working party. *J Pediatr Urol.* (2016) 12:229.e1–7. doi: 10.1016/j.jpurol.2016.04.007
6. Zamfir Snykers C, De Plaen E, Vermersch S, Lopez M, Khelif K, Luyckx S, et al. Laparoscopic pyeloplasty for ureteropelvic junction obstruction in infants under 1 year of age a good option? *Front Pediatr.* (2019) 7:352. doi: 10.3389/fped.2019.00352
7. Vemulakonda V, Yiee J, Wilcox DT. Prenatal hydronephrosis: postnatal evaluation and management. *Curr Urol Rep.* (2014) 15:430. doi: 10.1007/s11934-014-0430-5
8. Liu D, Zhou H, Ma L, Zhou X, Cao H, Tao T, et al. Comparison of laparoscopic approaches for dismembered pyeloplasty in children with ureteropelvic junction obstruction: critical analysis of 11-year experiences in a single surgeon. *Urology.* (2017) 101:50–5. doi: 10.1016/j.urology.2016.10.007
9. Lima M, Ruggeri G, Messina P, Tursini S, Destro F, Mogiatti M. One-trocar-assisted pyeloplasty in children: an 8-year single institution experience. *Eur J Pediatr Surg.* (2015) 25:262–8. doi: 10.1055/s-0034-1372459
10. Piaggio LA, Franc-Guimond J, Noh PH, Wehry M, Figueroa TE, Barthold J, et al. Transperitoneal laparoscopic pyeloplasty for primary repair of ureteropelvic junction obstruction in infants and children: comparison with open surgery. *J Urol.* (2007) 178:1579–83. doi: 10.1016/j.juro.2007.03.159
11. Esposito C, El Ghoneimi A, Yamataka A, Rothenberg S, Bailez M, Ferro M, et al. Work-related upper limb musculoskeletal disorders in paediatric laparoscopic surgery. A multicenter survey. *J Pediatr Surg.* (2013) 48:1750–6. doi: 10.1016/j.jpedsurg.2013.01.054
12. Villemagne T, Fourcade L, Camby C, Szwarc C, Lardy H, Leclair MD. Long-term results with the laparoscopic transposition of renal lower pole crossing vessels. *J Pediatr Urol.* (2015) 11:174.e1–7. doi: 10.1016/j.jpurol.2015.04.023
13. Polok M, Chrzan R, Veenboer P, Beyerlein S, Dik P, Klijn A, et al. Nondismembered pyeloplasty in a pediatric population: results of 34 open and laparoscopic procedures. *Urology.* (2011) 78:891–4. doi: 10.1016/j.urology.2011.04.039

14. Parente A, Angulo JM, Romero RM, Rivas S, Burgos L, Tardáguila A. Management of ureteropelvic junction obstruction with high-pressure balloon dilatation: long-term outcome in 50 children under 18 months of age. *Urology*. (2013) 82:1138–43. doi: 10.1016/j.urology.2013.04.072

15. Corbett HJ, Mullassery D. Outcomes of endopyelotomy for pelviureteric junction obstruction in the paediatric population: a systematic review. *J Pediatr Urol*. (2015) 11:328–36. doi: 10.1016/j.jpurol.2015.08.014

16. Parente A, Perez-Egido L, Romero RM, Ortiz R, Burgos L, Angulo JM. Retrograde endopyelotomy with cutting balloon™ for treatment of ureteropelvic junction obstruction in infants. *Front Pediatr*. (2016) 4:72. doi: 10.3389/fped.2016.00072

17. Chandrasekharam VV. Laparoscopic pyeloplasty in infants: single-surgeon experience. *J Pediatr Urol*. (2015) 11:272.e1–5. doi: 10.1016/j.jpurol.2015.05.013

18. Blanc T, Muller C, Abdoul H, Peev S, Paye-Jaouen A, Peycelon M, et al. Retroperitoneal laparoscopic pyeloplasty in children: long-term outcome and critical analysis of 10-year experience in a teaching center. *Eur Urol*. (2013) 63:565–72. doi: 10.1016/j.eururo.2012.07.051

19. Minnillo BJ, Cruz JA, Sayao RH, Passerotti CC, Houck CS, Meier PM, et al. Long-term experience and outcomes of robotic assisted laparoscopic pyeloplasty in children and young adults. *J Urol*. (2011) 185:1455–60. doi: 10.1016/j.juro.2010.11.056

20. Badawy H, Saad A, Fahmy A, Dawood W, Aboulfotouh A, Kamal A, et al. Prospective evaluation of retroperitoneal laparoscopic pyeloplasty in children in the first 2 years of life: is age a risk factor for conversion? *J Pediatr Urol*. (2017) 13:511.e1–4. doi: 10.1016/j.jpurol.2017.03.025

21. Cundy TP, Harley SJD, Marcus HJ, Hughes-Hallett A, Khurana S. Global trends in paediatric robot-assisted urological surgery: a bibliometric and progressive scholarly acceptance analysis. *J Robot Surg*. (2018) 12:109–15. doi: 10.1007/s11701-017-0703-3

22. Xu N, Chen SH, Xue XY, Zheng QS, Wei Y, Jiang T, et al. Comparison of retrograde balloon dilatation and laparoscopic pyeloplasty for treatment of ureteropelvic junction obstruction: results of a 2-year follow-up. *PLoS ONE*. (2016) 11:e0152463. doi: 10.1371/journal.pone.0152463

23. Badawy H, Zoaier A, Ghoneim T, Hanno A. Transperitoneal versus retroperitoneal laparoscopic pyeloplasty in children: randomized clinical trial. *J Pediatr Urol*. (2015) 11:122.e1–6. doi: 10.1016/j.jpurol.2014.11.019

24. Wu Y, Dong Q, Han P, Liu L, Wang L, Wei Q. Meta-analysis of transperitoneal versus retroperitoneal approaches of laparoscopic pyeloplasty for ureteropelvic junction obstruction. *J Laparoendosc Adv Surg Tech A*. (2012) 22:658–62. doi: 10.1089/lap.2011.0508

25. Braga LH, Pace K, DeMaria J, Lorenzo AJ. Systematic review and meta-analysis of robotic-assisted versus conventional laparoscopic pyeloplasty for patients with ureteropelvic junction obstruction: effect on operative time, length of hospital stay, postoperative complications, and success rate. *Eur Urol*. (2009) 56:848–57. doi: 10.1016/j.eururo.2009.03.063

26. Cundy TP, Harling L, Hughes-Hallett A, Mayer EK, Najmaldin AS, Athanasiou T, et al. Meta-analysis of robot-assisted vs conventional laparoscopic and open pyeloplasty in children. *BJU Int*. (2014) 114:582–94. doi: 10.1111/bju.12683

27. Taktak S, Llewellyn O, Aboelsoud M, Hajibandeh S, Hajibandeh S. Robot-assisted laparoscopic pyeloplasty versus laparoscopic pyeloplasty for pelvi-ureteric junction obstruction in the paediatric population: a systematic review and meta-analysis. *Ther Adv Urol*. (2019) 11:1756287219835704. doi: 10.1177/1756287219835704

28. Varda BK, Wang Y, Chung BI, Lee RS, Kurtz MP, Nelson CP, et al. Has the robot caught up? National trends in utilization, perioperative outcomes, and cost for open, laparoscopic, and robotic pediatric pyeloplasty in the United States from 2003 to 2015. *J Pediatr Urol*. (2018) 14:336.e1–8. doi: 10.1016/j.jpurol.2017.12.010

29. Reinhardt S, Ifaoui IB, Thorup J. Robotic surgery start-up with a fellow as the console surgeon. *Scand J Urol*. (2017) 51:335–8. doi: 10.1080/21681805.2017.1302990

30. Behan JW, Kim SS, Dorey F, De Filippo RE, Chang AY, Hardy BE, et al. Human capital gains associated with robotic assisted laparoscopic pyeloplasty in children compared to open pyeloplasty. *J Urol*. (2011) 186:1663–7. doi: 10.1016/j.juro.2011.04.019

31. Seideman CA, Sleeper JP, Lotan Y. Cost comparison of robot-assisted and laparoscopic pyeloplasty. *J Endourol*. (2012) 26:1044–8. doi: 10.1089/end.2012.0026

32. Cardona-Grau D, Bayne CE. Featuring: has the robot caught up? National trends in utilization, perioperative outcomes, and cost for open, laparoscopic, and robotic pediatric pyeloplasty in the United States from 2003 to 2015. *J Pediatr Urol*. (2018) 14:210–1. doi: 10.1016/j.jpurol.2018.05.013

33. Gkegkes ID, Mamais IA, Iavazzo C. Robotics in general surgery: a systematic cost assessment. *J Minim Access Surg*. (2017) 13:243–55. doi: 10.4103/0972-9941.195565

34. Baek M, Silay MS, Au JK, Huang GO, Elizondo RA, Puttmann KT, et al. Does the use of 5 mm instruments affect the outcomes of robot-assisted laparoscopic pyeloplasty in smaller working spaces? A comparative analysis of infants and older children. *J Pediatr Urol*. (2018) 14:537.e1–6. doi: 10.1016/j.jpurol.2018.06.010

35. Boysen WR, Gundeti MS. Robot-assisted laparoscopic pyeloplasty in the pediatric population: a review of technique, outcomes, complications, and special considerations in infants [published correction appears in pediatr surg int 2017. *Pediatr Surg Int*. (2017) 33:925–35. doi: 10.1007/s00383-017-4082-7

36. Simforoosh N, Abedi A, Hosseini Sharifi SH, Poor Zamany NKM, Rezaeetalab GH, Obayd K, et al. Comparison of surgical outcomes and cosmetic results between standard and mini laparoscopic pyeloplasty in children younger than 1 year of age. *J Pediatr Urol*. (2014) 10:819–23. doi: 10.1016/j.jpurol.2014.01.026

37. Tanaka ST, Grantham JA, Thomas JC, Adams MC, Brock JW III, Pope JC IV. A comparison of open vs laparoscopic pediatric pyeloplasty using the pediatric health information system database–do benefits of laparoscopic approach recede at younger ages? *J Urol*. (2008). 180:1479–85. doi: 10.1016/j.juro.2008.06.044

38. Rappaport BA, Suresh S, Hertz S, Evers AS, Orser BA. Anesthetic neurotoxicity–clinical implications of animal models. *N Engl J Med*. (2015) 372:796–7. doi: 10.1056/NEJMp1414786

39. Andropoulos DB. Effect of anesthesia on the developing brain: infant and fetus. *Fetal Diagn Ther*. (2018) 43:1–11. doi: 10.1159/000475928

40. Kajbafzadeh AM, Tourchi A, Nezami BG, Khakpour M, Mousavian AA, Talab SS. Miniature pyeloplasty as a minimally invasive surgery with less than 1 day admission in infants. *J Pediatr Urol*. (2011) 7:283–8. doi: 10.1016/j.jpurol.2011.02.030

41. Ruiz E, Soria R, Ormaechea E, Lino MM, Moldes JM, de Badiola FI. Simplified open approach to surgical treatment of ureteropelvic junction obstruction in young children and infants. *J Urol*. (2011) 185:2512–6. doi: 10.1016/j.juro.2011.01.012

42. Chacko JK, Koyle MA, Mingin GC, Furness PD III. The minimally invasive open pyeloplasty. *J Pediatr Urol*. (2006) 2:368–72. doi: 10.1016/j.jpurol.2006.05.001

43. Gatti JM, Amstutz SP, Bowlin PR, Stephany HA, Murphy JP. Laparoscopic vs open pyeloplasty in children: results of a randomized, prospective, controlled trial. *J Urol*. (2017) 197:792–7. doi: 10.1016/j.juro.2016.10.056

44. Wang MK, Li Y, Selekman RE, Gaither T, Arnhym A, Baskin LS. Scar acceptance after pediatric urologic surgery. *J Pediatr Urol*. (2018) 14:175.e1–6. doi: 10.1016/j.jpurol.2017.11.018

45. Barbosa JA, Barayan G, Gridley CM, Sanchez DC, Passerotti CC, Houck CS, et al. Parent and patient perceptions of robotic vs open urological surgery scars in children. *J Urol*. (2013) 190:244–50. doi: 10.1016/j.juro.2012.12.060

9

Early Robotic-Assisted Laparoscopic Pyeloplasty for Infants under 3 Months with Severe Ureteropelvic Junction Obstruction

Pin Li[1†], Huixia Zhou[1,2*†], Hualin Cao[1,3†], Tao Guo[4], Weiwei Zhu[4], Yang Zhao[4,5], Tian Tao[1], Xiaoguang Zhou[1], Lifei Ma[1], Yunjie Yang[2,6] and Zhichun Feng[1]

[1] Department of Pediatric Urology, Bayi Children's Hospital, Affiliated of the Seventh Medical Center of People's Liberation Army General Hospital, Beijing, China, [2] The Second School of Clinical Medicine, Southern Medical University, Guangzhou, China, [3] Department of Urology, Nan Xi Shan Hospital of Guangxi Zhuang Autonomous Region, Guilin, China, [4] Medical School of Chinese People's Liberation Army, Beijing, China, [5] Department of Pediatrics, The Third Medical Center of People's Liberation Army General Hospital, Beijing, China, [6] Department of Urology, The Affiliated Nanhai Hospital of the Southern Medical University, Foshan, China

*Correspondence:
Huixia Zhou
huixia99999@163.com

†These authors have contributed equally to this work

Objective: To present our primary experience of robotic-assisted laparoscopic pyeloplasty (RALP) for severe ureteropelvis junction obstruction (UPJO) infants under 3 months.

Methods: We performed a retrospective study of 9 infants under 3 months who underwent RALP for severe UPJO between April 2017 and March 2019 in our center. The severe UPJO was defined as infants with severe hydronephrosis (Society of Fetal Urology grades III or IV, anteroposterior diameter >3 cm or split renal function <40% or T 1/2 >20 min) involving bilateral, solitary kidney, or contralateral renal hypoplasia UPJO at the same time. All clinical, perioperative, and postoperative information was collected.

Results: There were four bilateral UPJO cases, two solitary kidney UPJO cases and three unilateral UPJO with contralateral renal hypoplasia cases included. One single surgeon performed RALP on all of the infants. The mean age of the infants was 1.62 ± 0.54 months. The mean operative time was 109.55 ± 10.47 min. The mean estimated blood loss was 19.29 ± 3.19 ml, and the mean length of hospital stay was 5.57 ± 0.73 days. According to the ultrasonography results, all patients had a significant recovery of renal function at 12 months after the operation.

Conclusions: To maximize the protection of renal function, early RALP is a safe and feasible option for the treatment of severe UPJO in infants under 3 months.

Keywords: robotic-assisted laparoscopic pyeloplasty, infant, hydronephrosis, ureteropelvic junction obstruction, RALP

INTRODUCTION

Ureteropelvic junction obstruction (UPJO) is one of the major causes of infant hydronephrosis (1). The management of UPJO has evolved from open pyeloplasty (OP), laparoscopic pyeloplasty (LP), and robotic-assisted laparoscopic pyeloplasty (RALP) (2, 3). Well-established evidence has demonstrated that LP or RALP not only has success rates equal to those of OP

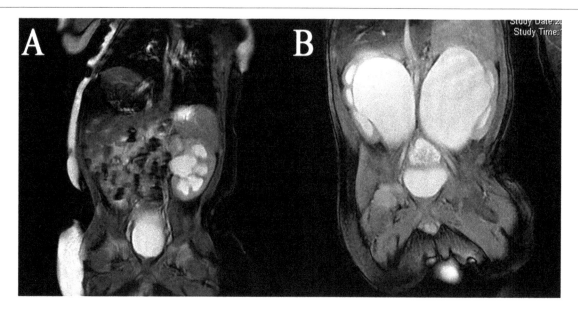

FIGURE 1 | MRI result of a **(A)** Unilateral UPJO with contralateral renal dysplasia; **(B)** bilateral severe UPJO.

but also has the advantages of minimal invasiveness, better cosmesis, less post-operative pain, decreased length of hospital stay, and early recovery[1] (4, 5). In general, the management of hydronephrosis included conservative observation and surgical invention. The clinical decision making usually depends on the rate of hydronephrosis severity. There is still no consensus on the optimal intervention time to perform the surgery, however; whether through conservative or surgical treatment, the ultimate goal is to maximally protect renal function.

Severe UPJO generally refers to bilateral UPJO, a solitary kidney with UPJO, or UPJO with contralateral renal dysplasia. In these complex situations, the selection of conservative observation, conservative nephrostomy, or early minimal invasive pyeloplasty is a problem, especially for very young children under 3 months of age. It is widely acknowledged that pyeloplasty for an infant under 1 year of age or under 10 kg of weight is a challenging procedure that requires more elaborate techniques to decrease the number of complications and lessen operating time to reduce the negative effect of anesthesia (6, 7). In this retrospective study, we summarize our initial experience with conducting RALP on nine severe UPJO infants under 3 months of age.

METHODS AND MATERIALS

Patients

Nine infants 0.8–2.6 months old (mean age 1.62 months) presented with severe UPJO confirmed by ultrasonography screening and were referred to our center from April 2017 to March 2019. The inclusion criteria of this study included age

<3 months, severe hydronephrosis defined as grade III and IV dilation as defined by the Society for Fetal Urology (SFU), anteroposterior diameter (APD) more than 3 cm, impaired split renal function <40%, along with one of the following three conditions: bilateral UPJO, solitary kidney UPJO, or unilateral severe UPJO with contralateral renal dysplasia. Exclusion criteria were UPJO with megaureters, vesicoureteral reflux, posterior urethral valve, or the existence of other structural anomalies. The diagnosis was based on ultrasonography, magnetic resonance urography (MRU) (**Figure 1**), voiding cystourethrography (VCUG), radionuclide, and 99mTc-mercaptoacetyltriglycine (MAG3) diuretic renography results. Perioperative demographic information was also recorded. All patients underwent robotic-assisted laparoscopic pyeloplasty (RALP) with one single surgeon. The Clavien-Dindo classification system was used to evaluate the postoperative complications. This study was undertaken with the approval of the Seventh Medical Center of PLA General Hospital Institutional Ethics Committee. All patients' parents have signed the written consent forms.

Surgical Technique

After routine preoperative preparation and anesthesia, pnuemoperitoneum was established and maintained at 6–8 mmHg pressure. All ports were placed under direct vision included one 8.5 mm camera trocar, one 8-mm trocar and one 5-mm trocar. One or two additional assistant 3-mm trocars were placed at the lateral 3 cm of the midpoint of the Pfannenstiel line, to improve the efficient of the suture (**Figure 2**). For left side cases, the transmesenteric approach was adopted while the dilated renal pelvis was located at the inside of the descending colon. For right side cases, we selected the paracolic sulci approach. Then we carefully dissected the proximal ureter and renal pelvis while preserving the ureteral blood supply. The

---
[1]The laparoscopic pyeloplasty: is there a role in the age of robotics? Accessed May 6, 2020. https://www.ncbi.nlm.nih.gov/pubmed/25455171

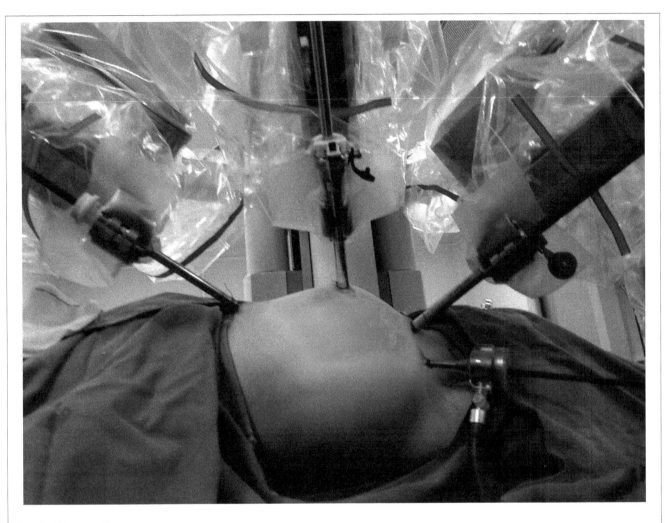

FIGURE 2 | Trocar position appearance.

pelvis was cut above the obstruction tissue and trimmed by a percutaneous hitch stich to stabilize it and facilitated the anastomosis. After spatulated the distal ureter after excision of the obstruction segment, we sutured the lowest point of the aperistaltic ureteral segment and the pelvis end with a running 6-0 PDS-II. Then the posterior wall of the ureter was closed through continuous suture. Before the anterior anastomoses were started with a second running 6-0 PDS II suture, a double-J ureteral stent (COOK, USI-512, Ireland) was placed antegrade. At last, we closed the mesenterium or peritoneum with a 5-0 absorbing suture. For the bilateral pyeloplasty infants, we performed one sided RALP and nephrostomy for the other side. After 1 week interval, we performed RALP for the contralateral UPJO in the same way.

Postoperative Management

The infants restarted general oral feeding after they had recovered from anesthesia. The double-J stent was removed under general anesthesia 6–8 weeks after the operation

by cystoscopy. Ultrasonography, radionuclide, and diuretic renography examinations were repeated the 6th and 12th months after surgery.

Statistical Analysis

Continuous data were presented as the mean $\pm$ STD and range. Functional outcomes were compared using the Student t-test or chi-square test. All statistical analyses were performed in the R software environment (version 3.6.3; http://r-project.org/), and $p < 0.05$ was considered significant in all statistical analyses.

RESULTS

The baseline clinical data of the nine infants were shown in **Table 1**. All operations were performed successfully without conversion to open surgery. No serious intraoperative complication happened. The perioperative findings were summarized in **Table 2**. Two patients with postoperative infection (Clavien-Dindo Grade II Complications) were

TABLE 1 | Patient characteristics.

Description	No.
Patient	9
Age at surgery, month, mean ± SD (range)	1.62 ± 0.54 (0.8–2.6)
Gender, No. male/female	6/3
Diagnosis	
Solitary kidney with UPJO	2
UPJO with contralateral renal dysplasia	3
Bilateral UPJO	4
APD (mm), mean ± SD(range)	4.06 ± 0.73(3.4–5.3)
SFU Grade III/IV	4/9
Split renal function	0.36 ± 0.04
Renography T1/2 >20 min	8

TABLE 2 | Perioperative outcomes.

Description	No.
Estimated blood loss	19.29 ± 3.19(15–30)
Operation time	109.55 ± 10.47(92–138)
Conversion to open surgery	0
Foley catheter indwelling days	1.86 ± 0.64
Length of hospital stay	5.57 ± 0.73
Complications Clavien-Dindo	
I and II	2
III and IV	0

TABLE 3 | Preoperative and follow-up characteristics.

Description	Pre-operation	6th month	12th month	p-value
APD (mm)	4.06 ± 0.73	0.97 ± 0.16	0.86 ± 0.12	<0.01
Split renal function	0.36 ± 0.04	0.53 ± 0.05	0.58 ± 0.04	<0.01
Renography T1/2 <10 min	0	8	9	<0.01

managed conservatively by intravenous antibiotics. No patient suffered Clavien III or IV complications. The mean time for Foley catheter removal was 1.86 ± 0.64 days.

According to the follow-up data listed in **Table 3**, the renal pelvis APD decreased to 0.97 ± 0.16 cm in the 6th month after surgery, which was significantly smaller than perioperative APD ($p < 0.01$). Radionuclide renography results showed that the split renal function had a great improvement in 6 months and slightly increased in 12 months. Diuretic renography revealed that 8 out of 9 patients have a T 1/2 time <10 min in the 6th month after surgery. In the 12th month examination, all of the 9 patients' T 1/2 times were <10 min.

DISCUSSION

Open dismembered pyeloplasty has been the gold standard treatment for UPJO for decades with overall success rates of more than 90% (8). Since first reported in 1993, laparoscopic pyeloplasty has been demonstrated as a safe and effective treatment for UPJO (9). Two years later, pediatric laparoscopic

pyeloplasty was introduced by Peters et al. (10). While limited by the small space for instrument movement and trocar placement, the use of laparoscopic and robotic-assisted laparoscopic is well-described (11, 12). Recently, more and more literature has proved that laparoscopic pyeloplasty or robotic-assisted laparoscopic pyeloplasty has not only the same success rate as open pyeloplasty, but also shorter hospitalization stay, faster recovery time, and better cosmetic appearance (13–16).

Meanwhile, the management of hydronephrosis in children has greatly changed during the last 20 years. In the 1990s, Ransley et al. (17) reported that early pyeloplasty may not be of greater benefit than observed or delayed surgery. After radiological imaging studies had become available for clinical evaluation, the value of split renal function and T1/2 was greatly improved for deciding the optimal time for surgical treatment (18). According to the results of a study conducted by Onen et al., (19) they only recommended surgical intervention for renal deterioration (decreased split renal function or progressive hydronephrosis). However, Tabari et al. (20) revealed that early pyeloplasty could benefit infants <1 year old suffering from severe but asymptomatic hydronephrosis better than conservative management through a prospective interventional study. In their study, they compared the functional outcomes of open pyeloplasty on a group of infants and conservative management of infants. They found that the group of infants who had early surgery have lower SFU grade and larger cortical thickness than the conservative group. According to the EAU Guidelines 2020, increased APD, SFU grade III or IV, split renal function <40%, or decrease >10% in follow-up and poor drainage function could be indications for asymptomatic UPJO.

For infants under 1 year old or even under 3 months, there are numerous challenges for surgical intervention so that whether to perform surgery is controversial. In 2006, Kutikov et al. (21) reported that transperitoneal laparoscopic pyeloplasty for UPJO in eight infants under 6 months old is technically possible. Zamfir Snykers et al. (22) also draw a similar conclusion in their research. Simforoosh et al. (14) compared the surgical outcomes of standard and minilaparoscopic pyeloplasty in children younger than 1 year of age. They believed that both of these approaches had the same effect while the minilaparoscopic technique could be more cosmetically pleasing and less invasive (14). In a retrospectively study, Turner et al. (23) assessed the effect of laparoscopic pyeloplasty performed in 29 infants 2–11 months old. Their experience revealed a success rate with minimal morbidity (23). In a multi-institutional trial, Daniel et al. (16) collected perioperative data of 60 patients underwent RALP by six surgeons and described an excellence success rate and a low complication rate in this cohort. Shukla et al. (24) summarized their experience about RALP and compared outcomes between infants aged <1 year and older children. They found that there were no significant differences in length of hospital stay and complications or failure rates in infants compared to older children, and they called for the adaptation of RALP for the entire pediatric patient population. Andolfi et al. (6) conducted a systematic review to compare whether

RALP is superior to conventional LP. They selected 19 original articles and 5 meta-analyses and concluded that RALP could decrease operative times, shorten the length of hospital stay, and reduce the complication rates while having the same success rates comparable to LP.

Conventional laparoscopy has a significant learning curve and is technically challenging for many surgeons compared to robot-assisted laparoscopy. Undoubtedly, the robotic-assisted technique can facilitate a shorter learning curve and act as a bridge between the open and endoscopic approaches. In these years, pediatric RALP has become a viable minimally invasive surgical option for UPJO children with some reports on its efficacy, safety, and cosmetic effect (15, 25, 26). Our team has also presented our experiences of transumbilical multi-stab laparoscopic pyeloplasty for infants younger than 3 months. On this basis, we performed RALP for these severe hydronephrosis patients under 3 months in this cohort.

This study included nine infants (thirteen sides) ranging from 0.8 to 2.6 months old who underwent transperitoneal RALP. All of the patients were diagnosed prenatally and had regular examinations after birth. As the hydronephrosis lasted and became even worse, we decided to intervene early with these patients because of our previous experience with the children who had undergone RALP. For the infants who were sensitive to the CO_2 pressure, we usually selected 6–8 mmHg to establish the existence of pneumoperitoneum. To expand the operating space as much as possible, we lifted and fixed robotic arm numbers 1 and 2. We have also explored several port positions for infants and finally selected the strategy described in this article as it could provide the most operating space and the least skin wounds. To reduce the incidence of anastomosis obstruction and improve success rates, several techniques were applied in RALP, including the way to identify the axis of renal calyx as the kidney axis and started the anastomosis at the lowest point of the renal pelvis and ureter, which was also described in our previously published literature (27). For the bilateral UPJO cases, we performed two RALPs at one-week intervals, but not side by side, as bilateral RALP had longer operating time and higher stent blockage risk. During the hospitalizations, no anesthesia complications were observed. Our clinical experience indicated that these techniques are important to facilitate RALP and improve success rates and decrease postoperative complications (27). According to follow-up data from the 6th and 12th months after operation, the primary outcomes were positive. T1/2 results showed no obstruction of the ureter after 12 months. The cosmetic appearance was also satisfactory although in our study the quantitative evaluation was not. Compared with our previous published study about our early experience of using LP for infants younger than 3 months (28), RALP (including docking time) has a longer operation time (109.55 vs. 75 min), same length of stay (5.57 vs. 6 d) and the same success rate. LP has a litter advantage on the cosmetic effect, but the learning curve of RALP is significantly decreased.

The limitations of this study include its retrospective nature, lack of randomization and design with no control group, small patient sample size, use of a single center, the lack of more than one surgeon with experience with RALP, and the focus only on primary outcomes within 1 year. These factors limit us from drawing more conclusions on the management of severe hydronephrosis. Despite the existence of these limitations, we believe that our study provides new insight into the application of the robotic technique in infant surgery. It confirms that RALP has the advantage of being minimally invasive and could be used to protect the renal function of severe UPJO patients under 3 months as early as possible.

CONCLUSION

Early RALP is a safe and feasible option for the treatment of severe UPJO infants under 3 months. However, further controlled prospective study is still necessary to determine the ultimate role of RALP in the management of young infants with UPJO.

AUTHOR CONTRIBUTIONS

Conceptualization: PL and HZ. Data curation and Investigation: PL and HC. Formal analysis: PL and TG. Funding acquisition and Project administration: HZ. Methodology: LM. Resources: TT, XZ, and LM. Software: WZ and YZ. Supervision: ZF and HZ. Validation: YY. Visualization: PL, HC, and TG. Writing—original draft: PL and HC. Writing—review and editing: HZ. All authors contributed to the article and approved the submitted version.

REFERENCES

1. Hashim H, Woodhouse CRJ. Ureteropelvic junction obstruction. *Eur. Urol. Suppl.* (2012) 11:25–32. doi: 10.1016/j.eursup.2012.01.004
2. Mufarrij PW, Woods M, Shah OD, Palese MA, Berger AD, Thomas R, et al. Robotic dismembered pyeloplasty: a 6-year, multi-institutional experience. *J. Urol.* (2008) 180:1391–6. doi: 10.1016/j.juro.2008.06.024
3. Shah KK, Louie M, Thaly RK, Patel VR. Robot assisted laparoscopic pyeloplasty: a review of the current status. *Int. J. Med. Rob. Comp. Assist. Surg.* (2007) 3:35–40. doi: 10.1002/rcs.122
4. Huang Y, Wu Y, Shan W, Zeng L, Huang L. An updated meta-analysis of laparoscopic versus open pyeloplasty for ureteropelvic junction obstruction in children. *Int. J. Clin. Exp. Med.* (2015) 8:4922–31.
5. Tasian GE, Casale P. The robotic-assisted laparoscopic pyeloplasty: gateway to advanced reconstruction. *Urol. Clin. North Am.* (2015) 42:89–97. doi: 10.1016/j.ucl.2014.09.008
6. Andolfi C, Adamic B, Oommen J, Gundeti MS. Robot-assisted laparoscopic pyeloplasty in infants and children: is it superior to conventional laparoscopy? *World J. Urol.* (2020) 38:1827–33. doi: 10.1007/s00345-019-02943-z
7. He Y, Song H, Liu P, Sun N, Tian J, Li M, et al. Primary laparoscopic pyeloplasty in children: a single-center experience of 279 patients and analysis

of possible factors affecting complications. *J. Pediatr. Urol.* (2020) 16:331.e1–e11. doi: 10.1016/j.jpurol.2020.03.028

8. Siqueira Jr TM, Nadu A, Kuo RL, Paterson RF, Lingeman JE, Shalhav AL. Laparoscopic treatment for ureteropelvic junction obstruction. *Urology.* (2002) 60:973–8. doi: 10.1016/S0090-4295(02)02072-1

9. Schuessler WW, Grune MT, Tecuanhuey LV, Preminger GM. Laparoscopic dismembered pyeloplasty. *J. Urol.* (1993) 150:1795–9. doi: 10.1016/S0022-5347(17)35898-6

10. Peters CA, Schlussel RN, Retik AB. Pediatric laparoscopic dismembered pyeloplasty. *J. Urol.* (1995) 153:1962–5. doi: 10.1016/S0022-5347(01)67378-6

11. Tasian GE, Wiebe DJ, Casale P. Learning curve of robotic assisted pyeloplasty for pediatric urology fellows. *J. Urol.* (2013) 190:1622–7. doi: 10.1016/j.juro.2013.02.009

12. Atug F, Woods M, Burgess SV, Castle EP, Thomas R. Robotic assisted laparoscopic pyeloplasty in children. *J. Urol.* (2005) 174(4 Part 1):1440–2. doi: 10.1097/01.ju.0000173131.64558.c9

13. Dangle PP, Kearns J, Anderson B, Gundeti MS. Outcomes of infants undergoing robot-assisted laparoscopic pyeloplasty compared to open repair. *J. Urol.* (2013) 190:2221–7. doi: 10.1016/j.juro.2013.07.063

14. Simforoosh N, Abedi A, Hosseini Sharifi SH, Nk MP, Rezaeetalab GH, Obayd K, et al. Comparison of surgical outcomes and cosmetic results between standard and mini laparoscopic pyeloplasty in children younger than 1 year of age. *J. Pediatr. Urol.* (2014) 10:819–23. doi: 10.1016/j.jpurol.2014.01.026

15. Barbosa JA, Kowal A, Onal B, Gouveia E, Walters M, Newcomer J, et al. Comparative evaluation of the resolution of hydronephrosis in children who underwent open and robotic-assisted laparoscopic pyeloplasty. *J. Pediatr. Urol.* (2013) 9:199–205. doi: 10.1016/j.jpurol.2012.02.002

16. Avery DI, Herbst KW, Lendvay TS, Noh PH, Dangle P, Gundeti MS, et al. Robot-assisted laparoscopic pyeloplasty: multi-institutional experience in infants. *J. Pediatr. Urol.* (2015) 11:139.e1–e5. doi: 10.1016/j.jpurol.2014.11.025

17. Ransley PG, Dhillon HK, Gordon I, Duffy PG, Dillon MJ, Barratt TM. The postnatal management of hydronephrosis diagnosed by prenatal ultrasound. *J. Urol.* (1990) 144(2 Part 2):584–7. doi: 10.1016/S0022-5347(17)39528-9

18. Ross SS, Kardos S, Krill A, Bourland J, Sprague B, Majd M, et al. Observation of infants with SFU grades 3–4 hydronephrosis: worsening drainage with serial diuresis renography indicates surgical intervention and helps prevent loss of renal function. *J. Pediatr. Urol.* (2011) 7:266–71. doi: 10.1016/j.jpurol.2011.03.001

19. Onen A, Jayanthi V, Koff S. Long-term followup of prenatally detected severe bilateral newborn hydronephrosis initially managed nonoperatively. *J. Urol.* (2002) 168:1118–20. doi: 10.1016/S0022-5347(05)64604-6

20. Tabari AK, Atqiaee K, Mohajerzadeh L, Rouzrokh M, Ghoroubi J, Alam A, et al. Early pyeloplasty versus conservative management of severe ureteropelvic junction obstruction in asymptomatic infants. *J. Pediatr. Surg.* 55:1936–40. doi: 10.1016/j.jpedsurg.2019.08.006

21. Kutikov A, Resnick M, Casale P. Laparoscopic pyeloplasty in the infant younger than 6 months—is it technically possible? *J. Urol.* (2006) 175:1477–9. doi: 10.1016/S0022-5347(05)00673-7

22. Zamfir Snykers C, De Plaen E, Vermersch S, Lopez M, Khelif K, Luyckx S, et al. Is laparoscopic pyeloplasty for ureteropelvic junction obstruction in infants under 1 year of age a good option? *Front. Pediatr.* (2019) 7:352. doi: 10.3389/fped.2019.00352

23. Turner RM, Fox JA, Tomaszewski JJ, Schneck FX, Docimo SG, Ost MC. Laparoscopic pyeloplasty for ureteropelvic junction obstruction in infants. *J. Urol.* (2013) 189:1503–7. doi: 10.1016/j.juro.2012.10.067

24. Kawal T, Srinivasan AK, Shrivastava D, Chu DI, Van Batavia J, Weiss D, et al. Pediatric robotic-assisted laparoscopic pyeloplasty: does age matter? *J. Pediatr. Urol.* (2018) 14:540.e1–e6. doi: 10.1016/j.jpurol.2018.04.023

25. Sukumar S, Roghmann F, Sood A, Abdo AA, Menon M, Sammon JD, et al. Correction of ureteropelvic junction obstruction in children: national trends and comparative effectiveness in operative outcomes. *J. Endourol.* (2014) 28:592–8. doi: 10.1089/end.2013.0618

26. Cundy TP, Harling L, Hughes-Hallett A, Mayer EK, Najmaldin AS, Athanasiou T, et al. Meta-analysis of robot-assisted vs conventional laparoscopic and open pyeloplasty in children. *BJU Int.* (2014) 114:582–94. doi: 10.1111/bju.12683

27. Liu D, Zhou H, Ma L, Zhou X, Cao H, Tao T, et al. Comparison of laparoscopic approaches for dismembered pyeloplasty in children with ureteropelvic junction obstruction: critical analysis of 11-year experiences in a single surgeon. *Urology.* (2017) 101:50–5. doi: 10.1016/j.urology.2016.10.007

28. Zhou H, Liu X, Xie H, Ma L, Zhou X, Tao T, et al. Early experience of using transumbilical multi-stab laparoscopic pyeloplasty for infants younger than 3 months. *J. Pediatr. Urol.* (2014) 10:854–8. doi: 10.1016/j.jpurol.2013.12.025

10

Meta-Analysis of the Efficacy of Laparoscopic Pyeloplasty for Ureteropelvic Junction Obstruction via Retroperitoneal and Transperitoneal Approaches

Fengming Ji[†], Li Chen[†], Chengchuang Wu[†], Jinrong Li, Yu Hang and Bing Yan*

Kunming Children's Hospital, Kunming, China

*Correspondence:
Bing Yan
yanbing29@q163.com

[†] These authors have contributed equally to this work

Objective: This study aimed to evaluate the clinical efficacy of laparoscopic pyeloplasty (LP) for ureteropelvic junction obstruction (UPJO) via retroperitoneal and transperitoneal approaches.

Method: A systematic literature search on keywords was undertaken using PubMed, Cochrane Library, Embase, China Nation Knowledge (CNKI), and Wanfang. The eligible literature was screened according to inclusion and exclusion criteria. Meta-analysis was performed by using RevMan 5.0 software.

Results: According to the inclusion and exclusion criteria, 12 studies were identified with a total of 777 patients. Four hundred eight patients were treated with retroperitoneal laparoscopic pyeloplasty (RLP), and 368 patients were treated with transperitoneal laparoscopic pyeloplasty (TLP). The meta-analysis results showed that the two approaches were similar in terms of presence of postoperative hospital stay, postoperative complication, the rate of conversion, and recurrence ($p > 0.05$). The operative time in the TLP group was significantly shorter than the RLP group (MD = 16.6; 95% CI, 3.40–29.80; $p = 0.01$). The duration of drainage was significantly shorter (MD = −1.06; 95% CI, −1.92 to −0.19; $p = 0.02$), and the score of postoperative visual analog score (VAS) was significantly lower in the RLP group than in the TLP group (MD = −0.52; 95% CI, −0.96 to −0.08; $p = 0.02$).

Conclusion: Both approaches have good success rates and low postoperative complication rates. RLP provides a shorter duration of drainage and lower VAS score, but it takes more operative time than TLP.

Keywords: ureteropelvic junction obstruction, laparoscopic, pyeloplasty, retroperitoneal, transperitoneal

BACKGROUND

With the popularity of prenatal ultrasound, the rate of diagnosis of hydronephrosis has increased in fetal and prenatal. There are many causes of hydronephrosis such as ureteropelvic junction obstruction (UPJO), vesicoureteral reflux (VUR), or ureterovesical junction obstruction. Ureteropelvic junction obstruction (UPJO) is the most common cause of congenital hydronephrosis (1). The standard surgical technique is dismembered pyeloplasty (Anderson–Hynes procedure) for UPJO, which was first performed successfully by Anderson and Hynes in 1949. It has the obvious advantages for long stenosis segment, presence of stones, and crossing vessels (2). With the continuous development of modern minimally invasive technology, laparoscopic pyeloplasy (LP) has become a more beneficial choice for the patients with UPJO than open surgery because of the advantages of excellent visualization, minimal trauma, rapid postoperative recovery, good cosmetic result, and a nearly successful rate compared with open pyeloplasy (3, 4). LP can be performed though retroperitoneal and transperitoneal approaches. To compare the advantages and disadvantages of the two approaches, this study consulted relevant literature and performed a meta-analysis.

METHODS
Search Strategy

We searched PubMed, Embase, CNKI, and Wanfang. Studies were restricted to English and Chinese language published before January 1, 2020. The following search terms were used using the Boolean operator terms "AND" and "OR": "laparoscopic pyeloplasty," "laparoscopic disconnected pyeloplasty," "Ureteropelvic junction obstruction," "UPJO," "retroperitoneal," and "transperitoneal."

Inclusion Criteria and Exclusion Criteria
Inclusion Criteria

(1) Interventions: laparoscopic ureteroplasty was performed through retroperitoneal and transperitoneal approaches. (2) Intervention subjects: unilateral UPJO patients. (3) Outcomes: postoperative time, hospital stay, postoperative complication, duration of drainage, visual analog score (VAS), the rate of conversion, and recurrence. (4) Study types—randomized controlled studies or retrospective studies. (5) For the studies published by the same unit, the latest one would be included.

Exclusion Criteria

(1) Approaches involved only retroperitoneal or transperitoneal. (2) The intervention subjects included patients with bilateral UPJO. (3) Outcome cannot be obtained. (4) Full text is unavailable. (5) The treatment includes robotic-assisted surgery and open surgery. (6) Literature with a quality evaluation result of <7 or low quality according to the Newcastle–Ottawa Scale (NOS) quality evaluation scale (5) and the Cochrane Collaboration's tool (6).

Study Selection and Quality Evaluation

In selecting studies for inclusion, a review of all relevant article titles and abstracts were conducted before an examination of the full published texts. Two professional reviewers reviewed the articles for eligibility and quality and extracted the data independently. Data were collected on standard collection tables. Extracted data included author's name, nation, published year, study type, patients' characteristics, and relevant outcomes. Disagreement was resolved by consensus with the intervention of a third reviewer.

For the quality assessment, the Newcastle–Ottawa Scale (NOS) quality evaluation scale and the Cochrane Collaboration's tool were used for non-randomized controlled trials and randomized controlled studies, respectively.

Statistical Analysis

All meta-analyses were carried out in RevMan 5.0 software, and $p < 0.05$ meant the difference was statistically significant. The continuous variables were described by standardized mean difference (SMD) and 95% confidence interval (95% CI), and the dichotomous variables were described by odds ratio (OR) and 95% CI. Evaluated by Q-test, heterogeneity was considered if $p > 0.1$ or $I < 50\%$, and the random effect model was adopted. If $p < 0.1$ or $I > 50\%$, it indicates that there was heterogeneity, and the fixed effect model was adopted. For the continuous variables, if only the median and value range were provided in the included studies, the mean and standard deviation were calculated according to the formula of Hozo (7).

RESULT
Study Characteristics

A total of 44 studies were retrieved. According to the inclusion and exclusion criteria, there were 12 studies that were included in the present study, of which 7 studies were in English, and 5 studies were in Chinese. A total of 777 patients were involved among the 12 studies, 408 patients were treated with RLP, and 369 patients were treated with TLP (The basic characteristics of the included studies are shown in **Table 1**, and the search process of the studies is shown in **Figure 1**).

Meta-Analysis Results
Operative Time

There were 12 studies that reported the operative time of the two groups. The heterogeneity test result was $p < 0.0001$, $I = 94\%$, and the random effect model was adopted. The meta-analysis result showed that there was significant difference in the operative time between the two groups (MD = 16.60; 95% CI, 3.40–29.80; $p = 0.01$) (**Figure 2**).

Postoperative Hospital Stay

There were 12 studies that reported the postoperative hospital stay of the two groups. The heterogeneity test result was $p < 0.0001$, $I = 91\%$, and the random effect model was adopted. The meta-analysis result showed that there was no significant difference in hospital stay between the two groups (MD = −0.21; 95% CI, −0.54–0.12; $p = 0.21$).

TABLE 1 | The basic characteristics of the included literature.

References	Nation	Year	Study type	RLP/TLP				
				Side: eft/right	Sex: male/female	Age:	Mean follow-up period	Quality evaluation
Abunaz et al. (8)	France	1999/10–2008/10	RS	14:17/16:18	12:19/15:19	36.94 ± 17.92/37.11 ± 16.75	48.9	8
Badawy et al. (9)	Egypt	2010/06–2012/09	RCT	/	11:8/14:5	/	10	High
Hemal et al. (10)	India	1999/10–2002/03	RS	4:8/7:5	8:4/9:3	26.3 ± 10.46/22.9 ± 9.87	11	9
Liu (11)	China	2012/09–2017/09	RS	20:8/21:9	17:11/18:12	27.12 ± 4.56/28.43 ± 3.25	/	9
Qadri and Khan (12)	India	2000/01–2009/08	RS	16:19/5:7	25:10/8:4	27.3 ± 11/32 ± 10.18	22/48	9
Shen et al. (13)	China	2012/04–2017/03	RCT	26:17/23:20	29:14/31:12	38.18 ± 3.05/39.11 ± 3.01	/	High
Shoma et al. (14)	Egypt	2002/02–2006/01	RCT	14:6/11:9	10:10/11:9	34 ± 15/29 ± 13	20/23	High
Singh et al. (15)	India	2008/01–2012/12	RCT	31:25/30:26	32:24/30:26	24.93 ± 3.94/24.79 ± 3.96	31	High
Xu and Li (16)	China	2013/01–2015/01	RCT	/	27:13/26:14	26.45 ± 4.45/26.34 ± 4.35	20	High
Zhai et al. (17)	China	2011/06–2015/05	NRCT	31:25/27:15	34:22/28:14	30.8 ± 12.8/27.2 ± 11.9	26/24	9
Zhang (18)	China	2010/01–2012/12	RS	22:18/24:16	22:18/28:12	22.41 ± 5.18/26.67 ± 4.59	18	7
Zhu et al. (19)	China	2009–2011	RS	16:12/13:9	16:12/9:13	30.6 ± 13.5/37.5 ± 8.25	11/10	8

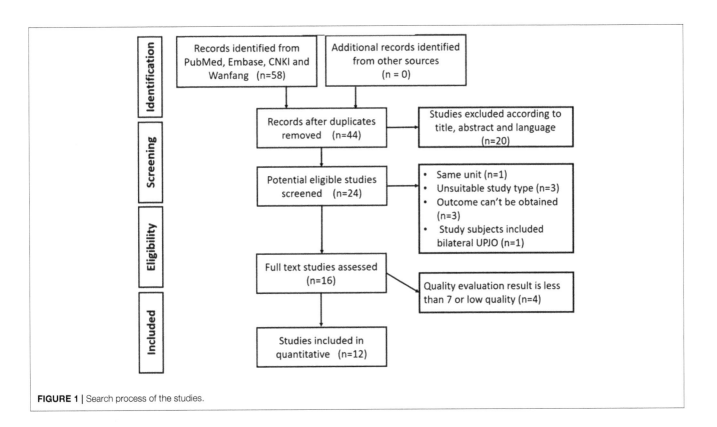

FIGURE 1 | Search process of the studies.

Duration of Drainage

There were four studies reported the duration of drainage of the two groups. The heterogeneity test result was $p < 0.0001$, $I = 87\%$, and the random effect model was adopted. The meta-analysis result showed that there was significant difference in the duration of drainage between the two groups (MD $= -1.06$; 95% CI, -1.92 to -0.19; $p = 0.02$) (**Figure 3**).

Visual Analog Score

There were four studies that reported the VAS of the two groups. The heterogeneity test result was $p < 0.0001$, $I = 94\%$, and the random effect model was adopted. The meta-analysis result showed that there was a significant difference in the VAS between the two groups (MD $= -0.52$; 95% CI, -0.96 to -0.08; $p = 0.02$) (**Figure 4**).

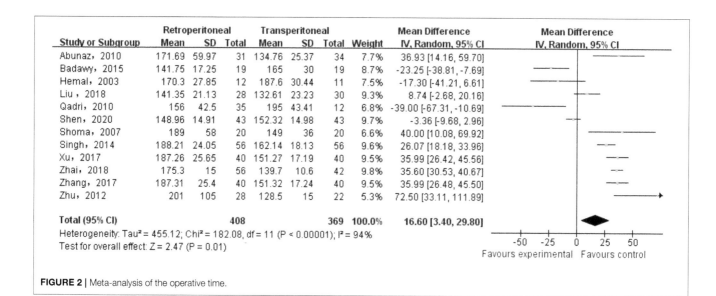

FIGURE 2 | Meta-analysis of the operative time.

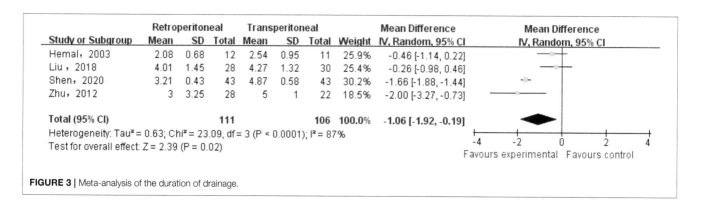

FIGURE 3 | Meta-analysis of the duration of drainage.

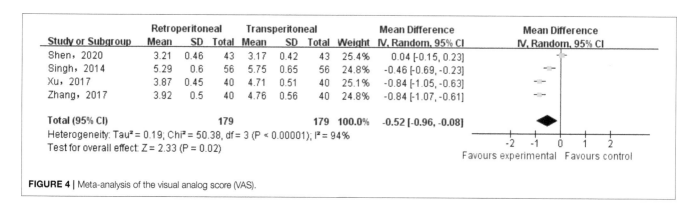

FIGURE 4 | Meta-analysis of the visual analog score (VAS).

Postoperative Complication

There were seven studies that reported the postoperative complication of the two groups. The heterogeneity test result was $p = 0.51$, $I = 0\%$, and the fixed effect model was adopted. The meta-analysis result showed that there was no significant difference in the postoperative complication between the two groups (OR = 1.19; 95% CI, 0.62–2.28; $p = 0.60$).

Conversion Rate

There were six studies that reported the conversion rate of the two groups. The heterogeneity test result was $p = 0.36$, $I = 7\%$, and the fixed effect model was adopted. The meta-analysis result showed that there was no significant difference in the conversion rate between the two groups (OR = 1.86; 95% CI, 0.67–5.16; $p = 0.23$).

Meta-Analysis of the Efficacy of Laparoscopic Pyeloplasty for Ureteropelvic Junction Obstruction...

73

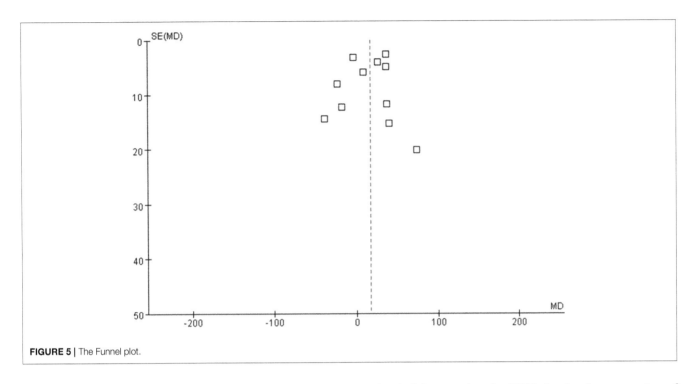

FIGURE 5 | The Funnel plot.

Recurrence

There were six studies that reported the recurrence of the two groups. The heterogeneity test result was $p = 0.99$, $I = 0\%$, and the fixed effect model was adopted. The meta-analysis result showed that there was no significant difference in the recurrence between the two groups (OR $= 1.23$; 95% CI, 0.55–2.74; $p = 0.62$).

Publication Bias

In the bias analysis, the effect index SMD was used as the abscissa axis and SE (SMD) as the vertical axis to draw an inverted funnel plot (see **Figure 5**). The results showed that the funnel plot was not completely symmetrical on the left and right, suggesting that there might be publication bias in the included literatures in this study.

DISCUSSION

UPJO is a common disease in pediatric urology with an incidence of about 1/2,000 in newborns, and the ratio of the men to women is 2∼3:1 (20). UPJO usually reduces the free flow of urine from the renal pelvis to the ureter, causing dilation of the renal pelvis and calyces and hydronephrosis (21). Ureteropelvic junction stenosis, crossing vessel, and ureteropelvic junction valve and stone are also important causes of UPJO. Ureteropelvic junction stenosis is the most important cause of congenital UPJO in newborns, which can impair renal function and eventually lead to renal parenchymal atrophy (22). Lack of smooth muscle, collagen deposition, increased connective tissue, and decrease in the proportion of interstitial cells of the Cajal are the pathological characteristics of ureteropelvic junction stenosis. According to the study of Bady et al. (23), the stenosis segment is related to the increase in acetylcholinesterase activity and norepinephrine response.

Surgical intervention for UPJO is aimed at removing of obstruction segment, relieving of pain, and preserving of renal function (4, 24). There are many indices that have been used to identify the need for surgery, such as SFU grade 3 or 4, continued expansion of the renal pelvis collection system, a renal cortex <5 mm, a single kidney with decrease in GFR, and symptom of pain (25, 26). Regrettably, there has been no reliable criterion that could be used in risk stratification and decision making with UPJO. Most researches support that the reduction in cortical thickness and increased severity of hydronephrosis are important signs of fibrosis of renal parenchyma and reduced glomerular numbers (27); however, in the study of Huang et al., (28) it was pointed out that the degree of hydronephrosis did not significantly correlate with the number of affected glomeruli. Mercapto-acetyl-triglycine and dimercaptosuccinic acid can objectively reflect the degree of kidney damage, but they usually need sedation and repeated evaluation in infants or younger children. Pavlaki et al. (29) proved that the level of urinary NGAL and serum cystatin C are remarkably decreased from the preoperative to the postoperative period, and they could be reliable biomarkers to distinguish the kidney condition among patients with severe and mild hydronephrosis.

There are many methods for treating UPJO, including endopyeloplasty, endopyelotomy, and pyeloplasty, but pyeloplasty is the most reliable, which is currently recognized as the gold standard for the treatment of UPJO (30). Up to now, the overall success rate of the open pyeloplasty is over 90%, and the recurrence of postoperative hydronephrosis usually occurs within 2 years after the operation. Chow et al. (24) pointed out that preoperative renal function <30%, history of endopyelotomy, and early urinary leakage were the risk factors for surgical failure.

According to the results of the meta-analysis, there were no significant difference between the two approaches on postoperative hospital stay, complications, conversion rate, and recurrence. RLP took more operative time than TLP, and the difference was statistically significant (MD = 16.60; 95% CI, 3.40–29.80; $p = 0.01$). Since the transperitoneal approach requires to cut the mesentery through the medial or lateral colon to enter the retroperitoneal cavity, it takes more time to expose the pelvis. Wu et al. (31) believed that the retroperitoneal approach will be more conducive to shortening the operative time with the familiarity of the surgeon with the anatomy of the retroperitoneal cavity. According to the results of the present study, RLP can significantly shorten the time of postoperative drainage and reduce the score of postoperative VAS (MD = −1.06; 95% CI, −1.92 to −0.19; $p = 0.02$; MD = −0.52; 95% CI, −0.96 to −0.08; $p = 0.02$), which may be related to the shorter route of retroperitoneal approach, with less interference to abdominal organs, faster recovery of gastrointestinal function, and low incidence of intestinal obstruction.

Open pyeloplasty has been widely accepted as the prior choice for UPJO, with a success rate of >90% in most reports (32). Since the LP in adults and children were first successfully performed in 1993 and 1995, respectively, it has gradually replaced open pyeloplasty as the preferred option for UPJO (33, 34). Most researchers support that LP is beneficial and advantageous to old patients, but for infants younger than 6 months, opinions are different (35, 36).

Nowadays, the application of laparoscopy in pediatric urology has been developed for 30 years. Laparoscopy seems to be an established technique for children. LP may be applied with transperitoneal and retroperitoneal approach. TLP can provide a larger space for free movement of instruments and intraoperative suturing. Meanwhile, the anatomical marks are easier to identify for surgeons. However, due to the stimulation of urine to the intestinal and the disturbed abdominal cavity, the rate of bowel-related complications, including abdominal organ injury and postoperative intestinal obstruction, is increased (1). Which surgical method is better is still controversial; some scholars argued that if the renal pelvis dilated more than 6 cm, with large or multiple renal stones, pelvic kidney, or horseshoe kidney, TLP was easier and safer than RLP (37). Because the infants have a high sensitivity at CO_2 effects, theoretically, increased intra-abdominal pressure and hypothermia, TLP seems to be safer for infants to decrease the intra-abdominal pressure and hypothermia through shortening of the operative time (36, 38). Unfortunately, postoperative hypercapnia was not reported in the literature included in the study.

In terms of TLP, the surgical approach remains controversial too. TLP included paracolic sulci approach and mesentery approach, and the option of surgical procedure usually depends on the location of the lesion. Due to the right renal pelvis and ureter, which are often located at the right colic flexure, UPJO on the right is recommended with the optimal paracolic sulci approach. During the operation, only the peritoneum of the lateral side of the right colon is cut, and the right colon is pushed medially to expose the renal pelvis and ureter. Due to the left colic flexure position, which is higher, covering the kidney, and the mesenteric just covering the left UPJ, the left mesentery approach is not only helpful in identifying the renal pelvis but also can avoid excessive dissection and dissociation of the left descending colon and perirenal fascia, shorten the operation time, relieve surgical trauma, relieve postoperative pain, and accelerate postoperative recovery (39, 40).

There were some limitations to this study that should be noted. On the one hand, not all of the studies included were RCT; it caused an inevitable selection bias in the study. On the other hand, there was limited documentation of follow-up; of the 10 studies assessed, 2 studies gave no length of follow-up and 3 studies published on a follow-up of <12 months. It affected the outcome of the long-term postoperative complications.

CONCLUSION

RLP and TLP have the same results in postoperative complications, conversion rate, and recurrence, but RLP has potential benefit to make the patients recover faster after the operation as it can reduce the time of postoperative drainage and postoperative VAS. It is hard to say which approach is better because RLP takes more operative time and needs a longer learning curve, so the surgeon should choose the appropriate operation according to personal preference and experience during the early practice. For experienced surgeons, RLP seems to be a more beneficial choice for patients.

AUTHOR CONTRIBUTIONS

FJ collected and analyzed data and drafted the original manuscript. LC collected data and participated in to amend the manuscript. CW collected and analyzed data. JL collected data. YH analyzed data. BY designed present study and amended the manuscript. All authors contributed to the article and approved the submitted version.

REFERENCES

1. Zhang S, Li J, Li C, Xie X, Ling F, Liang Y, et al. Evaluation of the clinical value of retroperitoneal laparoscopic pyeloplasty in the treatment of ureteropelvic junction obstruction in infants: a single-center experience involving 22 consecutive patients. *Medicine.* (2019) 98:e17308. doi: 10.1097/MD.00000000000 17308

2. Villemagne T, Fourcade L, Camby C, Szwarc C, Lardy H, Leclair M. Long-term results with the laparoscopic transposition of renal lower pole crossing vessels. *J Pediatr Urol.* (2015) 11:174.e1–7. doi: 10.1016/j.jpurol.2015. 04.023

3. Piaggio LA, Corbetta JP, Weller S, Dingevan RA, Duran V, Ruiz J, et al. Comparative, prospective, case-control study of open versus laparoscopic pyeloplasty in children with ureteropelvic junction obstruction: long-term results. *Front Pediatr.* (2017) 5:10. doi: 10.3389/fped.2017. 00010

4. Chen JC, Zhang QL, Wang YJ, Cui X, Chen L, Zhang JQ, et al. Laparoscopic disconnected pyeloplasty to treat ureteropelvic junction obstruction (UPJO) in children. *Med Sci Monit.* (2019) 25:9131–7. doi: 10.12659/MSM. 918164

5. Stang A. Critical evaluation of the newcastle-Ottawa scale for the assessment of the quality of nonrandomized studies in meta-analyses. *Eur J Epidemiol.* (2010) 25:603–5. doi: 10.1007/s10654-010-9491-z

6. Cumpston M, Li T, Page MJ, Chandler J, Welch VA, Higgins JP, et al. Updated guidance for trusted systematic reviews: a new edition of the cochrane handbook for systematic reviews of interventions. *Cochrane Database Syst Rev.* (2019) 10:ED000142. doi: 10.1002/14651858. ED000142

7. Hozo SP, Djulbegovic B, Hozo I. Estimating the mean and variance from the median, range, and the size of a sample. *BMC Med Res Methodol.* (2005) 5:13. doi: 10.1186/1471-2288-5-13

8. Abuanz S, Gamé X, Roche JB, Guillotreau J, Mouzin M, Sallusto F, et al. Laparoscopic pyeloplasty: comparison between retroperitoneoscopic and transperitoneal approach. *Urology.* (2010) 76:877–81. doi: 10.1016/j.urology.2009.11.062

9. Badawy H, Zoaier A, Ghoneim T, Hanno A. Transperitoneal versus retroperitoneal laparoscopic pyeloplasty in children: randomized clinical trial. *J Pediatr Urol.* (2015) 11:122.e1–6. doi: 10.1016/j.jpurol.2014. 11.019

10. Hemal AK, Goel R, Goel A. Cost-effective laparoscopic pyeloplasty: single center experience. *Int J Urol.* (2003) 10:563–8. doi: 10.1046/j.1442-2042.2003.00706.x

11. Liu SK. A comparison of the clinical effects of different approaches to laparoscopic pyeloplasty for ureteropelvic junction obstruction. (2018). doi: 10.13188/2380-0585.1000021

12. Qadri SJ, Khan M. Retroperitoneal versus transperitoneal laparoscopic pyeloplasty: our experience. *Urol Int.* (2010) 85:309–13. doi: 10.1159/000319395

13. Shen HF, Dong Y, Liu XZ, Huang W, Qin ZC. Clinical effect of transperitoneal and retroperitoneal laparoscopic pyeloplasty on the treatment of ureteropelvic junction obstruction. *J Clin Urology.* (2020) 117–20.

14. Shoma AM, El Nahas AR, Bazeed MA. Laparoscopic pyeloplasty: a prospective randomized comparison between the transperitoneal approach and retroperitoneoscopy. *J Urol.* (2007) 178:2020–4; discussion 2024. doi: 10.1016/j.juro.2007.07.025

15. Singh V, Sinha RJ, Gupta DK, Kumar V, Pandey M, Akhtar A. Prospective randomized comparison between transperitoneal laparoscopic pyeloplasty and retroperitoneoscopic pyeloplasty for primary ureteropelvic junction obstruction. *JSLS.* (2014) 18. doi: 10.4293/JSLS.2014.00366

16. Xu W, Li YX. Effect study of transperitoneal vesus retroperitoneal laparoscopic pyeloplasty for ureteropelvic junction obstruction1. *Chin Prac Med.* (2017) 46–7.

17. Zhai ZZ, Shang PF, Zhang X, Yue ZJ, Wang JJ, Wang ZZ, et al. Comparison of laparoscopic retroperitoneal and peritoneal approaches in the treatment of ureteropelvic junction obstruction. *Chin J Min Inv Sur.* (2018) 405–8.

18. Zhang H. Comparison between transperitoneal laparoscopic pyeloplasty and retroperitoneoscopic pyeloplasty for ureteropelvic junction obstruction. *Chin Med Eng.* (2017) 36–39.

19. Zhu H, Shen C, Li X, Xiao X, Chen X, Zhang Q, et al. Laparoscopic pyeloplasty: a comparison between the transperitoneal and retroperitoneal approach during the learning curve. *Urol Int.* (2013) 90:130–5. doi: 10.1159/ 000343989

20. Kohno M, Ogawa T, Kojima Y, Sakoda A, Johnin K, Sugita Y, et al. Pediatric congenital hydronephrosis (ureteropelvic junction obstruction):

medical management guide. *Int J Urol.* (2020) 27:369–76. doi: 10.1111/iju. 14207

21. Zhu H, Wang J, Deng Y, Huang L, Zhu X, Dong J, et al. Use of double-J ureteric stents post-laparoscopic pyeloplasty to treat ureteropelvic junction obstruction in hydronephrosis for pediatric patients: a single-center experience. *J Int Med Res.* (2020) 48:1–8. doi: 10.1177/03000605209 18781

22. Li XD, Wu YP, Wei Y, Chen SH, Zheng QS, Cai H, et al. Predictors of recoverability of renal function after pyeloplasty in adults with ureteropelvic junction obstruction. *Urol Int.* (2018) 100:209–15. doi: 10.1159/0004 86425

23. Babu R, Vittalraj P, Sundaram S, Shalini S. Pathological changes in ureterovesical and ureteropelvic junction obstruction explained by fetal ureter histology. *J Pediatr Urol.* (2019) 15:240.e1–240.e7. doi: 10.1016/j.jpurol.2019.02.001

24. Chow AK, Rosenberg BJ, Capoccia EM, Cherullo EE. Risk factors and management options for the adult failed ureteropelvic junction obstruction repair in the era of minimally invasive and robotic approaches: a comprehensive literature review. *J Endourol.* (2020). doi: 10.1089/end.2019.0737

25. Weitz M, Portz S, Laube GF, Meerpohl JJ, Bassler D. Surgery versus non-surgical management for unilateral ureteric-pelvic junction obstruction in newborns and infants less than two years of age. *Cochrane Database Syst Rev.* (2016) 7:CD010716. doi: 10.1002/14651858. CD010716.pub2

26. Tabari AK, Atqiaee K, Mohajerzadeh L, Rouzrokh M, Ghoroubi J, Alam A, et al. Early pyeloplasty versus conservative management of severe ureteropelvic junction obstruction in asymptomatic infants. *J Pediatr Surg.* (2020) 55:1936–40. doi: 10.1016/j.jpedsurg.2019.08.006

27. Passoni NM, Peters CA. Managing ureteropelvic junction obstruction in the young infant. *Front Pediatr.* (2020) 8:242. doi: 10.3389/fped.2020. 00242

28. Huang WY, Peters CA, Zurakowski D, Borer JG, Diamond DA, Bauer SB, et al. Renal biopsy in congenital ureteropelvic junction obstruction: evidence for parenchymal maldevelopment. *Kidney Int.* (2006) 69:137–43. doi: 10.1038/sj.ki.5000004

29. Pavlaki A, Printza N, Farmaki E, Stabouli S, Taparkou A, Sterpi M, et al. The role of urinary NGAL and serum cystatin C in assessing the severity of ureteropelvic junction obstruction in infants. *Pediatr Nephrol.* (2020) 35:163–70. doi: 10.1007/s00467-019-04349-w

30. Desai MM, Desai MR, Gill IS. Endopyeloplasty versus endopyelotomy versus laparoscopic pyeloplasty for primary ureteropelvic junction obstruction. *Urology.* (2004) 64:16–21; discussion 21. doi: 10.1016/j.urology.2004. 02.031

31. Wu Y, Dong Q, Han P, Liu L, Wang L, Wei Q. Meta-analysis of transperitoneal versus retroperitoneal approaches of laparoscopic pyeloplasty for ureteropelvic junction obstruction. *J Laparoendosc Adv Surg Tech A.* (2012) 22:658–62. doi: 10.1089/lap. 2011.0508

32. Gatti JM, Amstutz SP, Bowlin PR, Stephany HA, Murphy JP. Laparoscopic vs. open pyeloplasty in children: results of a randomized, prospective, controlled trial. *J Urol.* (2017) 197:792–7. doi: 10.1016/j.juro.2016. 10.056

33. Schuessler WW, Grune MT, Tecuanhuey LV, Preminger GM. Laparoscopic dismembered pyeloplasty. *J Urol.* (1993) 150:1795–9. doi: 10.1016/S0022-5347(17)35898-6

34. Peters CA, Schlussel RN, Retik AB. Pediatric laparoscopic dismembered pyeloplasty. *J Urol.* (1995) 153:1962–5. doi: 10.1097/00005392-199506000-00079

35. Fuchs J, Luithle T, Warmann SW, Haber P, Blumenstock G, Szavay P. Laparoscopic surgery on upper urinary tract in children younger than 1 year: technical aspects and functional outcome. *J Urol.* (2009) 182:1561–8. doi: 10.1016/j.juro.2009.06.063

36. Erol I, Karamik K, Islamoglu ME, Ateş M, Savaş M. Outcomes of infants undergoing laparoscopic pyeloplasty: a single-center experience. *Urologia.* (2019) 86:27–31. doi: 10.1177/03915603188 02165

37. Khoder WY, Waidelich R, Ghamdi A, Schulz T, Becker A, Stief CG. A prospective randomised comparison between the transperitoneal and retroperitoneoscopic approaches for robotic-assisted pyeloplasty in a single surgeon, single centre study. *J Robot Surg.* (2018) 12:131–7. doi: 10.1007/s11701-017-0707-z

38. Zamfir Snykers C, De Plaen E, Vermersch S, Lopez M, Khelif K, Luyckx S, et al. Is laparoscopic pyeloplasty for ureteropelvic junction obstruction in infants under 1 year of age a good option. *Front Pediatr.* (2019) 7:352. doi: 10.3389/fped.2019.00352

39. Gupta NP, Mukherjee S, Nayyar R, Hemal AK, Kumar R. Transmesocolic robot-assisted pyeloplasty: single center experience. *J Endourol.* (2009) 23:945–8. doi: 10.1089/end.2008.0430

40. Zacchero M, Volpe A, Billia M, Tarabuzzi R, Varvello F, Angelis PD. Transmesenteric approach for left transperitoneal renal surgery: technique and experience. *J Laparoendosc Adv Surg Tech A.* (2012) 22:176–9. doi: 10.1089/lap.2011.0395

11

Embryology and Morphological (Mal) Development of UPJ

Ali Avanoglu[1]* and Sibel Tiryaki[2]

[1] Division of Pediatric Urology, Department of Pediatric Surgery, Ege University, Izmir, Turkey, [2] Gaziantep Maternity and Children's Hospital, Pediatric Urology, Gaziantep, Turkey

*Correspondence:
Ali Avanoglu
ali.avanoglu@gmail.com

Kidney parenchyma and collecting system arise from two different embryologic units as a result of a close interaction between them. Therefore, their congenital abnormalities are classified together under the same heading named CAKUT (congenital abnormalities of the kidney and urinary tract). The pathogenesis of CAKUT is thought to be multifactorial. Ureteropelvic junction obstruction (UPJO) is the most common and most investigated form of CAKUT. Despite years of experimental and clinical research, and the information gained on the embryogenesis of the kidney; its etiopathogenesis is still unclear. It involves both genetic and environmental factors. Failure in development of the renal pelvis, failure in the recanalization of ureteropelvic junction, abnormal pyeloureteral innervation, and impaired smooth muscle differentiation are the main proposed mechanisms for the occurrence of UPJO. There are also single gene mutations like AGTR2, BMP4, Id2 proposed in the etiopathogenesis of UPJO.

Keywords: ureteropelvic junction obstruction, embryology, genetics, congenital anomalies of the kidney and urinary tract, BMP4

INTRODUCTION

The role of embryology in medical education is often underrated. Even clinicians dealing with congenital abnormalities consider in-depth knowledge on embryology unnecessary. Studies about urinary tract obstruction date back to forties (1), but there is still scarce information on how ureteropelvic junction obstruction (UPJO) develops. We believe, clinicians and embryologists shall work together to obtain further progress. The aim of this review is to demystify the current knowledge on the embryo-pathogenesis of UPJO to clinicians to promote future research.

THE CONCEPT OF CAKUT

Congenital anomalies of the kidney and urinary tract (CAKUT) refer to all the developmental abnormalities of kidney and ureter (2). The concept of CAKUT is based on the close interaction of the ureteric bud and metanephric mesenchyme in the development of kidney and ureter.

The main steps in the formation of the metanephric kidney and ureter are; formation of the ureteric bud from the Wolffian duct, its dorsal growth into the caudal portion of the nephric cord and branching of the ureter when it invades the mesenchyme. This appositional growth continues until the formation of the terminal nephrons in 32nd week in human embryo (3).

Experimental studies with knock-out mice support this interactive development delivering the renal parenchymal and ureteric abnormalities together. In fact, most popular theory about this close interaction by Mackie and Stephens was even earlier than these. They hypothesized that the association of renal parenchymal abnormalities with vesicoureteral reflux and other ureteric abnormalities were the result of initial ectopic budding of the ureter (4).

CAKUT accounts for one of the most frequent congenital abnormalities detected by routine fetal sonography (5), but the spectrum is wide. Ureteropelvic junction obstruction is the most common form of CAKUT with an estimated incidence of 1/1,000–1,500 (6).

THEORIES ON UPJO PATHOGENESIS

The first theory was obliteration-recanalization by Ruano-Gil and Tejedo-Mateu which they raised on their findings on 45 normal human embryos of 5–55 mm (7). They said the ureter becomes obstructed beginning when the fetus is 14 mm, this process starts in the middle zone and progresses to the entire lumen, and then recanalization occurs after the fetus is 22 mm (7). Later, Alcaraz et al. also supported the existence of an obstructive phenomena of the ureter with their study on human and rat embryos (8); however, showed that this obstruction site didn't reach the ureteropelvic junction. After that, obstruction-recanalization theory to explain UPJO was abandoned by the majority. Also others think this obstruction phenomenon can only be the collapse of the ureter before the passage of the urine (2).

Other early studies about the subject were pathological analyses of the specimens with UPJO. They all noted the changes in the ureteropelvic junction (UPJ) without attribution to the etiology (9). Zhang et al. were also researchers who analyzed UPJO specimens. They showed that UPJs were thicker with enlarged muscularis propria, increased perifascicular fibrosis and inflammation in cases with intrinsic UPJO (10). They also couldn't make a statement whether these changes were causative but showed that they were not apparent in the extrinsic cases.

Miyazaki et al. showed angiotension type 1 lacking mice failed to develop a renal pelvis (11). They also showed hypoplastic smooth muscle and lacking peristalsis in the ureters of mutant mice. Reminding the results of Miyazaki's experimental study, Kajbafzadeh et al. showed increased smooth muscle cell apoptosis and collagen fibers while a decreased number of nerve terminals in the UPJO specimens compared to normal ureteropelvic junctions from autopsies (12). These studies strongly suggest defective muscle and nerve structure in the site of obstruction, but it is still unknown if these are the causative changes or the results of the obstruction. Later, Yiee et al. compared intrinsic, and extrinsic cases focusing on the muscle distribution. Their findings support a causative role by revealing a different muscle density between them (13).

Chang et al. generated an animal model of UPJO with a mutation in a calcineurin protein subunit (14). The mutant mice had abnormal renal mesenchyme and lack of a funnel-shaped ureteropelvic junction. They showed no abnormality in the nerve distribution. They correlated abnormal

shape of the pelvis and faulty mesenchyme with abnormal pyeloureteral peristalsis which they concluded as the cause of UPJO.

Based on the studies about peristalsis, Lye et al. speculated that peristalsis in the urinary tract becomes more important in late gestation when the fetus stays upside down and urine travels against gravity. They concluded that failure of peristalsis results in a functional obstruction manifested by hydronephrosis (15).

In fact, none of the above studies describe the macroscopic findings of the surgeon which are as follows: mostly there is narrow but patent lumen, ureter inserts the pelvis in a level higher than ureter and pelvis first meet, they are attached to each other between these two levels and there is fibrotic tissue around. Stephen Koff has an interesting idea about this that he never published. He believes UPJO is a consequence of temporary vesicoureteral reflux during the fetal life. He says reflux disrupts the position of the ureter and UPJ, and then pelvic drainage. When this lasts long enough, it results in inflammation and the fibrotic attachments around and UPJO becomes permanent (Koff, personal communication).

Despite the above theories and two very interesting speculations, further studies are still required to reveal etiopathogenesis of UPJO.

THE GENETICS

CAKUT is thought to be multifactorial. There are familial cases with different occurrence, so genetic penetrance is regarded to be incomplete or variable. Also, there are several single gene mutations like Id2, PAX2, EYA, AGTR2, BMP4, SOX17, CHD1L, DSTYK proposed by the experimental and clinical studies about the etiopathogenesis of UPJO (16–19). However, mutations in these mostly results in more than one form of CAKUT. For example, mutant mice has a 3% chance of developing CAKUT when AGTR2 is inactivated, but it can be any type and happens randomly within the same pedigree (2).

Among these, Adamts1 and Id2 are reported to lead to a more restricted phenotype resembling human UPJO (17). Interestingly, the macroscopic morphology of the kidney of the Id2 knock-out mice even shows the high-insertion of the ureter into the pelvis (17).

BMP4 also has noteworthy features. It has an essential role in embryonic development shown by the fatality of the homozygous null mutations. Heterozygous mutation results, on the other hand, in multiple abnormalities including all types of CAKUT. It is also shown to cause ectopic budding of the ureter (like Mackie and Stephens described) (20). BMP4's role may seem too wide to explain UPJO alone; however, two screening studies showed its association with UPJO (21, 22). The study from China revealed BMP4 mutation in three cases with UPJO which were not apparent in the controls (21). Same study failed to show any specific mutation in Id2 gene. The other one from Brazil showed the association of BMP4 mutation with UPJO and multicystic dysplastic kidney (22).

Despite promising results of these papers, data to acknowledge a causative role of any gene is still lacking.

CONCLUSION

The etiopathogenesis and impacts of ureteropelvic junction obstruction has long been an interesting area for researchers.

Despite years of clinical and experimental research, there is no solid theory or genetic mutation to explain this frequent abnormality yet.

AUTHOR CONTRIBUTIONS

AA and ST contributed to the literature search and drafting the manuscript of this review.

REFERENCES

1. Peters CA. Obstruction of the fetal urinary tract. *J Am Soc Nephrol.* (1997) 8:653–63.
2. Ichikawa I, Kuwayama F, Pope JC, Stephens FD, Miyazaki Y. Paradigm shift from classic anatomic theories to contemporary cell biological views of CAKUT. *Kidney Int.* (2002) 61:889–98. doi: 10.1046/j.1523-1755.2002.00188.x
3. Saxen L. Ontogenesis of the vertebrate excretory system. In: Barlow P, Green P, Wylie C, editors. *Ontogenesis of the Kidney.* Cambridge: Cambridge University Press (1987). p. 13–8.
4. Mackie GG, Stephens FD. Duplex kidneys: a correlation of renal dysplasia with position of the ureteral orifice. *J Urol.* (1975) 114:274–80. doi: 10.1016/S0022-5347(17)67007-1
5. Caiulo VA, Caiulo S, Gargasole C, Chiriacò G, Latini G, Cataldi L, et al. Ultrasound mass screening for congenital anomalies of the kidney and urinary tract. *Pediatr Nephrol.* (2012) 27:949–53. doi: 10.1007/s00467-011-2098-0
6. Klein J, Gonzalez J, Miravete M, Caubet C, Chaaya R, Decramer S, et al. Congenital ureteropelvic junction obstruction: human disease and animal models. *Int J Exp Pathol.* (2011) 92:168–92. doi: 10.1111/j.1365-2613.2010.00727.x
7. Ruano Gil D, Coca Payeras A, Tejedo Mateu A. Obstruction and normal recanalization of the ureter in the human embryo. its relation to congenital ureteric obstruction. *Eur Urol.* (1975) 1:287–93.
8. Alcaraz A, Vinaixa F, Tejedo-Mateu A, Fores M, Gotzens V, Mestres C, et al. Obstruction and recanalization of the Ureter during embryonic development. *J Urol.* (1991) 145:410–6. doi: 10.1016/S0022-5347(17)38354-4
9. Starr NT, Maizels M, Chou P, Brannigan R, Shapiro E. Microanatomy and morphometry of the hydronephrotic obstructed renal pelvis in asyptomatic infants. *J Urol.* (1992) 148:519–24. doi: 10.1016/S0022-5347(17)36643-0
10. Zhang PL, Peters CA, Rosen S. Ureteropelvic junction obstruction: morphological and clinical studies. *Pediatr Nephrol.* (2000) 14:820–6. doi: 10.1007/s004679900240
11. Miyazaki Y, Tsuchida S, Nishimura H, Pope JC IV, Harris RC, McKanna JM, et al. Angiotensin induces the urinary peristaltic machinery during the perinatal period. *J Clin Invest.* (1998) 102:1489–97. doi: 10.1172/JCI4401
12. Kajbafzadeh AM, Payabvash S, Salmasi AH, Monajemzadeh M, Tavangar SM. Smooth muscle cell apoptosis and defective neural development in congenital ureteropelvic junction obstruction. *J Urol.* (2006) 176:718–23. doi: 10.1016/j.juro.2006.03.041
13. Yiee JH, Johnson-Welch S, Baker LA, Wilcox DT. Histologic differences between extrinsic and intrinsic ureteropelvic junction obstruction. *Urology.* (2010) 76:181–4. doi: 10.1016/j.urology.2010.02.007
14. Chang CP, McDill BW, Neilson JR, Joist HE, Epstein JA, Crabtree GR, et al. Calcineurin is required in urinary tract mesenchyme for the development of the pyeloureteral peristaltic machinery. *J Clin Invest.* (2004) 113:1051–8. doi: 10.1172/JCI20049
15. Lye CM, Fasano L, Woolf AS. Ureter myogenesis: putting teashirt into context. *J Am Soc Nephrol.* (2010) 21:24–30. doi: 10.1681/ASN.2008111206
16. dos Santos Junior ACS, de Miranda DM, Simões e Silva AC. Congenital anomalies of the kidney and urinary tract: an embryogenetic review. *Birth Defects Res C Embryo Today Rev.* (2014) 102:374–81. doi: 10.1002/bdrc.21084
17. Aoki Y, Mori S, Kitajima K, Yokoyama O, Kanamura H, Okada K, et al. Id2 haploinsufficiency in mice leads to congenital hydronephrosis resembling that in humans. *Genes Cells.* (2004) 9:1287–96. doi: 10.1111/j.1365-2443.2004.00805.x
18. Yerkes E, Nishimura H, Miyazaki Y, Tsuchida S, Brock JW, Ichikawa I. Role of angiotensin in the congenital anomalies of the kidney and urinary tract in the mouse and the human. *Kidney Int Suppl.* (1998) 54:75–7. doi: 10.1046/j.1523-1755.1998.06715.x
19. Vivante A, Kohl S, Hwang DY, Dworschak GC, Hildebrandt F. Single-gene causes of congenital anomalies of the kidney and urinary tract (CAKUT) in humans. *Pediatr Nephrol.* (2014) 29:695–704. doi: 10.1007/s00467-013-2684-4
20. Miyazaki Y, Ichikawa I. Ontogeny of congenital anomalies of the kidney and urinary tract, CAKUT. *Pediatr Int.* (2003) 45:598–604. doi: 10.1046/j.1442-200X.2003.01777.x
21. He JL, Liu JH, Liu F, Tan P, Lin T, Le XL. Mutation screening of BMP4 and Id2 genes in Chinese patients with congenital ureteropelvic junction obstruction. *Eur J Pediatr.* (2012) 171:451–456. doi: 10.1007/s00431-011-1561-z
22. Reis GS Dos, Simões E Silva AC, Freitas IS, Heilbuth TR, Marco LA De, Oliveira EA, et al. Study of the association between the BMP4 gene and congenital anomalies of the kidney and urinary tract. *J Pediatr.* (2014) 90:58–64. doi: 10.1016/j.jped.2013.06.004

12

Urinary Ultrasound and Other Imaging for Ureteropelvic Junction Type Hydronephrosis (UPJHN)

Ayse Kalyoncu Ucar[1]* and Sebuh Kurugoglu[2]

[1] Istanbul Kanuni Sultan Suleyman Training and Research Hospital, Istanbul, Turkey, [2] Istanbul University Cerrahpasa Faculty of Medicine, Istanbul, Turkey

*Correspondence:
Ayse Kalyoncu Ucar
aysekucar@gmail.com

Ultrasound is the main imaging study used to diagnose ureteropelvic junction (UPJ) obstruction. On ultrasound, abnormal dilatation of the pelvicalyceal system of varying degrees is seen, whereas the ureter is normal in caliber. A properly performed study provides essential information regarding laterality, renal size, thickness, and architecture of the renal cortex and degree of dilatation of the pelvicalyceal system. Doppler ultrasound may identify a crossing vessel, when present. This imaging method also has been used differentiating obstructive from non-obstructive hydronephrosis by renal arterial resistive index measurements. Abdominal radiographs may show soft tissue fullness, bulging of the flank, and displacement of bowel loops from the affected side. The voiding/micturating cystourethrogram helps exclude other causes of upper tract dilatation, including vesicoureteral reflux, urethral valves, and ureteroceles. Computerized Tomography angiography with multiplanar reformation and three-dimensional images may be used to depict suspected crossing vessels as a cause of UPJ obstruction in older children and adults. Magnetic Resonance Urography has progressed significantly in recent years due to the development of both hardware and software that are used to generate high-resolution images. This imaging technique currently allows for the detailed assessment of urinary tract anatomy, while also providing information regarding renal function, including differential renal function, and the presence or absence of obstructive uropathy.

Keywords: child, UPJ type hydronephrosis, ultrasonography, CT angiography, MR urography

INTRODUCTION

Ureteropelvic junction (UPJ) obstruction is the most common cause of pathologic obstructive hydronephrosis in children which is defined as a partial or complete obstruction of the flow of urine from the renal pelvis to the proximal ureter (1, 2). Many theories have been put forward to explain the pathophysiology; however, the cause is not clear. As an intrinsic cause of obstruction abnormally developed ureteral smooth muscle at the UPJ resulting in an aperistaltic segment is considered, while extrinsic obstruction is thought to be caused by an overlying renal vessel (3, 4). UPJ obstruction might lead to progressive damage to the renal function by increasing back pressure on the kidney (5). But the majority of cases resolve spontaneously without a real obstruction and renal damage. Especially in newborns and infants, hydronephrosis develops as a useful adaptation mechanism that protects the kidney from high pressure and damage secondary to the good compliance of the renal pelvis, not as a result of obstruction (6). Therefore, the differentiation of true obstruction from urinary tract dilatation is crucial to avoid unnecessary surgical intervention. All efforts are made to recognize which cases to follow and which ones to treat. Imaging methods play an important and crucial role at this point.

The purpose of this review is to discuss the radiological findings of hydronephrosis related to UPJ obstruction under the title of "ureteropelvic junction type hydronephrosis (UPJHN)," based mainly on ultrasonography and other imaging methods.

ULTRASONOGRAPHY

Ultrasonography (US) is the main imaging study used for evaluating the urinary system in the postnatal period in children with suspected or diagnosed prenatal hydronephrosis (7). This method has lots of advantages such as being safe and non-invasive, cheap, easily accessible in most institutions and also being repeatable with using no radiation exposure. The widespread use of antenatal US screening leads to a significant increase in the detection rate of UPJHN (8). All newborns

with a history of antenatal hydronephrosis should be evaluated by US in postnatal period (9). If US is performed in the first postnatal days, mild hydronephrosis may not be detected or the degree of hydronephrosis may appear milder than the fact due to transient dehydration as a result of physiological oliguria in the early postnatal period and subsequent polyuria. Therefore, it is more appropriate to perform the first urinary US examination usually after first week of birth (10, 11). However, in cases of bilateral hydronephrosis, severe hydronephrosis in a solitary kidney, elevated creatinine levels, urinary tract infection, suspected perforation, or posterior urethral valve, early neonatal US may require urgency. If postnatal US is normal, it should be repeated after 4–6 weeks (9). For instance, data in a study shows that 5% of patients requiring surgery for obstructive uropathies had abnormal US findings at 1 month of age despite normal US findings at 1 week of age (12).

A variety of (multifrequency) transducers are used in the evaluation of pediatric urinary tract. For standard pediatric exams, both use of convex probes ranging from 2.5 to 10 MHz and linear probes ranging from 5 to 17 MHz are advisable. High-frequency, high-resolution linear probes are necessary for evaluating details or for assessing neonatal patients. Each

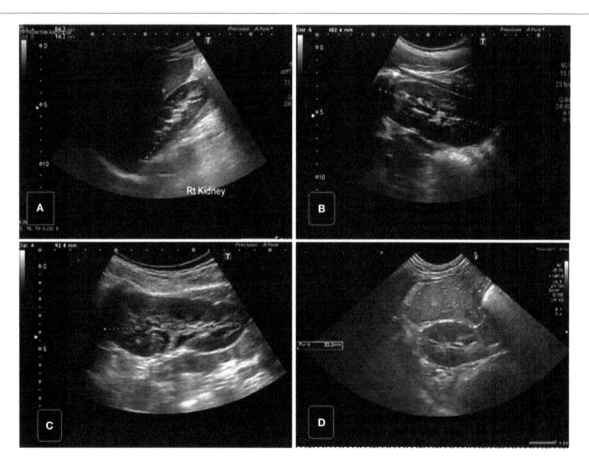

FIGURE 1 | Normal renal sonographic images obtained with convex probes. **(A)** Longitudinal US image of the right kidney demonstrating renal length and parenchymal thickness in supine position. **(B)** Longitudinal US image of the left kidney demonstrating renal length in supine position. **(C)** Longitudinal US image of the left kidney demonstrating renal length in prone position. **(D)** Transverse US image of the right kidney showing renal AP size.

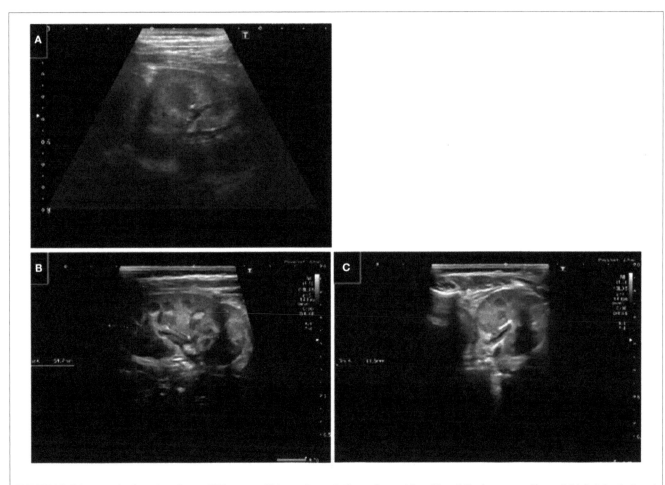

FIGURE 2 | US images using linear transducers. **(A)** Transverse US image demonstrating corticomedullary differentiation in prone position and detailed visualization of the parenchyma. **(B,C)** Renal longitudinal and transverse US images in prone position demonstrating physiologic medullary echogeneity with corticomedullary differentiation and uroepithelial thickening in pelvis.

kidney should be assessed both in transverse and longitudinal planes. In addition to supine and decubitus positions, prone position reduces the distance to the kidneys, increases image quality, provides better image quality, and enables the medullary structure to be better evaluated (13).

In the presence of UPJHN, US demonstrates multiple dilated calyces of uniform size which communicate with a dilated renal pelvis and abrupt narrowing at the level of the UPJ whereas the ureter is normal in caliber (14). Dilatation may vary depending on position, hydration, fullness of bladder, and kidney function. In the setting of dilatation, the patient should be reexamined after emptying bladder in order to assess the exact severity of dilatation. Since the position of the patient is one of the factors affecting hydronephrosis evaluation, the same position should be used for each follow-up measurement to make accurate comparisons (15).

In addition to ensuring an accurate determination of hydronephrosis, sonographic evaluation has an important role in determining the timing and necessity of other examinations. Since most unnecessary nuclear imaging and voiding cystourethrography examinations are mainly caused by inadequate or inaccurate information in US reports, a detailed and well-performed US can minimize unnecessary invasive tests that seriously concern children and their parents.

US examination provides essential information regarding laterality, kidney size, appearance (such as echogenicity, corticomedullary differentiation, cyst), parenchymal thickness, presence of pelvicalyceal dilatation (**Figure 1**) (7, 13, 16, 17). High frequency linear transducers maximize the sonographic resolution of the kidney enabling better evaluation of the medulla and cortex (**Figure 2**) (13). US also gives important information about contralateral kidney, ureter, and bladder. Due to the increased incidence of other congenital abnormalities of the urinary tract in patients with UPJ obstruction such as vesicoureteral reflux, renal duplication, ureterovesical obstruction, and bilateral UPJ obstruction (10%) (5, 18), a properly performed study should include all the necessary data. However, this is directly correlated to the practitioners training and experience.

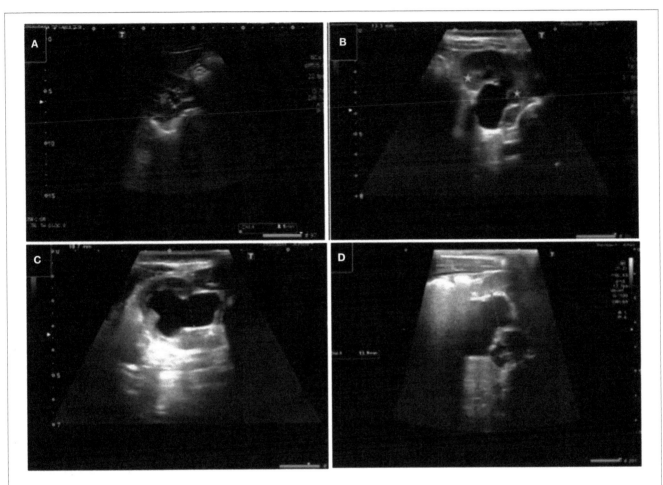

FIGURE 3 | Renal US images showing measurement of APRPD with different grades of hydronephrosis. **(A–D)** Samples of optimal APRPD measurements obtained within the confines of the renal cortex in transverse plane.

US examination is important to determine the exact level and severity of obstruction in patients with UPJHN, the appropriate treatment, and follow-up decision. This imaging method should be performed periodically at varying intervals according to the severity of hydronephrosis. The primary aim of treatment is to prevent or minimize renal damage and loss of function. In order to ensure the right decision regarding the necessity of surgery and follow- up, some measurements and grading systems have been developed (19–22). The most commonly approved sonographic measurement systems to assess hydronephrosis are the anterio-posterior renal pelvic diameter (APRPD), the Society for Fetal Urology (SFU) grading system, the Urinary Tract Dilation (UTD) system, and the Onen classification.

ANTERIO-POSTERIOR RENAL PELVIC DIAMETER

Anterio-posterior renal pelvic diameter (APRPD) is a quantitative parameter based on the measurement of the greatest diameter on US images acquired in a transverse plane

in order to assess the degree of dilatation of the renal pelvis (**Figure 3**) (22, 23). Monitoring the degree of pelvic dilatation is an important aspect of follow-up in UPJHN. Measurement of APRPD is commonly used as a comparable and sensitive parameter. But this measurement is not fully standardized among radiologists. The most common mistake is to measure the pelvis in longitudinal plane or from the widest extrarenal level (**Figure 4**). Even if the APRPD measurement is performed optimally, it may vary depending on the hydration status, the bladder being full/empty and the position where it is measured (supine or prone). Hydration can increase renal pelvic dilatation by causing fluctuation in bladder volume and an increase in fluid excretion (24, 25). Although there is no standard renal sonogram protocol regarding hydration status in the evaluation of pediatric hydronephrosis, the effect of hydration on the diameter of the pelvis has been well-documented (25). Hasch (26) recommended a fasting US scan in order to exclude a persistent hydronephrosis, as well as a reassessment after fluid intake so as not to overlook a case of intermittent hydronephrosis. However, performing this method on infants and younger children is not a simple task.

The accurate measurement of APRPD can be affected by patient position. According to Sharma et. al's study in many

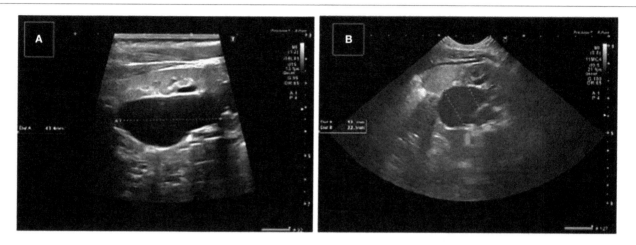

FIGURE 4 | Incorrect measurement of APRPD in longitudinal **(A)** and transverse **(B)** US images showing incorrect measurement at extrarenal level (arrow), correct measurement level is also shown.

cases the APRPD decreases when measured in the prone position (15). US done in the prone and supine positions can also help to differentiate non-obstructive dilatation from obstructive dilatation. While a non-obstructive dilated pelvis can drain better in the prone position, obstructive systems cannot. The measurement of APRPD in the supine and prone positions does not change in the setting of obstruction (15).

Besides the disadvantage of the dynamic nature of APRPD, it is not sufficient alone as it does not provide information about the presence of abnormal renal morphology, parenchymal integrity, or tension in the calices (27).

In some cases, there may be a serious difference between the measurement of APRPD and the actual degree of hydronephrosis, deeming it essential to indicate whether the pelvis is extrarenal or intrarenal, as the kidneys with extrarenal pelvis have lower parenchymal damage by keeping the pressure low for longer. If APRPD is measured from the extrarenal level, it may be perceived as having a more severe obstruction than in actuality (28–30). Therefore, measurement should be procured within the confines of the renal cortex in transverse plane. If the pelvis is located intrarenal, the maximum calyx diameter measurement becomes important in addition to the measurement of APRPD in patients with hydronephrosis. According to a recent study combining the presence of diffuse calyceal dilatation with standard APRPD grading, the first postnatal US provides more information for clinical management and improves the predictive probability of surgery (31). It is also reported in another study that pelvic dilatation with calyceal dilatation may be associated with worse postnatal outcomes than pelvic dilatation without calyceal dilation (32).

APRPD measurement has also a predictive importance in determining whether renal function loss occurs. Previous studies in neonates revealed that an APRPD of >6 mm implies obstruction, while a diameter >15 mm is highly accurate in distinguishing infants with severe uropathy (sensitivity and specificity, >90%) (33–36).

Dias et al. reported that combination of prenatal and postnatal APRPD, with cutoffs of 16 and 18 mm, respectively, was 100% sensitive and 86% specific for predicting surgical intervention for UPJ obstruction (33). Burgu et al. found that an APRPD of <20 mm correlated with the persistence of differential renal function. Stable or decreased APRPD on serial US examinations has predictive value to retained or improved function, postnatally (36). In Coplen's study, 15 mm threshold was used, with a 73% sensitivity and 82% specificity for predicting urological obstruction (37). In Sharifian et al.'s study the best APRPD cutoff to predict surgery was 15 mm (38). Dhillon et al. concluded that in the setting of preserved differential renal function (>40%), all patients in their study (n = 36) had APRPD of ≥40 mm and experienced renal deterioration requiring surgical intervention while no patients with renal pelvic diameters of <15 mm progressed to surgery (30).

SOCIETY FOR FETAL UROLOGY (SFU) GRADING SYSTEM

The SFU classification system was developed to replace the traditional grading system, which uses the subjective descriptors "mild," "moderate," and "severe." The SFU grading system is the most widely used grading system in assessment of hydronephrosis in the postnatal period (27).

The SFU grading system is a qualitative assessment of hydronephrosis in determining the degree of dilatation which describes the degree of hydronephrosis according to renal pelvic dilatation, calyceal dilatation, and the presence of cortical thinning. It is classified as grade 0 = no hydronephrosis, grade 1 = only visualized renal pelvis, grade 2 = dilatation of a few but not all calyces, grade 3 = dilatation of virtually all calyces, and grade 4 = dilatation of the renal pelvis and calyces in addition to parenchymal thinning (19). According to the SFU system the status of the calices is more important than the size of renal pelvis.

Although the SFU is a useful system, it can be influenced by the practitioner.

Some studies have demonstrated that the severity of hydronephrosis in the SFU grading system correlate with postnatal outcomes. Hydronephrosis with high SFU grades exhibit various features that result in a less predictable prognosis, whereas hydronephrosis with low SFU grades show good prognosis and resolve spontaneously (39). For example, Ross et al.'s study examined neonatally diagnosed patients with grade 3 or 4 hydronephrosis, who were followed up with serial diuretic renography. The study deduced that patients with grade 4 hydronephrosis were more susceptible to having impaired renal function or decreased drainage relative to patients with grade 3 hydronephrosis, making the former more likely to require surgical intervention (40).

SFU grading system has limitations such as being qualitative and subjective; the system is unable to consistently discern diffuse and segmental parenchymal thinning, and the difference between grade 3 and 4 disease remains unclear (41). Similarly, two separate cases that should have different management are defined in the same grade (SFU-4): hydronephrosis with a slightly thinned parenchyma, and a slightly reduced function with hydronephrosis with severely thinned parenchyma and a very severe loss of renal function. To address this shortfall, Sibai et al. (31) suggested the subcategorization of SFU grade 4 as two groups: segmental cortical thinning (grade 4A) and diffuse cortical thinning (grade 4B) (42). In the literature there are also some studies combining the SFU with APRPD (31, 43, 44). Dos Santos et al. proposed a grading system conjoining SFU and APRPD quartiles of <6, 6–9, 9–15, and >15 mm. They additionally included the presence of diffuse caliectasis as a factor in grading (31). In an another study, Longpre et al. offered that grade 4 hydronephrosis and a starting APRPD >29 mm holds predictive value for surgical intervention (44).

UTD CLASSIFICATION

Established in 2014, the Urinary tract dilation (UTD) classification system is a system developed by representatives from societies which specialize in the diagnosing and treatment of fetuses and children with hydronephrosis. The corresponding eight societies comprise the following: American College of Radiology, American Society of Pediatric Nephrology, Society for Fetal Urology, American Institute of Ultrasound in Medicine, Society for Maternal-Fetal Medicine, Society for Pediatric Radiology, Society for Pediatric Urology, and Society of Radiologists in Ultrasound (20).

The UTD classification system describes the urinary system with the use of six US findings: (1) APRPD, (2) calyceal dilation with distinction between central and peripheral calyces postnatally (central calyces in place of major calyces and peripheral calyces in place of minor calyces), (3) thickness of renal parenchyma, (4) appearance of renal parenchymal, (5) bladder abnormalities, and (6) ureteral abnormalities (20).

While there are only three antenatal subclassifications (normal, UTD A1, UTD A2–3), four subclassifications are defined in the postnatal period (normal, low risk (UTD P1); intermediate risk (UTD P2); and high-risk (UTD P3) (45).

The criteria of the postnatal classification are made regardless of the child's age. According to this classification system a normal kidney has an APRPD of <10 mm and should have no calyceal or ureteral dilation. If the APRPD measurement is between 10 and 15 mm or has central calyceal dilation, the urinary tract is classified as UTD P1. If the APRPD is >15 mm or peripheral calyces are dilated, it is classified as UTD P2. Classification is based on the most concerning US finding, if there is ureteral dilation with APRPD >10 mm it is evaluated as UTD P2. Accompanying with urinary tract dilation of either the renal parenchymal echogenicity, thickness or bladder is abnormal, it is upgraded to UTD P3 (45).

This classification system can be used in prenatal and postnatal evaluation with some advantages over SFU, since it also provides information about ureter and bladder. However, if the cause of hydronephrosis is only due to UPJ obstruction it is not advantageous to include these two parameters, and mentions of superiority would be unsubstantial. Its complicated nature is also a disadvantage for routine clinical practice.

ONEN CLASSIFICATION

In 2006, Onen proposed an alternative grading system by modifying the SFU grading system to display better the severity of dilatation and to enable easier follow-up in the prenatal and postnatal period evaluations. The system maintains that APRPD is affected by various factors and parenchymal thickness is a more important criterion and relies on the appearance of hydronephrotic kidney, the thickness of renal parenchyma, and the presence of caliceal dilatation. Regardless of the APDRP, severity of hydronephrosis is defined by the degree of caliceal dilatation and of renal parenchymal loss. Grade 1 represents pelvic dilatation alone, Grade 2 with calyceal dilation, Grade 3 with <50% loss of the renal parenchyma, and Grade 4 with severe loss of renal parenchyma (21). While the Onen grade 1 is a combination of SFU grades 1 and 2, SFU grade 4 is divided into two grades (<50% renal parenchymal loss as Onen grade 3; more than 50% renal parenchymal loss as Onen grade 4) (21, 46). The system has been upgraded. Findings such as the absence of corticomedullary differentiation, cortical parenchyma <3 mm, the loss of medullary parenchyma, and significant hyperechogenicity have also been defined AGS grade 4 (47). In our opinion these parenchymal details contribute significantly in the assessment of UPJ obstruction cases.

In addition to these classification systems, alternative several sonographic parameters have been proposed to assess the severity of the hydronephrosis such as pelvicalyceal area (48), parenchymal to pelvicalyceal area (hydronephrosis index) (49), calyx to parenchymal ratio (50), and pelvicalyceal volume using three dimensional (3D) US (51). These methods are more complicated to perform, neccessitate specialized software, therefore they are not commonly utilized in routine clinical practice.

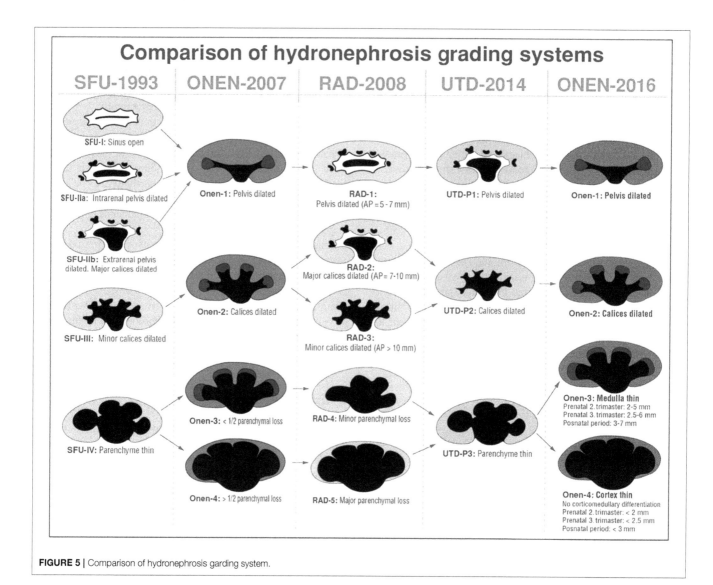

FIGURE 5 | Comparison of hydronephrosis garding system.

In the literature, many studies comparing these classification systems reported different results with some superiorities and predictive values for surgery (46, 52, 53). There is no definitive standardized imaging algorithm, classification systems, or consensus in terms of necessity of surgical intervention and follow-up (**Figure 5**). As a result, the current approach is mostly based on a physician's or institutional individual's practice. The decision for surgery is determined based mainly on the severity of hydronephrosis on US, impairment of kidney function in renal scintigraphy, unilaterality, or bilaterality of hydronephrosis and the presence of clinical symptoms including pain, infection, and renal stones (5, 21, 28, 53, 54). US is used as a primary diagnostic tool during follow up of hydronephrosis (7, 13, 17, 55). It is very important to accurately determine whether there is an increase in hydronephrosis on US. Hafez et al. showed the importance of US examination in the follow up of hydronephrosis patients (55). Worsening of hydronephrosis on two successive US scans is considered an indication for the necessity of surgery as it suggests deterioration in renal

functions (**Figure 6**) (54–56). In addition to worsening of hydronephrosis on follow-up US, it is very important to identify the findings that may develop secondary to urinary stasis such as infection or stone development (**Figure 7**). As management decisions are made based upon consecutive examinations, we suggest US scans be performed by the same practitioners with the same US device, under standardized circumstances and protocols.

In our institution according to the age and consciousness of the child we perform US examination with the bladder full and then emptied. By means of urinary US, drawing from the previous classification systems mentioned above, instead of using classification systems we report all the US measurements and findings of the patient's urinary tract such as; renal size (craniocaudal and axial), location of pelvis (intrarenal or extrarenal), APRPD, calyceal dilatation (central or peripheral), parenchymal thickness, the condition of the renal parenchyma (echogenicity of cortex and medulla, medullary compression, existence of cyst), ureter (caliber, peristalsis,

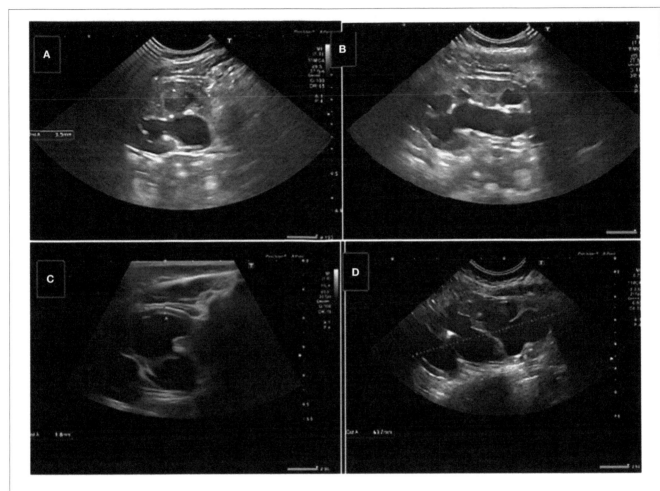

FIGURE 6 | Two consecutive US examinations in a 6-month-old girl with UPJ obstruction. **(A,B)** Baseline US images demonstrate decreased parenchymal thickness with pelvicalyceal dilatation. **(C,D)** Control (2 months later) US images showing significant decrease in renal parenchymal thickness with worsening pelvicalyceal dilatation. A new small echogenic focus suggesting microlithiasis is also present.

lateralization of the ureterovesical junction, ureteric jet), bladder (capasity, luminal echogenicity, and wall thickness), status of constipation, and possible accompanying urinary malformations. In a pediatric nephrourology council consisting of pediatric nephrologists, pediatric urosurgeons, pediatric radiologists, and nuclear medicine specialists, we discuss the children with all the data collected from the radiologic (prenatal, postnatal, and follow-up), and scintigraphic examinations, paying special attention to the patient's clinical status. A decision is then made for either surgical intervention or follow-up.

DOPPLER ULTRASONOGRAPHY

Color doppler US may identify a crossing vessel, when present. The UPJ obstruction due to crossing vessel is one of the extrinsic causes of obstruction that occurs at higher ages than intrinsic causes (3). These vessels usually supply the lower pole of the kidney and most of the time originate from the renal artery or

the aorta. Since its treatment is surgical, it is important to detect the presence of a crossing vessel.

Color doppler US might also allow to differentiate a dilated pelvicalyceal system from prominent vessels in the hilum of kidney. Furthermore, assessment of ureteric jets in the bladder can be used to differentiate obstructive causes of hydronephrosis from non-obstructive ones in children. In the presence of obstructive hydronephrosis, the frequency of ureteric jets on the affected side may be greatly reduced when compare with the contralateral normal side (57, 58).

Traditional US does not provide functional data about obstruction. With the use of pulsed doppler, obstructive hydroneprosis can be distinguished from non-obstructive hydronephrosis by renal arterial resistive index (RI) measurements (59, 60). RI is described as the peak systolic velocity minus the lowest diastolic velocity divided by the peak systolic velocity. Because of vasoconstriction caused by renin, angiotensin, and other hormones, diastolic arterial flow velocities are decreased and RI values are elevated in patients with obstructive hydronephrosis (61). A RI of >0.7

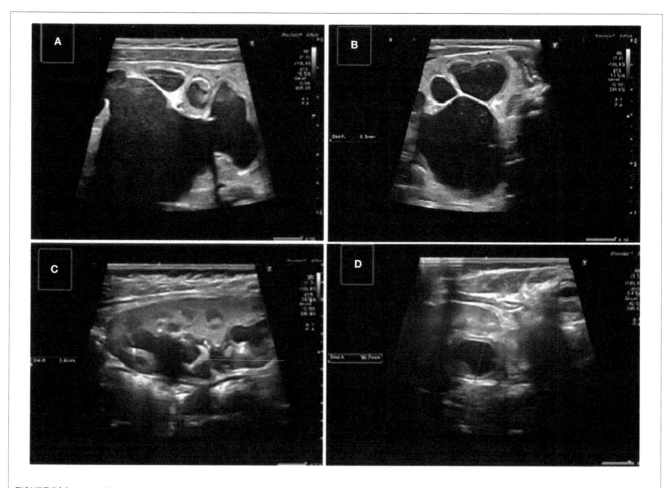

FIGURE 7 | Samples of important US findings in giving surgical desicion. **(A,B)** Longitudinal and transverse US images of the left kidney demonstrating severe pelvicaliyceal dilatation with serious parenchymal thinning, medullary compression, and echogeneity and luminal debris suggesting infection and/or cristalury. **(C)** Longitudinal US image showing pelvicalyceal dilatation with the presence of micro calculi, **(D)** Transverse US image showing uroepithelial thickening and layering of low-level debris consistent with pyonephrosis.

and a RI difference of >0.08 between kidneys in children are suggestive of renal obstruction, while a RI of <0.70 generally indicates non-obstructive dilation (59). An elevated RI is not a characteristic finding for obstruction, the value could be >0.70 without obstruction, in patients with renal parenchymal diseases. It should also be remembered that RI values may be higher than that of adults during the newborn and infant period (0.70–1.0). Furthermore, hypotension, a low heart rate, and dehydration can alter the RI values. Nevertheless, a normal RI values are still an important parameter in order to exclude obstruction (62).

ELASTOGRAPHY

US shear-wave elastography (SWE) with acoustic radiation force impulse technology, is a non-invasive, non-ionizing imaging method that might be used to evaluate the stiffness of tissues. In the presence of UPJ obstruction, back pressure from upper urinary tract obstruction may affect renal parenchymal

stiffness. A preclinical animal model investigation by Gennisson et al. (63) reported a progressive linear increase in renal stiffness related to increasing urinary pressure. Sohn et al. (64) found that SWE values were higher in kidneys with high-grade hydronephrosis than in normal kidney. In another study by Habibi et al. (65) showed different results: SWE values were higher in control kidneys compared with kidneys affected by UPJ obstruction. In Dillmann et al.'s study to distinguish obstructive hydronephrosis from non-obstructive ones was found no difference in SWE between two groups (66). In addition to limited experience with SWE technology to evaluate kidney, it is not a practical imaging method in the assessment of younger children and requires special application.

ABDOMINAL RADIOGRAPHS

Abdominal radiographs may show soft tissue fullness, bulging of the flank from the affected side and status of bowel loops (i.e., constipation). It may also demonstrate possible stone formation in the effected kidney and give information about the lumbosacral vertebraes.

VOIDING/MICTURATING CYSTOURETHROGRAM

As this imaging modality will be discussed in detail within the scope of this journal as a separate article, we want to mention only briefly.

The voiding/micturating cystourethrogram cannot evaluate the obstruction but enables to exclude other causes of hydronephrosis, including accompanying vesicoureteral reflux (VUR), urethral valves, and ureteroceles (67). VUR may coexist with UPJ obstruction in 8–14% of cases. Identification of VUR is important since children with concurrent VUR and UPJ obstruction may have increased risk for infection (68). Because of its invasive nature, radiation exposure, the risk of urinary tract infection after procedure, indications of voiding cystourethrography should be carefully determined. In the presence of bilateral hydronephrosis (or solitary kidney), duplicated system, small kidney, abnormal echogenicity, dilated ureter, ureterocele, suspected infravesical obstruction, and abnormal bladder voiding cystourethrogram should be performed (69).

INTRAVENOUS PYELOGRAPHY

Intravenous pyelography (IVP) or intravenous urography (IVU) has been the important imaging modality for assessment of the urinary tract (70). Although IVP indications have decreased with advances in imaging technology, it is still used in some centers where advanced imaging methods are limited. Dilatation of collecting system, with parenchymal changes in the nephrogram phase, and delay in excretion of contrast medium are characteristic findings of obstructive hydronephrosis (71). But IVP is not sufficient for visualization of poorly functioning kidneys which are severely blocked due to poor contrast excretion (72). It has some disadvantageous such as impaired image quality as a result of bowel gas, the risk of radiation exposure, contrast nephrotoxicity, and hypersensitivity reactions. It may also requires several radiographs with total examination time period extending up to many hours in cases of urinary tract obstruction.

COMPUTERIZED TOMOGRAPHY UROGRAPHY AND ANGIOGRAPHY

In spite of all advances, as a rule, computed tomography (CT) must be avoided in pediatric patients because of the x-ray content as much as possible (73). Despite ionizing radiation exposure, it can be useful in some specific indications in kidneys and urinary tract diseases in children (74). This method should be considered as a second line imaging technique in children; it can support the diagnosis after a comprehensive US evaluation including Doppler US. CT scan can detect the location and cause of obstruction such as crossing vessels

While maintaining the diagnostic value of CT examinations as in the ALARA principle, it should be aimed to minimize the dose of X-ray radiation as in the ALARA principle (75–77). For this purpose, the patient should be evaluated with age-adapted kVp and mAs values, multi-phase examinations should be avoided and appropriate amount of contrast, and delay time should be selected (77). If IV contrast medium administration injection is necessary, low or iso-osmolar and non-ionic iodinated ones should be administered and renal function must be checked prior to the examination. Children should be hydrated before the examination. Contrast agent dose may range from 1 and 4 ml/kg, generally 2 ml/kg (78). Since the scan times is shorter, sedation is not often needed.

Multidetector CT scanners allow for rapid and complete imaging of the urinary tract and comprehensive evaluation of the urinary system pathologies. Thin CT slices thickness of <1 mm provides optimal reconstruction in coronal and sagittal planes. The sagittal-coronal projections, additional 2D and 3D-reconstructions 3D-volume rendering and maximal intensity projection (MIP) images are very helpful in better visualizing the anatomy of the collecting system and as well the crossing vessel. Application of CT in the assessment of the urinary tract is called CT urography (CTU), vascular structures evaluation is called CT angiography (CTA).

CTU examination is used for imaging the kidneys and urinary tracts, where the excretory phase is mandatory (79). The triple-phase technique includes separate non-enhanced, contrast- enhanced, and excretory phases. Non-enhanced phase may be obtained to detect stones that may occur secondary to obstruction. On contrast enhanced excretory phased CT, the obstructed kidney demonstrates delayed opacifications, and excretions of contrast material. But it is essential to remember the increased radiation exposure risk of multi-phase studies in children. Therefore, several imaging protocols have been used in practice, in order to decrease radiation exposure such as split bolus technique (80). The contrast medium is administered in two parts, with a several minutes interval between the portions. A split bolus of the contrast agent, combining the parenchymal, and excretory phases may help to reduce the need for multiple phases in some conditions. In addition to ensuring that two examination phases during one scan, this protocol reduces the radiation dose while maintaining the diagnostic value of both phases (78, 80).

The arterial phase is very important and crucial in order to detect the crossing vessel and CTA with multiplanar reformatted and three-dimensional images are used to evaluate the cause of the crossing vessel as a cause of UPJ obstruction especially in older children (**Figure 8**) (81).

Although the radiation risk is well-known in pediatric patients, CTU, and CTA examinations provide important information both for anatomy and function of the urinary tract (renal parenchyma, collecting system, accessory vessel, stone formation, and contrast excretion) with higher acquisition speed especially in patients who are unable to undergo MRI or in center where MRI is not available.

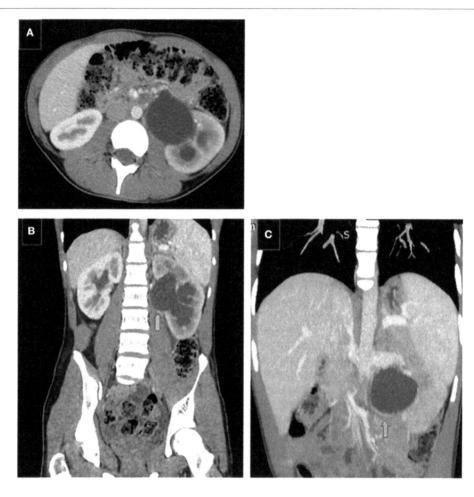

FIGURE 8 | Crossing aberrant renal artery causing left UPJ obstruction in a 14 year-old boy. **(A)** Axial and **(B)** coronal CT images showing left pelvicalyceal system dilatation with delayed nephrogram phase, pelvis is extrarenally located, dilatation is more prominent in the pelvis than calices, note the crossing vessel (arrow). **(C)** Coronal MIP image better demonstrates the crossing vessel as the cause of UPJ obstruction (aberrant lower pole artery) (arrows).

MAGNETIC RESONANCE UROGRAPHY

In recent years, Magnetic Resonance Urography (MRU) has substantially progressed due to the development of high-resolution image generating software and hardware. This imaging technique currently permits the detailed evaluation of complex renal and urinary tract anatomy, while also providing information regarding renal function, including differential renal function, and the presence or absence of obstructive uropathy without the use of ionizing radiation (82, 83). MRU has all the disadvantages of MRI, such as requiring sedation to prevent motion artifacts in younger children. The use of gadolinium, which may be the cause of nephrogenic systemic fibrosis in patients with low glomerular filtration rate (GFR), presence of a metallic prosthesis, staying 35–70 min in an enclosed area for claustrophobic patients and costs are other additional disadvantages (74).

MRU is a promising alternative method, being a single examination able to assess kidneys and the entire urinary tract as it combines both anatomic and functional information (84–86).

In addition to providing detailed anatomical and morphological information about the kidney, MRU enables the evaluation of the whole ureter course and identification of ectopic insertions and potential causes of obstruction (such as crossing vessel) (87, 88).

It is possible that a pediatric MRU be performed at 1.5 or 3 Tesla (T) in children of any age by using multi-element phased-array surface coils. 3 T magnets provide better image resolution, whereas 1.5 T magnets tend to provide more homogeneous fat saturation and are less susceptible to artifacts. A bladder catheter is placed, which permits for continual drainage of urine to avert patient discomfort and promote excretion and assessment of the urethra on imaging. The bladder catheter is first clamped to allow evaluation of the bladder, then the catheter is left to drain. A peripheral IV catheter is positioned to administer hydration, diuretic (usually furosemide) and IV contrast material (86).

MRU examination consists of two basic approaches. The first technique allows evaluation of the anatomical structures of the kidney, ureter, and bladder by using a diversity of T2-weighted pulse sequences (e.g., single shot fast spin echo, two-dimensional fast spin echo [2D] [FSE], and three-dimensional [3D] FSE) (74,

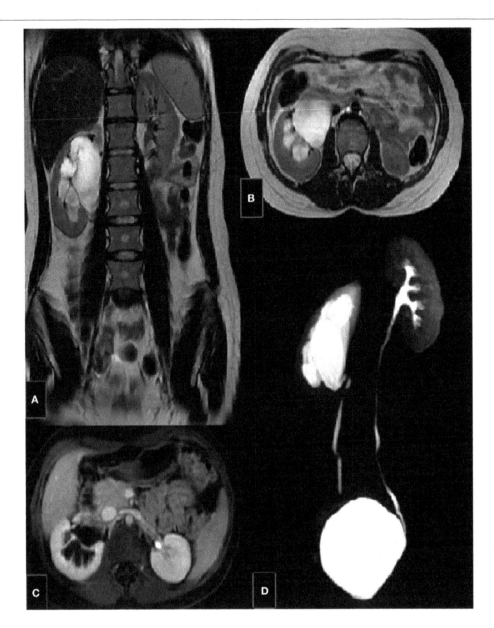

FIGURE 9 | Right UPJ obstruction in a 14-year-old girl. **(A,B)** T2-weighted fast spin-echo coronal (a) and axial (b) MR images showing right renal collecting system dilatation, pelvis is extrarenally located, the thickness of renal parenchyma is decreased and corticomedullary differentiaton is lost. **(C)** Axial post-contrast excretory phase showing delayed excretion in the right renal collecting system, notice the contrast material in the left pelvis. **(D)** MIP MR image showing UPJ obstruction with kinking and angulation at the UPJ and a normal caliber ureter, left kidney is normal.

86). It enables direct visualization of UPJ anatomic structures, assessing the degree of luminal narrowing, and determining the presence of UPJ kinking or tortuosity as well as the site of ureteral insertion on the renal pelvis (e.g., abnormally high insertion) (87, 88).

The second technique involves dynamic and delayed postcontrast MRU images that allow evaluation of renal perfusion (including imaging of renal arteries, quality of parenchymal enhancement, contrast material excretion into the renal collection systems, and ureters). Delayed postcontrast images can also be utilized in generating 2D

reformations that provide optimal visualization of relevant anatomic structures (e.g., the UPJ) and 3D reconstructions, including MIP and volume-rendered images, which provide an overview of urinary tract anatomic structures on a single image (**Figure 9**). This method also allows the measurement of differential renal function [based on the amount (volume) of enhancement of renal parenchyma or based upon glomerular filtration of contrast material] and time vs. signal intensity washout/excretion curves. Currently, accurate absolute quantification of glomerular filtration rate is not possible with MRU (89).

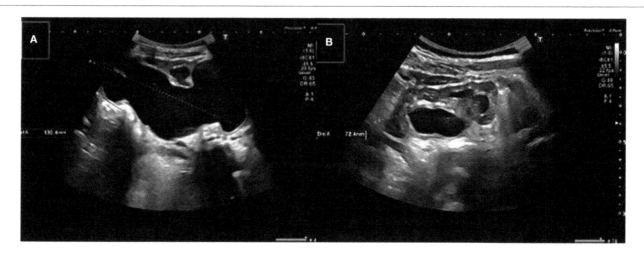

FIGURE 10 | (A) Longitudinal US image in a 1-month-old boy infant showing significant dilation of the pelvicalyceal system with parenchymal thinning **(B)** Control US image obtained after pyeloplasty demonstrates significant resolution of dilatation.

MRU is a promising imaging modality with superior anatomical and functional information in a single test free of the use of ionizing radiation and functional MRU might be able in the future to replace the renogram, because of the quality of the signal. However, due to difficulties of implementation in pediatric group, the absence of each center and the need to increase experience in this regard, it is not widely use yet.

POST-OPERATIVE EVALUATION

Many modalities have been used, US, IVP, radionucleotide scan (RS), and MRU to evaluate patients in postoperative period at various time intervals. US and RS are the most widely used investigations (90). As in pre-operative evaluation of UPJ obstruction, there is also no consensus about the follow-up approach and interval in the post-operative period. Studies suggest that follow-up can be performed with both US and RS at certain time intervals in the postoperative period which can direct the necessity of further investigations (91, 92). However, it is obvious that the US should be the first choice to avoid both radiation and urethral catheterization with an increased risk of urethral trauma and urinary system infections in pediatric patients. If there is suspicion about complications in post-operative periods such as urinary tract infections, pyelonephritis, urine extravasation, US is also the first imaging modality.

Properly performed US provides an accurate assessment of renal pelvis/caliceal dilatation, renal parenchymal thickness, echogenicity, and renal growth postoperatively. After successful pyeloplasty, renal function stabilization takes ~1 year and renal function may improve (**Figure 10**). If there is no problem in the early postoperative period, first control with urinary US may be performed 1 month after the operation. Persistance of the pelvicalyseal dilatation does not indicate continued obstruction (93). In this early post-operative period, significant

resolution of hydronephrosis should not be expected, no worsening, or a slight decrease in hydronephrosis can be sufficient (93). Because even if obstruction is surgically removed, the average time for the renal pelvis to regain flexibility is achieved around 2 years (21, 30). On the other hand, it should also be known that early improvement in dilatation on US could be due to surgical reduction of the renal pelvis rather than true improvement. Measurement of pelvis AP diameter and parenchymal thickness may be useful for follow-up but there is no cut-off value in pelvic diameter due to these factors mentioned above and the level of hydronephrosis is also affected by hydration or the amount of urine in the bladder. However, we can say that worsening or persistence of hydronephrosis, decrease in cortical thickness and clinical findings (i.e., colic pain, urinary tract infection) are not expected findings and should alert to determine the functional patency of the UPJ.

Although majority of surgical failures occur within 1 year after pyeloplasty, there are also cases reported later and failure rate has been described in published reports as 5–10% (94, 95). Serial renal US are recommended at 3, 6, and 12 months, and then annually for 2 years, with additional testing based on US and clinical presentation (95).

IVP was previously widely used to assess surgical success after pyeloplasty, although it is not preferred now. CT and MRU are other radiological options to assess surgical anastomoses (e.g., in the context of UPJ obstruction repair) and reimplanted ureters (96).

CONCLUSION

US is the main imaging study used to diagnose UPJ obstruction. This method has lots of advantages but does not provide functional information about the urinary tract. The question is to differentiate true obstruction from urinary tract dilatation which is very crucial in determining the treatment decision.

US examination provides essential information regarding laterality, kidney size, appearance (such as echogenicity, corticomedullary differentiation, cyst), parenchymal thickness, degree of obstruction. In order to provide right decision, necessity of surgery and standardization, grading, and classification systems have been developed. However, there is no definite consensus and worldwide accepted standard protocols and as a result current therapeutic approach is mostly based on US findings, follow-up results, clinical and scintigraphic findings, and dependent on physician or institutional individual practices. CT and MR are not routinely performed radiologic studies but are often reserved for special cases such as demonstration of an aberrant artery as the cause of obstruction.

AUTHOR CONTRIBUTIONS

All authors listed have made a substantial, direct and intellectual contribution to the work, and approved it for publication.

REFERENCES

1. Cohen HL, Kravets F, Zucconi W, Ratani R, Shah S, Dougherty D, et al. Congenital abnormalities of the genitourinary system. *Semin Roentgenol.* (2004) 39:282–303. doi: 10.1053/j.ro.2003.12.005
2. Gonzalez R, Schimke CM. Ureteropelvic junction obstruction in infants and children. *Pediatr Clin North Am.* (2001) 48:1505–18. doi: 10.1016/S0031-3955(05)70388-6
3. Yiee JH, Johnson-Welch S, Baker LA, Wilcox DT. Histologic differences between extrinsic and intrinsic ureteropelvic junction obstruction. *Urology.* (2010) 76:181–4. doi: 10.1016/j.urology.2010.02.007
4. Hosgor M, Karaca I, Ulukus C, Ozer E, Ozkara E, Sam B, et al. Structural changes of smooth muscle in congenital ureteropelvic junction obstruction. *J Pediatr Surg.* (2005) 40:1632–6. doi: 10.1016/j.jpedsurg.2005.06.025
5. Hashim H, Woodhouse CRJ. Ureteropelvic junction obstruction. *Eur Urol. Suppl.* (2012) 11:25–32 doi: 10.1016/j.eursup.2012.01.004
6. Koff SA. The beneficial and protective effects of hydronephrosis. *APMIS.* (2003) 111:7–12.
7. Epelman M, Victoria T, Meyers KE, Chauvin N, Servaes S, Darge K. Postnatal imaging of neonates with prenatally diagnosed genitourinary abnormalities: a practical approach. *Pediatr Radiol.* (2012) 42(Suppl 1):S124–41. doi: 10.1007/s00247-011-2177-1
8. Brown T, Mandell J, Lebowitz RL. Neonatal hydronephrosis in the era of sonography. *AJR Am J Roentgenol.* (1987) 148:959–63. doi: 10.2214/ajr.148.5.959
9. Sinha A, Bagga A, Krishna A, Bajpai M, Srinivas M, Uppal R, et al. Revised guidelines on management of antenatal hydronephrosis. *Indian J Nephrol.* (2013) 23:83–97. doi: 10.4103/0971-4065.109403
10. Wiener JS, O'Hara SM. Optimal timing of initial postnatal ultrasonography in newborns with prenatal hydronephrosis. *J Urol.* (2002) 168:1826–9. doi: 10.1016/S0022-5347(05)64423-0
11. Laing FC, Burke VD, Wing VW, Jeffrey RB Jr, Hashimoto B. Postpartum evaluation of fetal hydronephrosis: optimal timing for follow-up sonography. *Radiology.* (1984) 152:423–4. doi: 10.1148/radiology.152.2.6539930
12. Signorelli M, Cerri V, Taddei F, Groli C, Bianchi UA. Prenatal diagnosis and management of mild fetal pyelectasis implications for neonatal outcome and follow-up. *Eur J Obstet Gynecol Reprod Biol.* (2005) 118:154–9. doi: 10.1016/j.ejogrb.2004.04.023
13. Choi YH, Cheon JE, Kim WS, Kim IO. Ultrasonography of hydronephrosis in the newborn: a practical review. *Ultrasonography.* (2016) 35:198–211. doi: 10.14366/usg.15073
14. Siegel MJ. Urinary tract. In: Siegel MJ, editor. *Pediatric Sonography.* Philadelphia, PA: Lippincott Williams & Wilkins. (2011). p. 384–460.
15. Sharma G, Sharma A, Maheshwari P. Predictive value of decreased renal pelvis anteroposterior diameter in prone position for prenatally detected hydronephrosis. *J Urol.* (2012) 187:1839–43. doi: 10.1016/j.juro.2011.12.093
16. Rumack CM, Wilson SR, Charboneau JW. *Diagnostic Ultrasound.* 3rd ed. St. Louis, MO: Elsevier Health Sciences (2005). p. 16–20.
17. Paliwalla M, Park K. A practical guide to urinary tract ultrasound in a child: pearls and pitfalls. *Ultrasound.* (2014) 22:213–22. doi: 10.1177/1742271X14549795
18. Lebowitz AL, Blickman JG. The coexistence of ureteropelvic junction obstruction and reflux. *AJR.* (1983) 140:231–8. doi: 10.2214/ajr.140.2.231

19. Fernbach SK, Maizels M, Conway JJ. Ultrasound grading of hydronephrosis: introduction to the system used by the society for fetal urology. *Pediatr Radiol.* (1993) 23:478–80. doi: 10.1007/BF02012459
20. Nguyen HT, Benson CB, Bromley B, Campbell JB, Chow J, Coleman B, et al. Multidisciplinary consensus on the classification of prenatal and postnatal urinary tract dilation (UTD classification system). *J Pediatr Urol.* (2014) 10:982–98. doi: 10.1016/j.jpurol.2014.10.002
21. Onen A. An alternative grading system to refine the criteria for severity of hydronephrosis and optimal treatment guidelines in neonates with primary UPJ-type hydronephrosis. *J Pediatr Urol.* (2007) 3:200–5. doi: 10.1016/j.jpurol.2006.08.002
22. Nguyen HT, Herndon CD, Cooper C, Gatti J, Kirsch A, Kokorowski P, et al. The society for fetal urology consensus statement on the evaluation and management of antenatal hydronephrosis. *J Pediatr Urol.* (2010) 6:212–31. doi: 10.1016/j.jpurol.2010.02.205
23. Nguyen H. Degree of fetal renal pelvic dilatation predicts postnatal obstruction. *Nat Clin Pract Urol.* (2007) 4:10–11. doi: 10.1038/ncpuro0651
24. Angell SK, Pruthi RS, Shortliffe LD. The urodynamic relationship of renal pelvic and bladder pressures, and urinary flow rate in rats with congenital vesicoureteral reflux. *J Urol.* (1998) 160:150–6. doi: 10.1016/S0022-5347(01)63074-X
25. Peerboccus M, Damry N, Pather S, Devriendt A, Avni F. The impact of hydration on renal measurements and on cortical echogenicity in children. *Pediatr Radiol.* (2013) 43:155–65. doi: 10.1007/s00247-013-2748-4
26. Hasch E. Changes in renal pelvic size in children after fluid intake demonstrated by ultrasound. *Ultrasound Med Biol.* (1977) 2:287–90. doi: 10.1016/0301-5629(77)90028-X
27. Timberlake MD, Herndon CDA. Mild to moderate postnatal hydronephrosis - grading systems and management. *Nat Rev Urol.* (2013) 10:649–56. doi: 10.1038/nrurol.2013.172
28. Ulman I, Jayanthi VR, Koff SA. The long-term follow up of newborns with severe unilateral hydronephrosis initially treated non-operatively. *J Urol.* (2000) 164:1101–5. doi: 10.1097/00005392-200009020-00046
29. Onen A. The natural history and therapeutic approach of antenatally diagnosed primary UPJ-type hydronephrosis. *Turk J Pediatr Surg.* (2006) 20:33–8.
30. Dhillon HK. Prenatally diagnosed hydronephrosis: the great ormond street experience. *Br J Urol.* (1998) 81:39–44. doi: 10.1046/j.1464-410X.1998.0810s2039.x
31. Dos Santos J, Parekh RS, Piscione TD, Hassouna T, Figueroa V, Gonima P, et al. A new grading system for the management of antenatal hydronephrosis. *Clin J Am Soc Nephrol.* (2015) 10:1783–90. doi: 10.2215/CJN.12861214
32. Oktar T, Acar O, Atar A, Salabas E, Ander H, Ziylan O, et al. How does the presence of antenatally detected caliectasis predict the risk of postnatal surgical intervention? *Urology.* (2012) 80:203–6. doi: 10.1016/j.urology.2012.01.083
33. Dias CS, Silva JM, Pereira AK, Marino VS, Silva LA, Coelho AM, et al. Diagnostic accuracy of renal pelvic dilatation for detecting surgically managed ureteropelvic junction obstruction. *J. Urol.* (2013) 190:661–6. doi: 10.1016/j.juro.2013.02.014
34. Bouzada MC, Oliveira EA, Pereira AK, Leite HV, Rodrigues AM, Fagundes LA, et al. Diagnostic accuracy of postnatal renal pelvic diameter as a

predictor of uropathy: a prospective study. *Pediatr Radiol.* (2004) 34:798–804. doi: 10.1007/s00247-004-1283-8

35. Yiee J, Wilcox D. Management of fetal hydronephrosis. *Pediatr Nephrol.* (2008) 23:347–53. doi: 10.1007/s00467-007-0542-y

36. Burgu, B, Aydogdu O, Soygur T, Baker L, Snodgrass W, Wilcox D, et al. When is it necessary to perform nuclear renogram in patients with a unilateral neonatal hydronephrosis. *World J Urol.* (2012) 30:347–52. doi: 10.1007/s00345-011-0744-6

37. Coplen DE, Austin PF, Yan, Y, Blanco VM, Dicke JM. The magnitude of fetal renal pelvic dilation can identify obstructive postnatal hydronephrosis, direct postnatal evaluation management. *J Urol.* (2006) 176:724–7. doi: 10.1016/j.juro.2006.03.079

38. Sharifian M, Esfandiar N, Mohkam M, Dalirani R, Baban Taher E, Akhlaghi A. Diagnostic accuracy of renal pelvic dilatation in determining outcome of congenital hydronephrosis. *Iran J Kidney Dis.* (2014) 8:26–30.

39. Sidhu G, Beyene J, Rosenblum ND. Outcome of isolated antenatal hydronephrosis: a systematic review and metaanalysis. *Pediatr Nephrol.* (2006) 21:218–24. doi: 10.1007/s00467-005-2100-9

40. Ross SS, Kardos S, Krlll A, Dourland J, Sprague B, Majd M, et al. Observation of infants with SFU Grades 3–4 hydronephrosis: worsening drainage with serial diuresis renography indicates surgical intervention and helps prevent loss of renal function. *J Pediatr Urol.* (2011) 7:266–71. doi: 10.1016/j.jpurol.2011.03.001

41. Keays MA, Guerra LA, Mihill J, Raju G, Al-Asheeri N, Geier P, et al. Reliability assessment of society for fetal urology ultrasound grading system for hydronephrosis. *J Urol.* (2008) 180 (Suppl. 4):1680–2. doi: 10.1016/j.juro.2008.03.107

42. Sibai H, Salle JL, Houle AM, Lambert R. Hydronephrosis with diffuse or segmental cortical thinning: impact on renal function. *J. Urol.* (2001) 165:2293–5. doi: 10.1097/00005392-200106001-00019

43. Riccabona M, Avni FE, Blickman JG, Dacher JN, Darge K, Lobo ML, et al. Imaging recommendations in paediatric uroradiology: minutes of the ESPR workgroup session on urinary tract infection, fetal hydronephrosis, urinary tract ultrasonography and voiding cystourethrography, Barcelona, Spain, June 2007. *Pediatr Radiol.* (2008) 38:138–45. doi: 10.1007/s00247-007-0695-7

44. Longpre M, Nguan A, Macneily AE, Afshar K. Prediction of the outcome of antenatally diagnosed hydronephrosis: a multivariable analysis. *J Pediatr Urol.* (2012) 8:135–9. doi: 10.1016/j.jpurol.2011.05.013

45. Chow JS, Koning JL, Back SJ, Nguyen HT, Phelps A, Darge K. Classification of pediatric urinary tract dilation: the new language. *Pediatr Radiol.* (2017) 47:1109–15. doi: 10.1007/s00247-017-3883-0

46. Kim SY, Kim MJ, Yoon CS, Lee MS, Han KH, Lee MJ. Comparison of the reliability of two hydronephrosis grading systems: the society for foetal urology grading system vs. the Onen grading system. *Clin Radiol.* (2013) 68:484–90. doi: 10.1016/j.crad.2013.03.023

47. Onen A. Üreteropelvik bileşke darligi. *Çocuk Cerrahisi Dergisi.* (2016) 30:55–79. doi: 10.5222/JTAPS.2016.055

48. Cost GA, Merguerian PA, Cheerasarn SP, Shortliffe LM. Sonographic renal parenchymal and pelvicaliceal areas: new quantitative parameters for renal sonographic followup. *J Urol.* (1996) 156:725–9. doi: 10.1016/S0022-5347(01)65798-7

49. Shapiro SR, Wahl EF, Silberstein MJ, Steinhardt G. Hydronephrosis index: a new method to track patients with hydronephrosis quantitatively. *Urology.* (2008) 72:536–8. Discussion 8-9. doi: 10.1016/j.urology.2008.02.007

50. Imaji R, Dewan PA. Calyx to parenchyma ratio in pelviureteric junction obstruction. *BJU Int.* (2002) 89:73–7. doi: 10.1046/j.1464-410X.2002.02543.x

51. Riccabona M, Fritz GA, Schollnast H, Schwarz T, Deutschmann MJ, Mache CJ. Hydronephrotic kidney: pediatric three-dimensional US for relative renal size assessment initial experience. *Radiology.* (2005) 236:276–83. doi: 10.1148/radiol.2361040158

52. Braga LH, McGrath M, Farrokhyar F, Jegatheeswaran K, Lorenzo AJ. Associations of initial society for fetal urology grades and urinary tract dilatation risk groups with clinical outcomes in patients with isolated prenatal hydronephrosis. *J Urol.* (2017) 197:831–7. doi: 10.1016/j.juro.2016.08.099

53. Chalmers DJ, Meyers ML, Brodie KE, Palmer C, Campbell JB. Inter-rater reliability of the APD, SFU UTD grading systems in fetal sonography MRI. *J Pediatr Urol.* (2016) 12:305.e1-305.e5. doi: 10.1016/j.jpurol.2016.06.012

54. Onen A. The natural history and therapeutic approach of antenatally diagnosed primary UPJ-type hydronephrosis. *Turk J Pediatr Surg.* (2006) 20:33–8.

55. Hafez AT, McLorie G, Bagli D, Khoury A. Analysis of trends on serial ultrasound for high grade neonatal hydronephrosis. *J Urol.* (2002) 168:1518e21. doi: 10.1016/S0022-5347(05)64508-9

56. Onen A. Neonatal hydronephrosis. In: Onen A, editor. *Pediatric Surgery and Urology.* Istanbul: Nobel Tip Kitapevi (2006), p. 345–65.

57. De Bessa J Jr, Denes FT, Chammas MC, Cerri L, Monteiro ED, Buchpiguel CA, et al. Diagnostic accuracy of color Doppler sonographic study of the ureteric jets in evaluation of hydronephrosis. *J Pediatr Urol.* (2008) 4:113–7. doi: 10.1016/j.jpurol.2007.10.013

58. Cvitkovic Kuzmic A, Brkljacic B, Rados M, Galesic K. Doppler visualization of ureteric jets in unilateral hydronephrosis in children and adolescents. *Eur J Radiol.* (2001) 39:209–14. doi: 10.1016/S0720-048X(01)00329-1

59. Kessler RM, Quevedo H, Lankau CA, Ramirez-Seijas F, Cepero-Akselrad A, Altman DH, et al. Obstructive vs nonobstructive dilatation of the renal collecting system in children: distinction with duplex sonography. *AJR Am J Roentgenol.* (1993) 160:353–7. doi: 10.2214/ajr.160.2.8424349

60. Okada T, Yoshida H, Iwai J, Matsunaga T, Yoshino K, Ohtsuka Y, et al. Pulsed doppler sonography of the hilar renal artery: differentiation of obstructive from nonobstructive hydronephrosis in children. *J Pediatr Surg.* (2001) 36:416–20. doi: 10.1053/jpsu.2001.21607

61. Gilbert R, Garra B, Gibbons MD. Renal duplex Doppler ultrasound: an adjunct in the evaluation of hydronephrosis in the child. *J Urol.* (1993) 150:1192–4. doi: 10.1016/S0022-5347(17)35723-3

62. Shokeir AA, Provoost AP, Nijman RJM. Resistive index in obstructive uropathy. *Br J Urol.* (1997) 80:195–200. doi: 10.1046/j.1464-410X.1997.00243.x

63. Gennisson JL, Grenier N, Combe C, Tanter M. Supersonic shear wave elastography of *in vivo* pig kidney: influence of blood pressure, urinary pressure and tissue anisotropy. *Ultrasound Med Biol.* (2012) 38:1559–67. doi: 10.1016/j.ultrasmedbio.2012.04.013

64. Sohn B, Kim MJ, Han SW, Im YJ, Lee MJ. Shear wave velocity measurements using acoustic radiation force impulse in young children with normal kidneys versus hydronephrotic kidneys. *Ultrasonography.* (2014) 33:116–21. doi: 10.14366/usg.14002

65. Habibi H, Cicek R, Kandemirli S, Ure E, Ucar AK, Aslan M, et al. Acoustic radiation force impulse (ARFI) elastography in the evaluation of renal parenchymal stiffness in patients with ureteropelvic junction obstruction. *J Med Ultrason.* (2017) 44:167–72.1. doi: 10.1007/s10396-016-0760-7

66. Dillman JR, Smith EA, Davenport MS, DiPietro MA, Sanchez R, Kraft KH, et al. Can shear-wave elastography be used to discriminate obstructive hydronephrosis from nonobstructive hydronephrosis in children? *Radiology.* (2015) 277:259–67. doi: 10.1148/radiol.2015142884

67. Blickman JG. *Pediatric Urinary Tract Infection: Imaging Techniques With Special Reference to Voiding Cystoerethrography.* Rotterdam: Erasmus University (1991).

68. Silay MS, Spinoit AF, Bogaert G, Hoebeke P, Nijman R, Haid B, et al. Imaging for vesicoureteral reflux and ureteropelvic junction obstruction. *Eur Urol Focus.* (2016) 2:130–8. doi: 10.1016/j.euf.2016.03.015

69. Psooy K, Pike J. Investigation and management of antenatally detected hydronephrosis. *Can Urol Assoc J.* (2009) 3:69–72. doi: 10.5489/cuaj.1027

70. Platt JF. Urinary obstruction. *Radiol Clin North Am.* (1996) 34:1113–29.

71. Esmaeili M, Esmaeili M, Ghane F, Alamdaran A. Comparison between diuretic urography (IVP) and diuretic renography for diagnosis of ureteropelvic junction obstruction in children. *Iran J Pediatr.* (2016) 2:e4293. doi: 10.5812/ijp.4293

72. Tsai JD, Huang FY, Lin CC, Tsai TC, Lee HC, Sheu JC, et al. Intermittent hydronephrosis secondary to ureteropelvic junction obstruction: clinical and imaging features. *Pediatrics.* (2006) 117:139–46. doi: 10.1542/peds.2005-0583

73. Frush D, Donnelly LF, Rosen, NS. Computed tomography and radiation risks: what pediatric health care providers should know. *Pediatrics.* (2003) 112:951–7. doi: 10.1542/peds.112.4.951

74. Riccabona M, Avni FE, Dacher J-N, Damasio MB, Darge K, Lobo L, et al. ESPR uroradiology task force and ESUR paediatric working group: imaging and procedural recommendations in paediatric uroradiology, part III. minutes of the ESPR uroradiology task force minisymposium on intravenous urography,

uro-CT and MR-urography in childhood. *Pediatr Radiol.* (2010) 40:1315–20. doi: 10.1007/s00247-010-1686-7

75. Strauss KJ, Goske MJ, Kaste SC, Bulas D, Frush DP, Butler P, et al. Image gently: ten steps you can take to optimize image quality and lower CT dose for paediatric patients. *AJR Am J. Roentgenol.* (2010) 194:868–73. doi: 10.2214/AJR.09.4091

76. Thomas KE, Wang B. Age-specific effective doses for paediatric MSCT examinations at a large children's hospital using DLP conversion coefficients: a simple estimation method. *Pediatr Radiol.* (2008) 38:645–56. doi: 10.1007/s00247-008-0794-0

77. Basics of Radiation Protection for Everyday Use. *How to Achieve ALARA: Working Tips and Guidelines.* Geneva: WHO (2004).

78. Damasio MB, Darge K, Riccabona M. Multi-detector CT in the paediatric urinary tract. *Eur J Radiol.* (2013) 82:11181125 doi: 10.1016/j.ejrad.2011.12.005

79. Van Der Molen AJ, Cowan NC, Mueller-Lisse UG, Nolte-Ernsting CC, Takahashi S, Cohan RH. CT urography: definition, indications and techniques: a guideline for clinical practice. *Eur Radiol.* (2008) 18:4–17. doi: 10.1007/s00330-007-0792-x

80. Dillman JR, Caoili EM, Cohan RH, Ellis JH, Francis IR, Nan B, et al. Comparison of urinary tract distension and opacification using single-bolus 3-phase vs split-bolus 2- phase multidetector row CT urography. *J Comput Assist Tomogr.* (2007) 31:750–7. doi: 10.1097/RCT.0b013e318033df36

81. Mitsumori A, Yasui K, Akaki S, Togami I, Joja I, Hashimoto H, et al. Evaluation of crossing vessels in patients with ureteropelvic junction obstruction by means of helical CT. *Radiographics.* (2000) 20:1383–93, discussion 1393–1395. doi: 10.1148/radiographics.20.5.g00se061383

82. Darge K, Higgins M, Hwang TJ, Delgado J, Shukla A, Bellah R. Magnetic resonance and computed tomography in pediatric urology: an imaging overview for current and future daily practice. *Radiol Clin North Am.* (2013) 51:583–98 doi: 10.1016/j.rcl.2013.03.004

83. Perez-Brayfield MR, Kirsch AJ, Jones RA, Grattan-Smith JD. A prospective study comparing ultrasound, nuclear scintigraphy and dynamic contrast enhanced magnetic resonance imaging in the evaluation of hydronephrosis. *J Urol.* (2003) 170:1330–4. doi: 10.1097/01.ju.0000086775.66329.00

84. McDaniel BB, Jones RA, Scherz H, Kirsch AJ, Little SB, Grattan-Smith JD. Dynamic contrast-enhanced MR urography in the evaluation of pediatric hydronephrosis: Part 2, anatomic and functional assessment of ureteropelvic junction obstruction. *AJR Am J Roentgenol.* (2005) 185:1608–14. doi: 10.2214/AJR.04.1574

85. Zielonko J, Studniarek M, Markuszewski M. MR urography of obstructive uropathy: diagnostic value of the method in selected clinical groups. *Eur Radiol.* (2003) 13:802–9. doi: 10.1007/s00330-002-1550-8

86. Dickerson EC, Dillman JR, Smith EA, Di Pietro MA, Lebowitz RL, Darge K. Pediatric MR urography: indications, techniques, and approach to review. *RadioGraphics.* (2015) 35:1208–30 doi: 10.1148/rg.2015140223

87. Wong MCY, Piaggio G, Damasio MB, Molinelli C, Ferretti SM, Pistorio A, et al. Hydronephrosis and crossing vessels in children: optimization of diagnostic-therapeutic pathway and analysis of color Doppler ultrasound and magnetic resonance urography diagnostic accuracy. *J Pediatr Urol.* (2018) 14:68:1–6. doi: 10.1016/j.jpurol.2017.09.019

88. Parikh KR, HammerMR, Kraft KH, Ivančić V, Smith EA, Dillman JR. Pediatric ureteropelvic junction obstruction: can magnetic resonance urography identify crossing vessels? *Pediatr Radiol.* (2015) 45:1788–95. doi: 10.1007/s00247-015-3412-y

89. Piepsz A, Ismaili K, Hall M, Collier F, Tondeur M, Ham H. How to interpret a deterioration of split function? *Eur Urol.* (2005) 47:686–90. doi: 10.1016/j.eururo.2004.10.028

90. Salem YH, Majd M, Rushton HG, Belman AB. Outcome analysis of pediatric pyeloplasty as a function of patient age, presentation and differential renal function. *J Urol.* (1995) 154:1889–93. doi: 10.1016/S0022-5347(01)66819-8

91. Kis E, Verebely T, Kovi R, Máttyus I. The role of ultrasound in the follow-up of postoperative changes after pyeloplasty. *Pediatr Radiol.* (1998) 28:247–9. doi: 10.1007/s002470050342

92. Amling CL, O'Hara SM, Wiener JS, Schaeffer CS, King LR. Renal ultrasound changes after pyeloplasty in children with ureteropelvic junction obstruction: long-term outcome in 47 renal units. *J Urol.* (1996) 156:2020–4.

93. Lim DJ, Walker RD. Management of the failed pyeloplasty. *J Urol.* (1996) 156:738–40. doi: 10.1016/S0022-5347(01)65801-4

94. Helmy TE, Sarhan OM, Hafez AT, Elsherbiny MT, Dawaba ME, Ghali AM, et al. Surgical management of failed pyeloplasty in children: single-center experience. *J Pediatr Urol.* (2009) 5:87–9. doi: 10.1016/j.jpurol.2008.09.001

95. Thomas JC, DeMarco RT, Donohoe JM, Adams MC, Pope JC IV, Brock JW III. Management of the failed pyeloplasty: a contemporary review. *J Urol.* (2005) 174:2363–6. doi: 10.1097/01.ju.0000180420.11915.31

96. Kirsch, AJ, McMann LP, Jones RA, Smith EA, Scherz HC, Grattan-Smith JD. (2006) Magnetic resonance urography for evaluating outcomes after pediatric pyeloplasty. *J. Urol.* 176:1755–61. doi: 10.1016/j.juro.2006.03.115

13

Variations in the Density and Distribution of Cajal Like Cells Associated with the Pathogenesis of Ureteropelvic Junction Obstruction

U. M. J. E. Samaranayake [1,2], Y. Mathangasinghe [2,3*], U. A. Liyanage [2], M. V. C. de Silva [4], M. C. Samarasinghe [5], S. Abeygunasekera [6], A. K. Lamahewage [6] and A. P. Malalasekera [2]

[1] Department of Anatomy, Faculty of Medicine, Sabaragamuwa University of Sri Lanka, Ratnapura, Sri Lanka, [2] Department of Anatomy, Faculty of Medicine, University of Colombo, Colombo, Sri Lanka, [3] Proteostasis and Neurodegeneration Laboratory, Australian Regenerative Medicine Institute, Monash University, Clayton, VIC, Australia, [4] Department of Pathology, Faculty of Medicine, University of Colombo, Colombo, Sri Lanka, [5] Department of Surgery, Faculty of Medicine, University of Colombo, Colombo, Sri Lanka, [6] Lady Ridgeway Hospital for Children, Colombo, Sri Lanka

*Correspondence:
Y. Mathangasinghe
yasith@anat.cmb.ac.lk

Introduction: Cajal like cells (CLCs) in the upper urinary tract have an ability to generate coordinated spontaneous action potentials and are hypothesized to help propel urine from renal pelvis into the ureter. The objective of this review was to describe the variations in the density and distribution of CLCs associated with ureteropelvic junction obstruction (UPJO).

Materials and Methods: Studies comparing the density and distribution of CLCs in the human upper urinary tract in patients with UPJO and healthy controls were included in this systematic review. We searched online electronic databases; Ovid MEDLINE, Scopus, PubMed and Cochrane reviews for the studies published before October 31, 2020. A meta-analysis was conducted to compare the density of CLCs at the ureteropelvic junction (UPJ) in patients with UPJO and matched controls.

Results: We included 20 and seven studies in the qualitative and quantitative synthesis, respectively. In majority (55%) CLCs were located between the muscle layers of the upper urinary tract. The CLC density in the UPJ gradually increased with aging in both healthy subjects and patients with UPJO. The pooled analysis revealed that the density of CLCs at the UPJ was significantly low in patients with UPJO compared to the controls (SMD = −3.00, 95% CI = −3.89 to −2.11, $p < 0.01$).

Conclusions: The reduction in CLC density at the UPJ in patients with UPJO suggests a contribution from CLCs in the pathogenesis of UPJO. Since age positively correlates with CLC density, it is imperative to carefully match age when conducting case control studies comparing the CLC density and distribution.

Protocol Registration Number: CRD42020219882.

Keywords: interstitial cells of Cajal, Cajal like cells, ureteropelvic junction obstruction, density, aging

INTRODUCTION

Primary ureteropelvic junction obstruction (UPJO) is the most common congenital abnormality causing hydronephrosis in children (1) which affects 1 in 750–1,500 newborns annually (2–4). Structurally, the UPJO is characterized by a narrowed segment of the ureteropelvic junction (UPJ) containing atrophied smooth muscles and a hypertrophied segment proximal to the obstruction with increased collagen deposition (5). The widely accepted theory for the pathogenesis of UPJO is the disruption of coordinated unidirectional smooth muscle contractions, leading to dampening of peristaltic waves that propels urine downward from the renal pelvis to the ureter (6). Nevertheless, the exact mechanism of how these unidirectional contractions are coordinated in healthy ureteropelvic junction remains a mystery. Nearly a century ago Santiago Ramón y Cajal discovered a cell, later named in his honor, which has a regulatory role in smooth muscle contractility. These cells form a plexus that runs between the gut muscle layers, with processes extending from the ganglion cells of Auerbach plexus and nerve terminals residing on the plasmalemma of smooth muscle cells (7). These cells express c-kit (CD177) encoding receptor tyrosine kinase in their cytoplasmic membrane, which allow visualization of them using immunostaining (8). Reduction in the density of intestinal Cajal cells was later found to be associated with motility disorders of the gastrointestinal system such as congenital pyloric stenosis, achalasia cardia, Hirschsprung's disease and chronic intestinal pseudo obstruction (9–12).

Huizinga and Faussone-Pellegrini (13) reported the presence of different subtypes of Cajal cells, termed Cajal like cells (CLCs), outside the gastrointestinal tract with unique ultrastructural characteristics that help distinguish them from other cell types expressing c-kit such as mast cells, glial cells and melanocytes. The CLCs in the urinary tract have a stellate shape or a fusiform cell body with two distinct dendrites (14, 15). Subsequently, CLCs were identified in many organs including urinary tract, vagina, blood vessels and glands (13, 16, 17). The CLCs in the upper urinary tract in guinea pigs generate and amplify action potentials both in the renal pelvis and the ureter (18, 19), suggesting a unique role of CLCs in maintaining a unidirectional flow of urine at the UPJ (20, 21). With the discovery of an intrinsic motility action of the human UPJ (20), the CLCs were considered to be the pacemaker regulating the expulsion of urine at the UPJ. Nonetheless, the postulated role of CLCs in the pathogenesis of UPJO was challenged since the early studies failed to demonstrate a consistent decrease in the density of the CLCs at the UPJ in patients with UPJO (22, 23). These contradicting results led to further studies that primarily focused on the functions of the CLCs which generated clues on the pathogenesis of UPJO.

Despite decades of research, the exact pathogenic mechanism (s) of primary UPJO remains enigmatic. In this review, we provide a comprehensive analysis of the density and distribution of CLCs in the upper urinary tract associated with the UPJO and mechanistic insights to the pathophysiology of this disease. Moreover, we critically evaluate the methodological inaccuracies of certain studies which may have led to false assumptions regarding the association of the density of the CLCs at the UPJ with the UPJO.

MATERIALS AND METHODS

Protocol and Registration

We conducted a systematic review and meta-analysis according to the Preferred Reporting Items for Systematic Reviews and Meta-Analyses (PRISMA) guidelines (24). The study protocol was documented in advance in the International Prospective Register of Systematic Reviews (PROSPERO) online database (protocol registration number: CRD42020219882).

Eligibility Criteria

Studies comparing the density and/or distribution of CLCs in the human upper urinary tract in patients with UPJO and controls were included in this systematic review. Only the studies comparing the density of CLCs at the UPJ in patients with UPJO and matched controls were included in the quantitative synthesis. Case reports and animal studies on CLCs were excluded.

Information Sources and Search Strategy

We searched online electronic databases; Ovid MEDLINE (Medical Literature Analysis and Retrieval System), Scopus, PubMed and Cochrane reviews. To obtain additional information, we conducted a manual search of the reference list of the selected articles. The online search strategy was generated by YM. The search comprised of studies listed up to October 31, 2020. We did not set search limits. The PubMed search strategy is provided in **Table 1**.

Study Selection

Two independent reviewers (US and YM) assessed the eligibility in an unbiased standardized manner. A third reviewer (AM) was involved in case of any disagreements. We screened the total hits obtained by reading "title" and "abstract." We excluded studies that failed to satisfy the inclusion criteria at this stage. Next, we read the full text of each selected paper to extract data. All relevant articles published in languages other than English were translated into English language before screening. The reviewers determined the final group of articles to be included in the review after an iterative consensus process.

Data Collection Process

We developed a data extraction sheet, pilot-tested it on three randomly selected studies that were consistent with the inclusion criteria and revised it accordingly. One reviewer (US) extracted data from the included studies using this standardized form and another reviewer (YM) checked for the accuracy of data extraction. We extracted the following data from each study: (a) study details (author, country and year published), (b) sample characteristics (age of the study population and sample size), (c) methods (detection and/or quantification of CLC distribution and density) and (d) results (distribution of CLCs in a cross section and along the upper urinary tract and the density of CLCs with its association with disease status (UPJO vs. healthy subjects), age and postoperative outcomes).

TABLE 1 | The PubMed search strategy.

	Search string
1	Ureteropelvic
2	Pelviureteric
3	Pyeloureteric
4	Kidney
5	Urology*
6	Disease, urinary tract*
7	Ureter
8	Ureteral obstruction*
9	Interstitial cell of Cajal like cell*
10	Interstitial Cells of Cajal*
11	Telocytes*
12	1 or 2 or 3 or 4 or 5 or 6 or 7 or 8
13	9 or 10 or 11
14	12 and 13

MeSH terms are indicated by asterisks (*).

Ureteropelvic junction was defined as the junction between the renal pelvis and the ureter (20). Despite no clear external feature to locate the UPJ (20, 25), the internal appearance of crowding of mucosal folds forming characteristic "mucosal rosettes" allows its precise localization (20), whereas pathological UPJs in patients with UPJO is visualized intra-operatively as a valve-like appearance (26) preceding a narrowed segment with interrupted development of circular muscle fibers (27). Distribution of CLCs was defined as the location of the CLCs in different layers in the cross section of the ureter or along the upper urinary tract (UPJ, renal pelvis, or ureter). Density was defined as the total number of CLCs per high power field of an optical microscope. We resolved discrepancies in the extracted data by discussion, involving a third reviewer (AM) when necessary. We contacted the corresponding authors of the published manuscripts to obtain additional data such as the age distribution of their study populations and data sets of the measurements.

Risk of Bias in Individual Studies

The methodological quality and the risk of bias of the included studies were assessed independently by two authors (US and YM) using Joanna Briggs Institute (JBI) Critical Appraisal Tool (28). Each criterion was evaluated as "Yes," "No," or "Other" (unclear/not applicable). Overall rating was provided for each study based on the items rated with an affirmative answer and accordingly, the quality score was determined by the range 67–100 (good), 34–66 (average), and 0–33 (bad). The studies meeting the "good" scores were selected for the review.

Quantitative Analysis

We conducted a meta-analysis of studies comparing the density of CLCs at the UPJ in patients with UPJO and matched control. A random effects model was used for the comparisons. Heterogeneity was assessed using the χ^2 test on Cochrane's Q statistic and by I^2 statistic. The I^2 statistic was interpreted as follows: 0–40% might not be important; 30–60% may represent moderate heterogeneity; 50–90% may represent substantial heterogeneity; and 75–100% may represent considerable heterogeneity (29). When appropriate, sensitivity analyses were performed based on the sample size and the age distribution of the study samples to explore the sources of heterogeneity. Data were analyzed using RevMan version 5.4.1 (30). $p < 0.05$ was considered statistically significant in all analyses.

RESULTS

We found a total of 266 hits in the initial literature search, and after 50 duplicates were removed, 241 articles remained. We did not find additional articles after manual screening. We obtained full texts that had potential for the final review and included twenty of these studies in the final qualitative synthesis. **Figure 1** illustrates the PRISMA flow diagram of the search. The results of the qualitative synthesis are summarized in **Table 2**. Of them, five studies presented the density of CLC as an ordinal variable (e.g., low, medium, and high density) as opposed to a continuous variable *viz*, the absolute number of CLCs per high power field, hence were subsequently excluded from the quantitative synthesis. The reasons of excluding articles from the quantitative synthesis are provided in the **Supplementary Table 1**. The risk of bias assessment is provided in the **Supplementary Tables 2, 3**. Of the studies included in the qualitative synthesis, eleven were conducted exclusively among children, while eight pooled results of adults and children. One study did not provide the age distribution of the subjects. The studies were conducted in Turkey, Poland, India, Egypt, Belgium, Germany, Korea, Singapore, Iran, Romania, Ireland, and China.

Distribution of Cajal-Like Cells

Majority (11/20, 55%) of the studies found CLCs between the inner longitudinal and outer circular muscle layers or in close proximity to the muscle layers (7/20, 35%), while others found these cells to be present both in the lamina propria and serosal layers (1/20, 5%) in addition to the muscle layers (**Supplementary Table 4**).

The reported distribution of the CLCs in different parts of the upper urinary system were controversial. Wishahi et al. (44) reported that the CLC density gradually increased from renal pelvis to proximal ureter in healthy subjects, while two studies found a decrease in CLC density from UPJ to distal ureter (37, 41). Conversely, Metzger et al. (39) reported that the CLC density gradually increased from the pelvis to the intermediate ureter, and then reduced at the distal ureter, while Ven Der Aa et al. (14) could not find a statistically significant difference in CLC density between upper, mid and distal thirds of the ureter.

Most studies (31–33, 42, 45) reported a lower density of CLCs in the UPJ of the patients with UPJO compared to the controls (**Table 2**). On the contrary, Koleda et al. (23), and Kuvel et al. (22) found a comparatively higher density of CLCs at the UPJ in patients. How et al. (34) found no statistically significant difference between the CLC density in the UPJ between the cases and controls. Apoznanski et al. (1) explored the density of CLCs

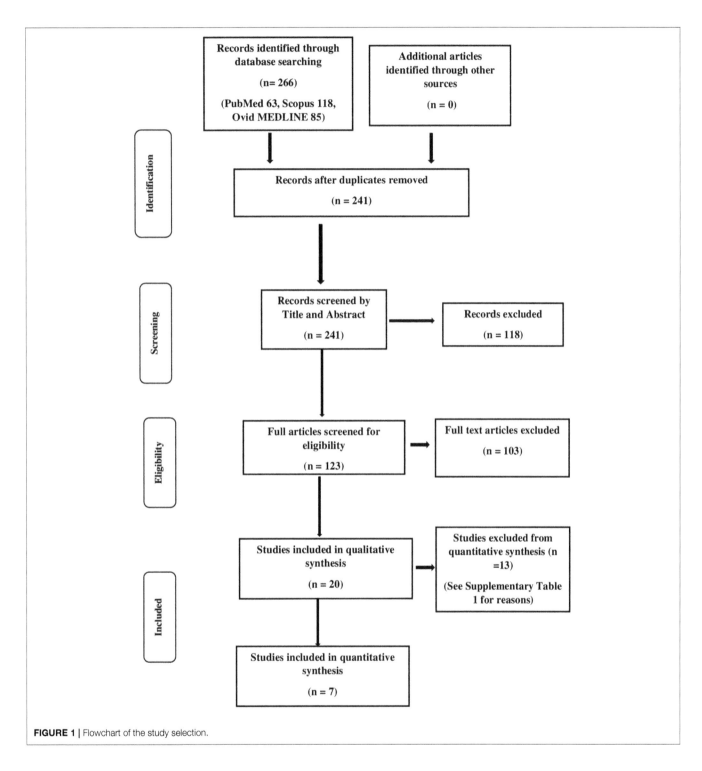

FIGURE 1 | Flowchart of the study selection.

in affected patients with UPJO by quantifying the density of CLCs in adjacent high-power fields of the UPJ and calculated the gradient of CLCs. They found no significant differences of the CLC gradient between cases and controls (1).

Age Related Changes in Cajal-Like Cells
The CLC density increases in the UPJ with the advancement of the gestational age of the fetal ureter (31). Nevertheless according to Koleda et al. (23) the density gradually decrease as the age advanced into childhood. Based on the studies included in the quantitative synthesis, a line diagram was drawn to illustrate the CLC density at the UPJ and we found an increase in CLC density with age in both healthy and those affected with UPJO (31, 32, 36, 42) (**Figure 2**). Further, the affected subjects consistently had a low CLC density compared to the healthy controls.

TABLE 2 | Summary of the studies included in the qualitative synthesis.

	Number of cases: control	Mean (± SD or range) age of cases: controls	Method of identification of CLCs	Area of CLCs distribution in ureter/UPJ	CLC density or distribution in cases	CLC density or distribution in controls	Conclusion of the study
Apoznanski et al., Poland (1)	7: 5	2.2 (0.7–5.2) years: 2.3 (0.2–7.4) years	CLC gradient at the UPJ in patients with UPJO and controls was compared using IHC. Eleven adjacent HPFs (400X magnification) were examined to determine the CLC gradient. Gradient was defined as a difference of cell number per HPF greater than one in adjacent fields. Gradient was analyzed in relation to the patient's age.	Inner border of muscle layer	CLC gradient at UPJ = 19 ($P = 0.087$, $r = -0.3927$)	CLCs gradient at UPJ = 10 ($P = 0.3753$, $r = 0.1689$)	No statistically significant difference in CLC distribution between cases and controls. No correlation between age of cases and the distribution of CLCs.
Babu et al., India (15)	31: 31	2.9 (±0.6) years	The difference of CLC density of the UPJ and the anastomotic end of ureter in children with UPJO undergoing pyeloplasty was analyzed. Association between post-operative outcome of the patients and the CLC density using IHC in 10 HPF (400X magnification) under light microscope was explored.	Not available	CLC density was significantly lower in the UPJ (mean = 5.3, SD = 2.3) compared to the anastomosed end of the ureter (mean = 12.4; SD = 5.1).		UPJ had a lower density of CLCs compared to the anastomotic end of the ureter in children with UPJO undergoing pyeloplasty. Resected ureter end with mean CLC density more than 10 per HPF had a better surgical outcome.
Babu et al., India (31)	31: 20	2.9 (±3.1) years: 4.9 (±4.1) years	CLC density at the narrowed segment in patients with UPJO and controls (UPJ segments obtained from patients undergoing nephrectomy) was compared using IHC (400X magnification). The correlation between CLC density at the UPJ of the normal fetuses (aborted due to maternal conditions or intrauterine death) and gestational age was explored.	Not available	Median CLC density of the narrowed UPJO segment per HPF was 5.1 (SD = 2.3).	Median CLC density of the normal ureter per HPF was 16.1 (SD = 8.3) Median CLC density of the fetal ureter per HPF was 5.0 (SD = 2.3)	CLC density at the narrowed segment in patients with UPJO was lower than that of the normal ureter. A positive correlation was found between the increasing gestational age and the CLC density ($r = 0.83$; $P < 0.001$) in the fetal ureter.
Balikci et al., Turkey (32)	63: 30	43.5 (2–72) years: 58.6 (38–82) years	Samples were obtained from multiple areas of the urinary tract in patients with hydronophroureter due to ureteric obstruction and controls. The CLC density was studied using IHC (400X magnification) at: renal pelvis lamina propria (RPLP), renal pelvis muscularis propria (RPMP), proximal ureter lamina propria (PULP), proximal ureter muscularis propria (PUMP).	Lamina propria and muscularis propria	CLCs density in; RPLP = 22(14–28) RPMP = 26(15–36) PULP = 12(9–20) PUMP = 17(10–23)	CLCs density in; RPLP = 32(26–42) RPMP = 42(34–64) PULP = 24(20–26) PUMP = 29(25–32)	CLC density in the renal pelvis and proximal ureter in cases was significantly low ($P < 0.001$) compared to the controls.
Eken et al., Turkey (33)	35: 7	3 (0.25–18) years: 29 (10–40) years (for light microscope)	CLC density at the UPJ in patients with UPJO and controls was compared using IHC and electron microscopy. CLC density per HPF (400X magnification) was graded as: 0–3 cells/HPF = sparse 4-8 cells/HPF = few >8 cells/HPF = many	Lamina propria and muscular layer	CLC density; Sparse = 8 (22.9%) Few = 26 (74.3%) Many = 1 (2.9%)	CLC density; Sparse = 0 Few = 0 Many = 7 (100%)	CLC density was significantly higher in the controls compared to cases ($P < 0.001$). CLCs of patients with UPJO had decreased number of mitochondria and caveolae compared to controls.
How et al., Singapore (34)	38: 20	2.1 (0.2–14) years: 4.0 (0.1–16) years	Level of CD117 staining was at the UPJ in patients with UPJO and controls was compared (400X and 100X magnifications)	Not available	Difference between cases and controls with CD117 staining; No difference in cases 30 (78.9%), Increased staining in cases 8 (21.1%), Decreased staining in cases 0 (0%).		There was no statistically significant difference of CD117 staining between cases and controls.

(Continued)

TABLE 2 | Continued

	Number of cases: control	Mean ± SD or (range) age of cases: controls	Method of identification of CLCs	Area of CLCs distribution in ureter/UPJ	CLC density or distribution in cases	CLC density or distribution in controls	Conclusion of the study
Inugala et al., India (35)	23: 2	1.1 (0.04–4) years: 0.6 years	The association between outcome of Anderson-Hynes pyeloplasty and CLC density in resected margin was assessed. CLC density per HPF (400X magnification) was graded as: 0–1 cell/HPF = negative 2–5 cells/HPF = + 6–10 cells/HPF = ++ >11 cells/HPF = + + +	Not available	CLC density at the UPJ in patients with good surgical outcomes: 0–1 cells = 12 (52.2%) 2–5 cells = 2 (8.7%) 6–10 cells = 7 (30.4%) >11 cells = 2 (8.7%) CLC density at the UPJ in patients with poor surgical outcomes: 0–1 cells = 1 (50%) 2–5 cells = 1 (50%) 6–10 cells = 0 >11 cells = 0		Having a high density of CLCs at the resection margin was associated with good surgical outcomes ($p = 0.001$).
Kart et al., Turkey (36)	11: 7	3.9 (±2.6) years: 3.6 (±3.8) years	CLC density at the UPJ in patients with UPJO and controls was compared using IHC (400X magnification)	Between Muscle layers	CLC density in cases per HPF was 1.75 (SD = 1.14)	CLC density in controls per HPF was 5.76 (SD = 2.99)	CLC density was significantly lower in cases compared to controls ($P < 0.01$).
Koleda et al., Poland (23)	20: 5	8.1 (0.7–16.8) years: 2.3 (0.2–7.4) years	CLC density at the UPJ in patients with UPJO and controls was compared using IHC. CLC density per HPF (400X magnification) was graded as: few (0 to 1), moderate (2 to 3), many (4 to 8) cells. The correlation between CLC density and age of the patients was explored.	Not available	Number of fields with few CLCs was significantly lower in cases than in controls ($P = 0.0122$). The number of fields with many CLCs was significantly higher in cases than in controls ($P = 0.0004$).		CLC density was significantly higher in cases compared to controls. CLC density of patients with UPJO decreased with aging ($r = -0.6167$, $P = 0.0038$).
Kuvel et al., Turkey (22)	32: 30	Not available	CLC density at the UPJ in patients with UPJO and controls was compared using IHC (400X magnification) Cases were classified according to location of sample obtained from the UPJ; Group Ia (proximal) Group Ib (intermediate) Group Ic (distal) segments	lamina propria (LP), muscularis propria (MP), and serosa (S) layers	CLC density in Group Ia was higher than Group Ib for LP, MP and for S layers. Group Ic had increased CLCs in LP and MP.	CLCs density in Group Ia was increased compared to controls for LP ($p < 0.05$) and S ($p < 0.01$). In intrinsic UPJO, CLCs were located more in LP and S compared to chronic UPJO.	An increased density of CLCs was observed in proximal segments of UPJ in intrinsic UPJO compared to normal subjects and chronic UPJO.
Lee et al., Korea (37)	8: 8	37 to 54 years age range	Two groups of specimens were studied: proximal group ≤5 cm from the UPJ, distal group ≥5 cm from UPJ. IHC was performed on the obtained tissues and observed under 400X magnification. Contractibility was assessed based on the dose dependent response of acetylcholine and norepinephrine.	Between inner longitudinal muscles and interface between inner longitudinal and outer circular muscle layers	CLCs were found abundantly in the proximal group. There were spontaneous contractions (3 to 4 contractions within 5 min) in the proximal group. Distal sections did not show any spontaneous contractions.	No CLCs were found in the distal group.	Spontaneous contractions in human ureter could be generated by CLCs in the proximal region. This action might be regulated by cholinergic and/or adrenergic systems.
Mehrazma et al., Iran (38)	25: 19	1.7 (0.1 to 8) years	CLC density at the UPJ in patients with UPJO and controls was compared using IHC (400X magnification)	Between the muscle layers	Mean CLC density per HPF was 14.5 (SD = 5.6)	Mean CLC density per HPF was 32.8 (SD = 11.9)	CLCs density was significantly low in cases compared to controls ($P < 0.001$).

(Continued)

TABLE 2 | Continued

	Number of cases: control	Mean ± SD or (range) age of cases: controls	Method of identification of CLCs	Area of CLCs distribution in ureter/UPJ	CLC density or distribution in cases	CLC density or distribution in controls	Conclusion of the study
Metzger et al., Germany (39)	56 ureter samples	Cadavers aged 54 (24–82) years and patients with renal tumours aged 49 (42–64) years	Samples were obtained from renal pelvis, and proximal, intermediate, and distal ureter. CLC density was assessed following IHC per HPF (200X magnification).	Lamina propria and muscularis propria	CLC density per HPF were: pelvis 13 (range 0.33 to 3.66) proximal ureter 10 (range 0 to 3.00) intermediate ureter 32 (range 0 to 6.66) distal ureter 22 (range 0.33 to 7.66).		CLC density was lower in the proximal ureter compared to the renal pelvis. The CLC density increased from proximal to intermediate ureter, and then decreased at the distal ureter.
Pande et al., India (40)	30: 7	0.7 (0.2–8) years: 2 (0.7–5) years	CLC density at the UPJ in patients with UPJO and controls was compared using IHC (under 400X magnification). Surgical outcome was assessed using ultrasonographs at 6-month post-operatively.	Not available	CLC density in cases per HPF was 4.86 (SD = 0.76)	CLC density in controls per HPF was 11.74 (SD = 0.86)	CLC density was significantly low in cases compared to controls (p = 0.04).
Prisca et al., Romania (41)	13	0.6 to 83 years	Samples were obtained from multiple areas of the urinary tract from the deceased with no evidence of UPJO. The obtained samples were categorized into following levels: upper urinary tract: 1st level- Kidney, 2nd level- Calyces, 3rd level- Pyelon, 4th level- UPJ, 5th level- Proximal ureter, 6th level- Middle ureter, 7th level- Distal ureter. IHC was performed and observed under HPF (400X magnification)	Between muscle layers	Median CLC density per HPF at levels; 2nd level- 6 (4 to 9) 3rd level- 5 (2 to 8) 4th level- 4 (2 to 7) 5th level- 3 (1 to 6) 6th level- 2 (1 to 5) 7th level- 2 (0 to 5)		In normal individuals, CLC density was high in the calyces and pyelon, while CLCs were scanty in the mid and distal ureter.
Senol et al., Turkey (42)	19: 12	116 ± 116 months: 279 ± 312 months	CLC density at the UPJ in patients with UPJO and controls was compared using IHC. CLC density per HPF (400X magnification) was graded as: very few (0 to 3), few (4 to 6) and many (>7) cells.	Closer to the inner longitudinal layer	CLC density in cases per HPF is 2.37 (SD = 2.19) Many – 1 (5.3%) Few – 5 (26.3%) Very few – 13 (68.4%)	CLC density in controls per HPF is 24.5 (SD = 9.73) All individuals had >7 CLCs per HPF.	Compared to controls cases had either no or few CLCs (p < 0.0001).
Solaris et al., Ireland (43)	19: 7	2.3 (0.2–12) years: 4.5 (0.9–9) years	CLC density at the UPJ in patients with UPJO and controls was compared using IHC. CLC density per HPF (400X magnification) was graded as: sparse (0 to 1), few (2 to 3), moderate (4 to 8), and many (>8).	Inner border of circular muscle layer	CLCs were sparse or absent (<2 per HPF).	CLC density was >8 per HPF (Grading: "many").	Patients with UPJO have a lower density of CLCs in the UPJ and renal pelvis compared to controls (p < 0.05).
Ven der Aa et al., Belgium (14)	44 (65 tissue samples)	39.7 (1–78) years in males, 16 (1–50) years in females	Tissue samples were obtained from renal pelvis, upper, middle, and lower ureter, vesicoureteral junction, bladder dome, bladder neck and urethra. IHC was performed and observed under HPF (400X and 200X magnifications).	Beneath urothelium and between muscle layers	Values not available	Values not available	CLC density was greater in pyelon compared to ureter. No significant difference in the CLC density was observed between upper, mid, and lower thirds of the ureter or between the longitudinal and circular muscle layers of the ureter.
Wishahi et al., Egypt (44)	7: 5	28 ± 10 years :52 ± 7 years	CLC density at the UPJ, PU and RP in patients with UPJO and controls were compared using IHC and transmission electron microscopy.	Between Muscular layers	CLC density was high in PU, moderate in RP, scanty or absent in UPJ.	CLC density was high in the PU, excess in RP, and moderate in the UPJ.	Patients with UPJO have a lower density of CLCs in the UPJ and renal pelvis compared to controls (p < 0.05).

(Continued)

TABLE 2 | Continued

	Number of cases: control	Mean ± SD or (range) age of cases: controls	Method of identification of CLCs	Area of CLCs distribution in ureter/UPJ	CLC density or distribution in cases	CLC density or distribution in controls	Conclusion of the study
Yang et al., China (45)	24: 21	0.25 to 12 years	CLC density at the UPJ in patients with UPJO and controls was compared using IHC (400X magnification)	Between muscle layers	Density of CLCs per HPF in cases was 0.207 (SD = 0.020).	Density of CLCs per HPF in controls was 0.262 (SD = 0.026).	CLC density at the UPJ was significantly lower in the cases compared to the controls (p < 0.05).

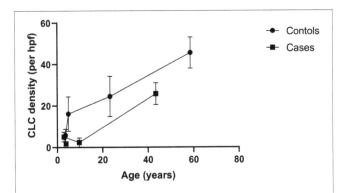

FIGURE 2 | A line diagram demonstrating the associations of density of Cajal like cells (CLCs) at the ureteropelvic junction and age. The diagram illustrates that the CLC density increases with age in both healthy and those affected with ureteropelvic junction obstruction. Data from four studies were used to create the chart (31, 32, 36, 42).

Cajal-Like Cell Contribution to Post-operative Outcome

Two studies exploring the association between the post-operative outcome of Anderson-Hynes pyeloplasty and the CLC density at the resected margin of ureter, showed that patients with a higher density of CLCs had a better surgical functional outcome (15, 35). Nevertheless, Pande et al. (40) found no correlation between the CLC density and the post-operative functional outcome.

Meta-Analysis

Seven studies reporting the mean difference of the density of CLC in the UPJ per high power field in patient with UPJO and controls were included in the meta-analysis. In the pooled analysis, the density of CLCs was significantly low in patients with UPJO (standardized mean difference = −3.00, 95% confidence interval = −3.89 to −2.11, p < 0.01) (**Figure 3**). The funnel plot of the selected studies is provided in the **Supplementary Figure 1**. We detected a considerable heterogeneity in this comparison (χ^2 = 41.03, I^2 = 85%, df = 6, p < 0.01). We performed a sensitivity analysis by including studies conducted on children only (aged <14 years) (n = 5) (31, 36, 38, 40, 45). The studies including both children (<2 years) and elders (>70 years) were excluded (32, 42). Nonetheless, the sensitivity analysis found a

standardized mean difference of −2.93 (95% CI = −4.14 to −1.73) with a considerable heterogeneity (χ^2 = 32.71, I^2 = 88%, df = 4, p < 0.01) (**Supplementary Figure 2**). We were unable to perform a subgroup analysis comparing pediatric and adult populations since none of the included studies had a homogeneous adult population. To explore the effect of sample sizes, we performed another sensitivity analysis after including studies with at least 10 samples per group (n = 5) (31, 32, 38, 42, 45). The results showed a standardized mean difference of −2.56 (95% CI = −3.14 to −1.97) with a substantial heterogeneity (χ^2 = 11.40, I^2 = 65%, df = 4, p < 0.01) (**Supplementary Figure 3**). Subsequently, we combined the two sensitivity analyses by including studies of children with a large sample size (as defined above) (n = 3) (31, 38). In this analysis we found a standardized mean difference of −2.11 (95% CI= −2.53 to −1.68) with no heterogeneity (χ^2 = 0.56, I^2 = 0%, df = 2, p < 0.01) (**Supplementary Figure 4**).

DISCUSSION

UPJO is the partial or intermittent blockage of urinary flow from the renal pelvis into the ureter, governed by either an anatomical derangement or in most instances a functional disturbance (5, 26, 46–48). About a decade ago, dilemma on the pathophysiology of UPJO brought myogenic theory to light, which suggests that uncoordinated muscular contractions at the UPJ leads to a functional obstruction of antegrade urine flow (49). The discovery of CLCs in the upper urinary tract which could propagate action potentials in the UPJ, intrigued researchers to investigate into their role in UPJO (49).

Cajal Like Cells in the Upper Urinary Tract

Ureteric wall consists of a transitional epithelium, lamina propria, inner longitudinal, and outer circular muscle layers and a serosa. In most studies, CLCs were located between the inner longitudinal and outer circular muscle layers (**Supplementary Table 4**). Few studies found CLCs in the lamina propria (14, 22, 39), while a single study detected CLCs in the serosa (22). Cajal cells in the intestines, are located near the myenteric plexus and submucosal plexus, between longitudinal and circular muscle layers, between inner and outer circular muscle layers and within interlamellar connective tissues of circular muscles (50). They are, however not often observed

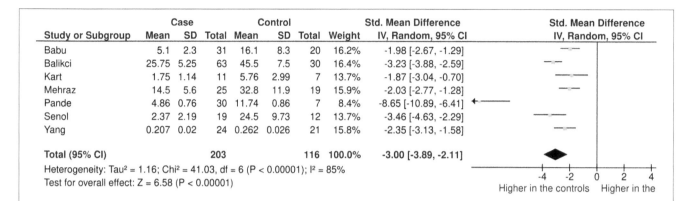

Study or Subgroup	Case Mean	Case SD	Case Total	Control Mean	Control SD	Control Total	Weight	Std. Mean Difference IV, Random, 95% CI
Babu	5.1	2.3	31	16.1	8.3	20	16.2%	-1.98 [-2.67, -1.29]
Balikci	25.75	5.25	63	45.5	7.5	30	16.4%	-3.23 [-3.88, -2.59]
Kart	1.75	1.14	11	5.76	2.99	7	13.7%	-1.87 [-3.04, -0.70]
Mehraz	14.5	5.6	25	32.8	11.9	19	15.9%	-2.03 [-2.77, -1.28]
Pande	4.86	0.76	30	11.74	0.86	7	8.4%	-8.65 [-10.89, -6.41]
Senol	2.37	2.19	19	24.5	9.73	12	13.7%	-3.46 [-4.63, -2.29]
Yang	0.207	0.02	24	0.262	0.026	21	15.8%	-2.35 [-3.13, -1.58]
Total (95% CI)			203			116	100.0%	**-3.00 [-3.89, -2.11]**

Heterogeneity: Tau² = 1.16; Chi² = 41.03, df = 6 (P < 0.00001); I² = 85%
Test for overall effect: Z = 6.58 (P < 0.00001)

FIGURE 3 | The study characteristics and standardized mean differences of the density of the interstitial cells of Cajal like cells at the ureteropelvic junction in patients with ureteropelvic junction obstruction and matched controls.

in serosa. Similarly, in ureter, CLCs are not readily located in the serosa in most instances but are present considerably more in the lamina propria. These cells are believed to play a coordinator role of impulse transmission between the sensory nerve endings and smooth muscle cells (18, 19), hence are located in areas richly innervated by sensory nerves. Ureteric innervation is to the muscular and subepithelial layers (51) where the nerve endings reside, therefore the deficiency in CLCs in serosal layer could be due to the lack of sensory nerve endings in the serosa.

Majority of the studies suggest that the overall CLC density at UPJ is reduced in individuals with UPJO compared to controls (33, 38, 40, 42, 45), which is consistent with the results of our quantitative synthesis. A constellation of gastrointestinal motility diseases including achalasia cardia (52) and Hirschsprung's disease (53) are associated with depletion of Cajal cells, while reduction of Cajal cell density in small intestinal segments of inflammation or obstruction significantly improves when treating the pathology causing inflammation or removal of obstruction (54, 55). Abstracting from this knowledge, a theory was postulated on the lack of CLCs in the UPJ as a contributor of failed peristaltic wave propagation across the UPJ in UPJO. However, the observational nature of these studies lacked the ability to derive a direct causation, but only an association. This putative role of CLCs was projected to doubt by Koleda et al. (23) and Kuvel et al. (22) with their description of an increase in the CLC density in the UPJ in affected individuals. Interestingly, in Koleda et al. (23) study, the age of the cases was markedly higher compared to the controls which could have contributed to the rising CLCs in cases, since there is a gradual increase of the CLC density with age in normal individuals as well as in patients with UPJO (**Figure 2**). Similarly, data was lacking on the age of the subjects in Kuvel et al. (22) study. Due to this reason, it may not be prudent to derive meaningful comparisons of the CLC density in cases and controls from the latter two studies. Although CLC density increases in the urinary tract with aging (**Figure 2**), the Cajal cell number and volume reduces steadily in colon and stomach (56). Furthermore, Cajal

cell loss and aging increases slow waves conduction velocity in the stomach (57) resulting in delayed gastric emptying. Nevertheless it is possible that other syncytial factors have an interdependent role with Cajal cells giving rise to slow wave velocity changes (57).

Though immunohistochemical studies have failed to establish differences of the expression levels of neuronal markers in UPJO (34), it is suggested that a defective innervation at the UPJ in intrinsic obstruction could contribute to increase in CLC density causing increased peristaltic activity as a result of an attempt to overcome peristaltic failure (22). In chronic UPJO from tumors or ureteric stones up-regulation of c-kit expression is not observed to overcome the obstruction (22). The excitatory impulses are generated from a single site of origin propelling urine into the ureter (58). However, when more than one impulse generator sites are present, they block the conduction of waves of excitation (58). This suggests that if there is a change in distribution of impulse generating CLCs in UPJ, it may contribute to alteration of impulse generation leading to intrinsic UPJO. This hypothesis is supported by a study conducted on rabbits where increased frequency of spontaneous mechanical activity of the UPJ was observed during obstruction (59). Researchers pondered on the distributional changes in CLCs in the pathogenesis of UPJO, to which Apoznanski et al. (1) answered by demonstrating no distributional gradient changes in the CLCs in UPJO compared to the age of the affected. However, this study included only seven cases. In addition, we noted that there is a marked deficiency in studies that embark on the distributive changes in the CLCs in affected and healthy UPJ.

CLCs do not possess a primary action potential generation ability in animals, but form a conduit for transmission of signals (60) (Animal study findings related to CLCs are summarized in **Supplementary Table 5**). Guinea pig renal system, which resembles similar anatomy to humans, shows pacemaker oscillations at the pelvicalyceal junction and UPJ, while oscillations are absent in the ureter (19). When the proximal pacemaker drive is blocked either by pharmacological means or by transection, the distal regions take over the waves of excitation (61), suggesting the presence of pacemaker potential generation mechanism in the mid and distal ureter. These findings corroborate the results of the human studies where CLCs, the potential pacemakers of the renal tract, are not restricted to the renal pelvis and UPJ, but also found in the mid and distal ureter to coordinate unidirectional peristaltic activity.

LIMITATIONS

Few studies (23, 33, 34, 43) could not be incorporated in the quantitative synthesis when the CLC density was not presented as a continuous variable with means and standard deviations as summary statistics. The marked variability of the study designs, especially the wide range of age and limited sample sizes contributed to the high heterogeneity of the quantitative synthesis.

QUALITY OF EVIDENCE

This systematic review followed the standard recommended methodology set out by PRISMA guidelines. Two reviewers independently assessed the studies for potential sources of bias and a standard approach of data extraction was employed, thus reducing the risk of performance bias in the review and data

extraction errors. PRISMA checklist of the review is presented in **Supplementary Table 6.**

CONCLUSIONS

Cajal like cells are predominantly distributed between the muscle layers of the upper urinary tract. However, the distribution of CLCs along the urinary tract from the renal pelvis toward the lower ureter is subjected to controversy. The CLC density at the UPJ is significantly low in patients with UPJO compared to the controls, suggesting a pivotal contribution by CLCs in the pathogenesis of UPJO. The CLC density gradually increases with aging in both healthy subjects and patients with UPJO, which could potentially bias the results of the anatomical studies when age is not strictly matched in cases and controls. Careful matching of age in cases and controls, avoiding large age ranges and using an adequate sample size are necessary when performing future studies.

ACKNOWLEDGMENTS

Authors thank the Faculty of Medicine, University of Colombo.

REFERENCES

1. Apoznanski W, Koleda P, Wozniak Z, Rusiecki L, Szydelko T, Kalka D, et al. The distribution of interstitial cells of Cajal in congenital ureteropelvic junction obstruction. *Int Urol Nephrol.* (2013) 45:607–12. doi: 10.1007/s11255-013-0454-7
2. Degheili JA, Termos S, Moussa M, Aoun B. Ureteropelvic junction obstruction: diagnosis, treatment and prognosis. In: *Advances in Medicine and Biology.* New York, NY: Nova Medicine and Health (2020). p. 75–7.
3. Nguyen HT, Benson CB, Bromley B, Campbell JB, Chow J, Coleman B, et al. Multidisciplinary consensus on the classification of prenatal and postnatal urinary tract dilation (UTD classification system). *J Pediatric Urol.* (2014) 10:982–98. doi: 10.1016/j.jpurol.2014.10.002
4. Gopal M, Peycelon M, Caldamone A, Chrzan R, El-Ghoneimi A, Olsen H, et al. Management of ureteropelvic junction obstruction in children—a roundtable discussion. *J Pediatric Urol.* (2019) 15:322–29. doi: 10.1016/j.jpurol.2019.05.010
5. Pinter A, Horvath A, Hrabovszky Z. The relationship of smooth muscle damage to age, severity of pre-operative hydronephrosis and post-operative outcome in obstructive uropathies. *Br J Urol.* (1997) 80:227–33. doi: 10.1046/j.1464-410X.1997.00311.x
6. Murnaghan G. The dynamics of the renal pelvis and ureter with reference to congenital hydronephrosis. *Br J Urol.* (1958) 30:321. doi: 10.1111/j.1464-410X.1958.tb03525.x
7. Cajal R. *Histologie du système nerveux de l'Homme et des Vertébrés.* Grand sympathique. Paris, Maloine (1911). p. 2.
8. Miliaras D, Karasavvidou F, Papanikolaou A, Sioutopoulou D. KIT expression in fetal, normal adult, and neoplastic renal tissues. *J Clin Pathol.* (2004) 57:463–6. doi: 10.1136/jcp.2003.013532

9. Huizinga JD, Thuneberg L, Vanderwinden, JM, Rumessen JJ. Interstitial cells of Cajal as targets for pharmacological intervention in gastrointestinal motor disorders. *Trends Pharmacol Sci.* (1997) 18:393–403. doi: 10.1016/S0165-6147(97)90668-4
10. Sanders KM, Ördög T, Koh S, Torihashi S, Ward S. Development and plasticity of interstitial cells of Cajal. *Neurogastroenterol Motil.* (1999) 11:311–38. doi: 10.1046/j.1365-2982.1999.00164.x
11. Vanderwinden JM, Rumessen JJ. Interstitial cells of Cajal in human gut and gastrointestinal disease. *Microsc Res Tech.* (1999) 47:344–60. doi: 10.1002/(SICI)1097-0029(19991201)47:5<344::AID-JEMT6>3.0. CO;2-1
12. Wedel T, Spiegler J, Soellner S, Roblick UJ, Schiedeck TH, Bruch HP, et al. Enteric nerves and interstitial cells of Cajal are altered in patients with slow-transit constipation and megacolon. *Gastroenterology.* (2002) 123:1459–67. doi: 10.1053/gast.2002. 36600
13. Huizinga JD, Faussone-Pellegrini MS. About the presence of interstitial cells of Cajal outside the musculature of the gastrointestinal tract. *J Cell Mol Med.* (2005) 9:468–73. doi: 10.1111/j.1582-4934.2005.tb00372.x
14. Van Der Aa F, Roskams T, Blyweert W, Ost D, Bogaert G, De Ridder D. Identification of kit positive cells in the human urinary tract. *J Urol.* (2004) 171:2492–6. doi: 10.1097/01.ju.0000125097.25475.17
15. Babu R, Vittalraj P, Sundaram S, Manjusha MP, Ramanan V, Sai V. Comparison of different pathological markers in predicting pyeloplasty outcomes in children. *J Pediatric Surg.* (2020) 55:1616–20. doi: 10.1016/j.jpedsurg.2019.08.015
16. Shafik A, El-Sibai O, Shafik I, Shafik AA. Immunohistochemical identification of the pacemaker cajal cells in the normal human vagina. *Arch Gynecol Obstet.* (2005) 272:13–6. doi: 10.1007/s00404-005-0725-3

17. Gherghiceanu M, Hinescu M, Andrei F, Mandache E, Macarie C, Faussone-Pellegrini MS, et al. Interstitial Cajal-like cells (ICLC) in myocardial sleeves of human pulmonary veins. *J Cell Mol Med.* (2008) 12:1777–81. doi: 10.1111/j.1582-4934.2008.00444.x

18. Constantinou C, Silvert M, Gosling J. Pacemaker system in the control of ureteral peristaltic rate in the multicalyceal kidney of the pig. *Investig Urol.* (1977) 14:440.

19. Klemm MF, Exintaris B, Lang RJ. Identification of the cells underlying pacemaker activity in the guinea-pig upper urinary tract. *J Physiol.* (1999) 519:867–84. doi: 10.1111/j.1469-7793.1999.0867n.x

20. Shafik A, Al-Sherif AM. Ureteropelvic junction: a study of its anatomical structure and function. *Eur Urol.* (1999) 36:150–7. doi: 10.1159/000067987

21. Lang RJ, Tonta MA, Zoltkowski BZ, Meeker WF, Wendt I, Parkington HC. Pyeloureteric peristalsis: role of atypical smooth muscle cells and interstitial cells of Cajal-like cells as pacemakers. *J Physiol.* (2006) 576:695–705. doi: 10.1113/jphysiol.2006.116855

22. Kuvel M, Canguven O, Murtazaoglu M, Albayrak S. Distribution of Cajal like cells and innervation in intrinsic ureteropelvic junction obstruction. *Arch Ital Urol Androl.* (2011) 83:128–32.

23. Koleda P, Apoznanski W, Wozniak Z, Rusiecki L, Szydelko T, Pilecki W, et al. Changes in interstitial cell of Cajal-like cells density in congenital ureteropelvic junction obstruction. *Int Urol Nephrol.* (2012) 44:7–12. doi: 10.1007/s11255-011-9970-5

24. Moher D, Liberati A, Tetzlaff J, Altman DG, Group P. Preferred reporting items for systematic reviews and meta-analyses: the PRISMA statement. *PLoS Med.* (2009) 6:e1000097. doi: 10.1371/journal.pmed.1000097

25. Standring S. *Gray's Anatomy: The Anatomical Basis of Clinical Practice.* Philadelphia: Elsevier (2020).

26. Foote J, Blennerhassett J, Wiglesworth F, Mackinnon K. Observations on the ureteropelvic junction. *J Urol.* (1970) 104:252–7. doi: 10.1016/S0022-5347(17)61710-5

27. Wein AJ, Kavoussi LR, Dmochowski R, Partin AW, Peters CA. *Campbell-Walsh Urology.* North York, ON: Elsevier (2020).

28. Moola S, Munn Z, Tufanaru C, Aromataris E, Sears K, Sfetcu R, et al. Chapter 7: systematic reviews of etiology and risk. *Joanna Briggs Institute Reviewer's Manual. The Joanna Briggs Institute.* (2017). p. 2019–05. doi: 10.46658/JBIRM-17-06

29. Higgins JP, Thomas J, Chandler J, Cumpston M, Li T, Page MJ, et al. *Cochrane Handbook for Systematic Reviews of Interventions.* John Wiley and Sons (2019). doi: 10.1002/9781119536604

30. The Cochrane Collaboration. *Review Manager (Revman)* [Computer Program]. Version 5.4.1 (2020).

31. Babu R, Vittalraj P, Sundaram S, Shalini S. Pathological changes in ureterovesical and ureteropelvic junction obstruction explained by fetal ureter histology. *J Pediatric Urol.* (2019) 15:e247. doi: 10.1016/j.jpurol.2019.02.001

32. Balikci Ö, Turunç T, Bal N. Çelik H, Özkardeş H. Comparison of Cajal-like cells in pelvis and proximal ureter of kidney with and without hydronephrosis. *Int Braz J Urol.* (2015) 41:1178–84. doi: 10.1590/S1677-5538.IBJU.2014.0427

33. Eken A, Erdogan S, Kuyucu Y, Seydaoglu G, Polat S, Satar N. Immunohistochemical and electron microscopic examination of Cajal cells in ureteropelvic junction obstruction. *Can Urol Assoc J.* (2013) 7:E311–6. doi: 10.5489/cuaj.1247

34. How GY, Chang KTE, Jacobsen AS, Yap TL, Ong CCP, Low Y, et al. Neuronal defects an etiological factor in congenital pelviureteric junction obstruction? *J Pediatric Urol.* (2018) 14:e57. doi: 10.1016/j.jpurol.2017.07.014

35. Inugala A, Reddy RK, Rao BN, Reddy SP, Othuluru R, Kanniyan L, et al. Immunohistochemistry in ureteropelvic junction obstruction and its correlation to postoperative outcome. *J Indian Assoc Pediatric Surg.* (2017) 22:129–33. doi: 10.4103/jiaps.JIAPS_254_16

36. Kart Y, Karakuş OZ, Ateş O, Hakgüder G, Olguner M, Akgür FM. Altered expression of interstitial cells of Cajal in primary obstructive megaureter. *J Pediatric Urol.* (2013) 9:1028–31. doi: 10.1016/j.jpurol.2013.02.003

37. Lee HW, Baak CH, Lee MY, Kim YC. Spontaneous contractions augmented by cholinergic and adrenergic systems in the human ureter. *Korean J Physiol Pharmacol.* (2011) 15:37–41. doi: 10.4196/kjpp.2011.15.1.37

38. Mehrazma M, Tanzifi P, Rakhshani N. Changes in structure, interstitial Cajal-like cells and apoptosis of smooth muscle cells in congenital ureteropelvic junction obstruction. *Iran J Pediatr.* (2014) 24:105–10. doi: 10.1097/01.PAT.0000454556.77877.27

39. Metzger R, Schuster T, Till H, Stehr M, Franke FE, Dietz HG, et al. Cajal-like cells in the human upper urinary tract. *J Urol.* (2004) 172:769–72. doi: 10.1097/01.ju.0000130571.15243.59

40. Pande T, Dey SK, Chand K, Kinra P. Influence of interstitial cells of cajal in congenital ureteropelvic junction obstruction. *J Indian Assoc Pediatric Surg.* (2020) 25:231–5. doi: 10.4103/jiaps.JIAPS_115_19

41. Prişcă RA, Loghin A, Gozar HG, Moldovan C, Moso T, Derzsi Z, et al. Morphological aspects and distribution of interstitial cells of Cajal in the human upper urinary tract. *Turk Patoloji Derg.* (2014) 30:100–4. doi: 10.5146/tjpath.2014.01242

42. Senol C, Onaran M, Gurocak S, Gonul II, Tan MO. Changes in Cajal cell density in ureteropelvic junction obstruction in children. *J Pediatric Urol.* (2016) 12:e85. doi: 10.1016/j.jpurol.2015.08.010

43. Solari V, Piotrowska AP, Puri P. Altered expression of interstitial cells of Cajal in congenital ureteropelvic junction obstruction. *J Urol.* (2003) 170:2420–2. doi: 10.1097/01.ju.0000097401.03293.f0

44. Wishahi M, Mehena A, Elganzoury H, Badawy M, Hafiz E, El-Leithy T. Telocytes and Cajal cells distribution in renal pelvis, ureteropelvic junction (UPJ), and proximal ureter in normal upper urinary tract and UPJ obstruction: reappraisal of the etiology of UPJ obstruction. *Folia Morphol.* (2020). doi: 10.5603/FM.a2020.0119

45. Yang X, Zhang Y, Hu J. The expression of Cajal cells at the obstruction site of congenital pelviureteric junction obstruction and quantitative image analysis. *J Pediatric Surg.* (2009) 44:2339–42. doi: 10.1016/j.jpedsurg.2009.07.061

46. Murakumo M, Nonomura K, Yamashita T, Ushiki T, Abe K, Koyanagi T. Structural changes of collagen components and diminution of nerves in congenital ureteropelvic junction obstruction. *J Urol.* (1997) 157:1963–8. doi: 10.1016/S0022-5347(01)64910-3

47. Sui G, Rothery S, Dupont E, Fry C, Severs N. Gap junctions and connexin expression in human suburothelial interstitial cells. *BJU Int.* (2002) 90:118–29. doi: 10.1046/j.1464-410X.2002.02834.x

48. Mut T, Acar Ö, Oktar T, Kiliçaslan I, Esen T, Ander H, et al. Intraoperative inspection of the ureteropelvic junction during pyeloplasty is not sufficient to distinguish between extrinsic and intrinsic causes of obstruction: correlation with histological analysis. *J Pediatric Urol.* (2016) 12:223.e221–223. e226. doi: 10.1016/j.jpurol.2016.02.016

49. Lang RJ, Hashitani H. Pacemaker mechanisms driving pyeloureteric peristalsis: modulatory role of interstitial cells. *Adv Exp Med Biol.* (2019) 1124:77–101. doi: 10.1007/978-981-13-5895-1_3

50. Veress B, Ohlsson B. Spatial relationship between telocytes, interstitial cells of Cajal and the enteric nervous system in the human ileum and colon. *J Cell Mol Med.* (2020) 24:3399–406. doi: 10.1111/jcmm.15013

51. Schulman C, Duarte-Escalante O, Boyarsky S. The autonomic innervation of the ureter and ureterovesical junction. In: Lutzeyer W, Melchior H, editors. *Urodynamics.* Berlin: Springer-Verlag (1973). p. 90–7. doi: 10.1007/978-3-642-65640-8_14

52. Gockel I, Bohl JR, Eckardt VF, Junginger T. Reduction of interstitial cells of Cajal (ICC) associated with neuronal nitric oxide synthase (n-NOS) in patients with achalasia. *Am J Gastroenterol.* (2008) 103:856–64. doi: 10.1111/j.1572-0241.2007.01667.x

53. Wang H, Zhang Y, Liu W, Wu R, Chen X, Gu L, et al. Interstitial cells of Cajal reduce in number in recto-sigmoid Hirschsprung's disease

and total colonic aganglionosis. *Neurosci Lett.* (2009) 451:208–11. doi: 10.1016/j.neulet.2009.01.015

54. Der T, Bercik P, Donnelly G, Jackson T, Berezin I, Collins SM, et al. Interstitial cells of Cajal and inflammation-induced motor dysfunction in the mouse small intestine. *Gastroenterology.* (2000) 119:1590–9. doi: 10.1053/gast.2000.20221

55. Chang IY, Glasgow NJ, Takayama I, Horiguchi K, Sanders KM, et al. Loss of interstitial cells of Cajal and development of electrical dysfunction in murine small bowel obstruction. *J Physiol.* (2001) 536:555. doi: 10.1111/j.1469-7793.2001.0555c.xd

56. Gomez-Pinilla PJ, Gibbons SJ, Sarr MG, Kendrick ML, Robert Shen K, Cima RR, et al. Changes in interstitial cells of cajal with age in the human stomach and colon. *Neurogastroenterol Motil.* (2011) 23:36–44. doi: 10.1111/j.1365-2982.2010.01590.x

57. Wang THH, Angeli TR, Ishida S, Du P, Gharibans A, Paskaranandavadivel N, et al. The influence of interstitial cells of Cajal loss and aging on slow wave conduction velocity in the human stomach. *Physiol Rep.* (2021) 8:e14659. doi: 10.14814/phy2.14659

58. Lammers W, Ahmad H, Arafat K. Spatial and temporal variations in pacemaking and conduction in the isolated renal pelvis. *Am J Physiol.* (1996) 270:F567–74. doi: 10.1152/ajprenal.1996.270.4.F567

59. Ekinci S, Ertunc M, Ciftci A, Senocak M, Buyukpamukcu N, Onur R. Evaluation of Pelvic contractility in ureteropelvic junction obstruction: an experimental study. *Eur J Pediatric Surg.* (2004) 14:93–9. doi: 10.1055/s-2004-815854

60. Mccloskey KD. Interstitial cells of Cajal in the urinary tract. *Handb Exp Pharmacol.* (2011) 2:233–54. doi: 10.1007/978-3-642-16499-6_11

61. Hurtado R, Bub G, Herzlinger D. The pelvis–kidney junction contains HCN3, a hyperpolarization-activated cation channel that triggers ureter peristalsis. *Kidney Int.* (2010) 77:500–8. doi: 10.1038/ki.2009.483

14

Grading of Hydronephrosis: An Ongoing Challenge

Abdurrahman Onen*

Section of Pediatric Urology, Department of Pediatric Surgery, Faculty of Medicine, Dicle University, Diyarbakir, Turkey

*Correspondence:
Abdurrahman Onen
aonenmd@gmail.com

The crucial point for prompt diagnostics, ideal therapeutic approach, and follow-up of hydronephrosis associated with UPJ anomalies in children is the severity of hydronephrosis. Such many hydronephrosis grading systems as AP diameter, SFU, radiology, UTD, and Onen have been developed to evaluate hydronephrosis severity in infants. Unfortunately, it is still an ongoing challenge and there is no consensus between different disciplines. AP diameter is a very dynamic parameter and is affected by many factors (hydration, bladder filling, position, respiration). More importantly, its measurement is very variable and misleading due to different renal pelvic configurations. The radiology grading system has the same grades 1, 2, and 3 as the SFU grading system with addition of the AP diameter for the first 3 grades. This grading system divides parenchymal loss into two different grades. Grade 4 represents mild parenchymal loss while grade 5 suggests severe parenchymal loss. However, it is operator dependent, is not decisive, and does not differentiate grades 4 and 5 clearly. All grades of SFU are very variable between operators and clinicians. UTD classification aims to put all significant abnormal urinary findings together including the kidney, ureter, and bladder and thus determines the risk level for infants with any urinary disease. Different renal deterioration risks occur depending on the mechanism of hydronephrosis. Therefore, SFU and UTD classification may result in significant confusion and misleading in determining the severity of hydronephrosis. SFU-4 and UTD-P3 represent a considerable range of severity of hydronephrosis. Both represent minimal thinning of the medullary parenchyma and severe thinning of the cortical parenchyma (cyst-like hydronephrotic kidneys) at the same grade. The wide definition of SFU-4 and UTD-P3 fails to indicate accurately the severity of hydronephrosis and thus significantly misleads from a prompt treatment. They do not suggest who need surgical treatment and who can safely be followed non-operatively. The anatomy and physiology of the 4 suborgans of the kidney (renal pelvis, calices, medulla, and cortex) are completely different from each other. Therefore, each part of the kidney affect and behave differently as a response to UPJ-type hydronephrosis (UPJHN) depending on the severity of hydronephrosis. The upgraded Onen hydronephrosis grading system has been developed based on this basic evidence both for prenatal and post-natal periods. The Onen grading system determines specific detailed findings of significant renal damage, which clearly show and suggest who can safely be followed conservatively from who will need surgical intervention for UPJHN. Neither AP diameter nor radiology, SFU, or UTD classification is the gold standard in determining the severity of hydronephrosis. All these grading systems are based on subjective parameters and are affected by many factors. They do not determine the exact severity of UPJHN and thus cause permanent renal damage due to a delay in surgical decision in some infants while they may cause an unnecessary surgery in others. The Onen grading system has resolved all disadvantages of other grading systems and promises a safer follow-up and a prompt treatment for UPJHN. It is an accurate and easily reproducible grading that has high sensitivity and specificity.

Keywords: children, hydronephrosis, ureteropelvic junction obstruction, grading, treatment, surgery

INTRODUCTION

Urinary ultrasound (US) is the best we have for the diagnosis and follow-up of both prenatal and post-natal hydronephrosis as a similar modality (1–11). It is non-invasive, easily available, fast, and low-cost; can be performed directly in bedside manner; and does not involve radiation. It shows the size of kidneys, thickness, and appearance of parenchyma (echogenicity, corticomedullary differentiation, cortical cysts), severity of hydronephrosis, ureteral dilation, and bladder anatomy (1, 2, 4–6, 9–11).

Ultrasound not only gives anatomic details but also gives some functional clues about the urinary system. It, therefore, provides excellent diagnostic accuracy. There are two important benefits of ultrasound: It determines the severity of hydronephrosis promptly and the time and necessity of other diagnostics (1, 3–6, 8, 10–12).

We need to determine specific criteria and risky findings suggestive of renal damage, which help clinicians to decide a prompt therapeutic approach. In this review, we will outline the most recent criteria to accurately determine the severity of hydronephrosis and thus predict who may develop renal damage and need intervention compared with who can safely be followed conservatively.

ANATOMO-PHYSIO-PATHOLOGY OF URETEROPELVIC JUNCTION TYPE HYDRONEPHROSIS (UPJHN)

The kidney has 2 main parts: The most important part is the renal parenchyma which does function and produce urine. The other is the pelvicaliceal system which collects and sends urine into the ureter. The renal parenchyma has two suborgans: medulla and cortex. The collecting system has two suborgans: renal pelvis and calices.

Two factors affect the kidney in infants with UPJHN: the compliance of renal pelvis and the degree of stenosis at UPJ. First, hydronephrosis develops as a protecting anatomic response. If the stenosis is severe and persists for a long period, then renal damage occurs as a functional response (1, 4, 11).

The anatomy and physiology of renal suborgans (renal pelvis, calices, medulla, and cortex) are completely different from each other. Therefore, each part affects and behaves differently as a response to UPJHN depending on the severity of hydronephrosis.

- *Renal pelvis*: The compliance of renal pelvis is very high in infants. It is particularly true for those who have extrarenal pelvic configuration due to their high expandability. The renal pelvis enlarges significantly to protect the renal parenchyma even in mild increase at renal pelvic pressure. Therefore, the risk of renal parenchymal damage is low and takes time in such infants comparatively. However, the risk of renal damage is high in those who have intra-renal pelvic configuration due to their low compliance.

- *Calices*: The expandability of calices is lower than that of the renal pelvis. Their compliance is low comparatively. Therefore, the dilation of calices means a greater degree (risk) of hydronephrosis compared to renal pelvic dilation alone. On the other hand, the calices enlarge to protect the renal parenchyma.

- *Medulla*: Its structure is somewhat similar to that of the lung. This part of the renal parenchyma is more expandable and compressed rapidly compared to the renal cortex. Depending on the degree of UPJ stenosis and time interval, the medulla becomes shorter and loses its pyramid form. The lower limit of the normal renal parenchymal thickness is 7.5 mm at the neonatal period, 8 mm at 1 year of age, and 10 mm at 2 years of age (10).

- *Cortex*: It is the most important functional part of the kidney. The normal thickness of the cortex is > 3 mm in infants. Its structure is somewhat similar to that of the liver, which is a relatively hard solid organ. Therefore, its compression or thinning means there is a significant risk of renal damage. In such cases, corticomedullary differentiation is lost and the thickness of the cortex decreases. It is an objective parameter because, opposite of the pelvicaliceal system, it is not affected from hydration, bladder filling, position, and respiration. The measurement points are not controversial and are not operator dependent. The renal parenchyma is measured at the thinnest point of the parenchyma on the longitudinal section of the kidney (1, 4, 5, 7, 10). It does not have intraobserver or interobserver variation (1, 10, 11, 13). Long-lasting cortical thinning is associated with low renal function and decrease in the number of nephrons (1, 4, 5, 11, 14). Therefore, the compressed and thinned cortex is suggestive of renal damage. The loss of more than half of the cortex (cortex thickness < 1.5 mm) is mostly associated with renal atrophy and irreversible renal damage.

The quality of the renal parenchyma which includes the *thickness* and *appearance* of the parenchyma is the most important and objective parameter to determine kidney exposure and thus the severity of hydronephrosis.

- *Thickness of the renal parenchyma*: Severe cortical damage (dilation, epithelial apoptosis, and atrophy of the renal tubules, and inflammation and fibrosis of the glomerulus) and decrease in glomerular filtration and renal function occur in infants, developing parenchymal loss due to severe UPJHN (14). The incidence of permanent functional loss is high (8–16%) while histopathological changes do not improve even after a successful pyeloplasty in infants with severe parenchymal loss which delayed surgery (1, 4, 5, 11, 15, 16). Loss of the renal cortex and reduced renal size are the result of tubular atrophy and correlate with chronic irreversible renal disease (15). The number of nephrons decreases, renal maturation is affected, and renal failure occurs in such cases (17).
- *Appearance of the renal parenchyma*: Hyperechogene parenchyme, cystic degeneration in the cortex, and loss of corticomedullary differentiation on ultrasound are findings suggesting significant renal damage, which are compatible with decrease in renal function on scintigraphy (1, 11). Cortical echogenicity is a parameter that correlates well with tubular atrophy and interstitial inflammation (15).

Another important parameter is the longitudinal length of both normal and hydronephrotic kidneys. The compensatory hypertrophy of the contralateral kidney (length > 20% of normal) means affected kidney worsening even if Onen-3 hydronephrosis is stable. The longitudinal length of the affected kidney should be higher than the normal value, depending on the severity of hydronephrosis. If the affected kidney length stays in the normal range despite severe hydronephrosis, it means the affected kidney undergoes atrophy.

HYDRONEPHROSIS GRADING SYSTEMS

Anterior–Posterior (AP) Diameter of Renal Pelvis (APDRP)

The measurement of the AP diameter of the renal pelvis is not standardized between different disciplines, and there is a consensus only in 64% of physicians (10, 18). Unfortunately, it is significantly operator dependent. Some sonographers measure the AP diameter at the largest point of the renal pelvis while others measure it at vertical plan. However, the APDRP is mostly measured at the parenchymal edge (hilus) during the transverse section of the kidney.

The renal pelvis and AP diameter is very dynamic; its measurement changes significantly depending on hydration, bladder filling, position (supine or prone), and respiration (1, 10, 12, 18, 19).

More importantly, its measurement is very variable and misleading due to different renal pelvic configurations. Hydronephrosis may be moderate even if the AP diameter is high in infants with extrarenal pelvic configuration. On the other hand, hydronephrosis may be very severe with significant parenchymal thinning even if the AP diameter is low in infants with intrarenal pelvic configuration. Therefore, if the

quality of parenchyma which is the most important factor in determining the degree of hydronephrosis is omitted and the AP diameter itself is accepted as the only finding for severity of hydronephrosis, then some infants may undergo an unnecessary surgery while some may result in permanent renal damage due to a delay for prompt surgery.

Disadvantages/limitations of APDRP:

- The rate of operator differences is very high
- AP diameter is low in dehydrated infants
- AP diameter is low in the empty bladder
- AP diameter is low in the expirium phase
- AP diameter is less ideally measured in supine position
- AP diameter (even low) is very risky in the presence of intrarenal pelvic configuration.

SFU Grading System

This grading system has been developed in 1993 (9) (**Figure 1**). It is quantitative and subjective. All grades of SFU are very variable between operators and clinicians (1, 4–6, 10, 11, 20–22). Therefore, it is not popular between disciplines other than pediatric urologists (1, 4, 5, 7, 10, 11, 19–21, 23–25).

Disadvantages/limitations of SFU

- *SFU-1 and SFU-2a*: Both indicate different degrees of renal pelvic dilation. Therefore, it is confusing and very difficult to differentiate each other (1, 2, 4). Moreover, follow-up, treatment, and prognosis of these two degrees are similar; all of them resolve spontaneously without renal damage (1, 2, 4, 5, 20).
- *SFU-2b and SFU-3*: Both represent different degrees of calyceal dilation. It is very operator dependent in differentiating the dilation of peripheral (minor) calices from those of central (major) calices due to a high discrepancy within and between raters for interpretation of the two types of calyceal dilation (26, 27). Therefore, it is subjective and confusing and it is very difficult to differentiate each other (1, 4).
- *SFU-3*: Although it represents only calyceal dilation, the pictures used for SFU-3 in the original article clearly show severe medullary thinning. This causes significant confusion among clinicians and radiologists.
- *SFU-4*: It represents minimal thinning of the medullary parenchyma (e.g., 6 mm) and severe thinning of the cortical parenchyma (e.g., 2 mm) and cyst-like hydronephrotic kidneys at the same grade (2). The wide definition of SFU-4 fails to demonstrate accurately the severity of hydronephrosis and thus significant misleads from a prompt treatment. It does not suggest who need surgery and who can safely be followed non-operatively. The first example (medulla thin) can safely be followed non-operatively while the second (cortex thin) clearly need surgery. This wide definition makes prognosis difficult to predict in UPJHN cases (1, 4–6, 8, 11, 28).

Radiology Grading System

The radiology grading system has partially been modified from SFU for post-natal use (7, 9) (**Figure 2**). It has the same grades 1, 2, and 3 as the SFU grading system (8, 14). In addition, it includes AP diameter for the grades 1, 2, and 3.

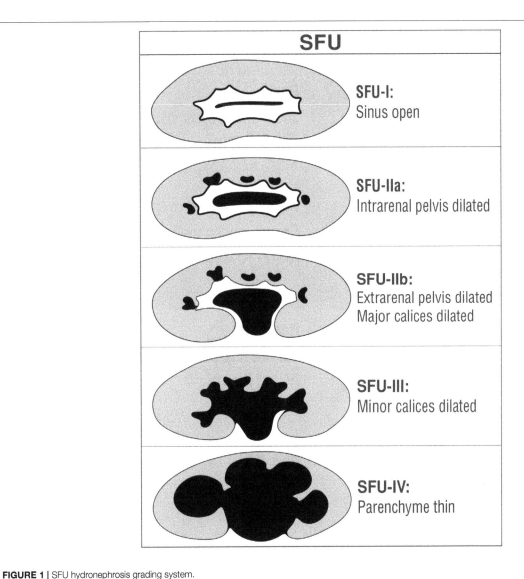

FIGURE 1 | SFU hydronephrosis grading system.

This grading system divides parenchymal loss into two different grades, suggesting the importance of the renal parenchyma to determine the severity of hydronephrosis which has a somewhat similar idea as in the Onen grading system (1, 4, 7). Grade 4 hydronephrosis represents mild parenchymal loss; grade 5, severe parenchymal loss.

Disadvantages/limitations of the radiology grading system

- *Radiology grades 1 and 2 (SFU-1 and SFU-2a):* Both indicate different degrees of renal pelvic dilation. Therefore, it is confusing and very difficult to differentiate each other (1, 2, 4). Moreover, follow-up, treatment, and prognosis of these two degree are similar; all of them resolve spontaneously without renal damage (1, 2, 4, 5, 20).
- *The usage of the AP diameter:* It makes this grading system even more confusing, because SFU grades and AP diameter are not parallel for many patients depending on different renal pelvic configurations. In addition, the AP diameter is affected

significantly by many factors as previously described in this review (1, 10, 12, 18, 19).
- *Radiology grades 4 and 5:* Grade 4 represents mild parenchymal loss, while grade 5 represents severe parenchymal loss. It is completely operator dependent, is not decisive, and does not differentiate grades 4 and 5 clearly. Therefore, between- and intra-rater reliability is low.

UTD Classification

UTD has been created retrospectively based on reviewing, combining, and summarizing the current literature (2) (**Figure 3**). It, therefore, is not an evidence-based grading system. Actually, it most likely has been modified from SFU and Onen grading systems (4, 9). It aims to put all significant abnormal urinary findings together including the kidney, ureter, and bladder and thus determines the risk level for a hydronephrotic infant with any kind urinary diseases. It

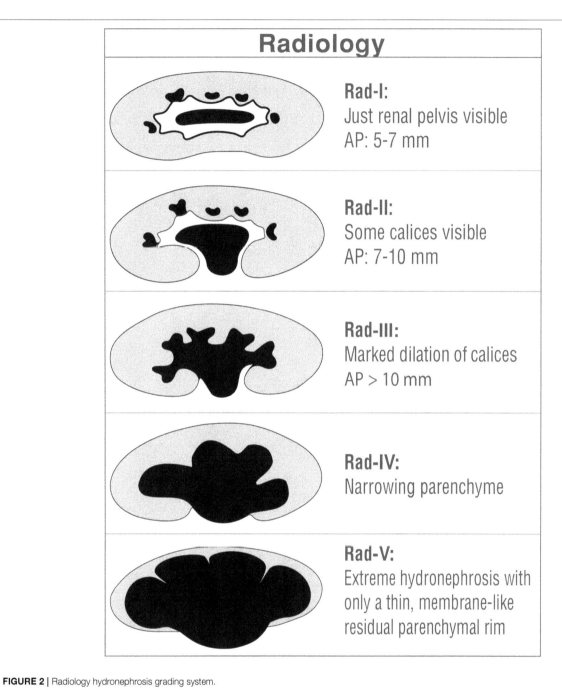

FIGURE 2 | Radiology hydronephrosis grading system.

includes such parameters as AP diameter of renal pelvis, central and peripheral calyceal dilation, renal parenchyma, ureteral abnormalities, and bladder abnormalities (2). All these findings are very important by themselves. However, the natural history, diagnosis, follow-up, treatment, and prognosis of urinary diseases are significantly different from each other depending on the etiopathology of hydronephrosis.

This classification suggests the general term "urinary tract dilation" to indicate ultrasound findings that include all ureteral and kidney dilations (2). It is clear that UPJ-type hydronephrosis,

UVJ-type hydroureteronephrosis, vesicoureteral reflux, bladder pathologies (ureterocele, diverticula, etc.), and posterior urethral valve cause hydronephrosis in very different ways. They may cause different levels and types of renal damage and prognosis (1, 4, 5). For example, Onen-3 (medulla thin) hydronephrosis due to UPJHN can be followed non-operatively while an infant with the same degree of hydronephrosis due to grade 5 reflux has a much higher risk of UTI, renal scar, and surgical need (1). Different renal deterioration risks occur depending on the mechanism of hydronephrosis. Therefore, UTD classification

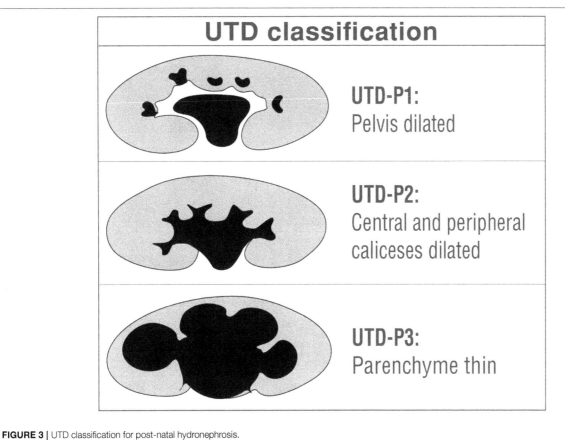

FIGURE 3 | UTD classification for post-natal hydronephrosis.

may result in significant confusion and mislead in determining the severity of hydronephrosis (1).

Disadvantages/limitations of UTD classification

- *Central and peripheral calices:* It is very operator dependent to differentiate the dilation of peripheral (minor) calices from those of central (major) calices due to a high discrepancy within and between raters for interpretation of the two types of calyceal dilation (26, 27). Therefore, it is subjective and confusing and is very difficult to differentiate each other (1, 4).
- *UTD-P3:* Like SFU, it represents minimal thinning of the medullary parenchyma (e.g., 6 mm) and severe thinning of the cortical parenchyma (e.g., 2 mm) and cyst-like hydronephrotic kidneys at the same grade (2). The wide definition of UTD-P3 fails to demonstrate accurately the severity of hydronephrosis and thus significant misleads from prompt treatment. It does not suggest who need surgical treatment and who can safely be followed non-operatively. The first example (medulla thin) can safely be followed non-operatively while the second (cortex thin) clearly need surgery. This wide definition makes prognosis difficult to predict in UPJHN cases (1, 4–6, 8, 11, 28).

Onen Grading System

This grading system has been developed for both prenatal and post-natal UPJHN (**Figure 4**). It is appropriate and applicable for both fetus and children, which standardize the language of the sonographers, clinicians, method of evaluation, and measurement of kidneys. The Onen grading system is terminologically simple and clear. Therefore, all disciplines including radiology, perinatology, pediatric nephrology, and pediatric urology can easily use not only for clinical practice but also for future researches.

The Onen grading system has evidence-based standardized objectives and reproducible parameters (4). It includes two categories of kidney findings. The first is dilation of the pelvicalyceal system; the second which is the most important category is the quality of the renal parenchyma (thickness and appearance) (1). This grading system divides thinning of the renal parenchyma into two grades: medullary thinning and cortical thinning. In addition, the appearance of the parenchyma (echogenicity, cortical cysts, corticomedullary differentiation) which is suggestive of renal damage is also taken into account in this grading system.

It was proposed on the basis of a well-known tight association between the severity of hydronephrosis and prognosis; renal deterioration may occur in severe hydronephrosis not timely and promptly treated (1, 4–6, 8, 11, 23, 29, 30). This grading system is beneficial in determining the possible risk of renal damage, surgical necessity, and prognosis in infants with UPJHN. Therefore, such cases can safely be followed based on this grading

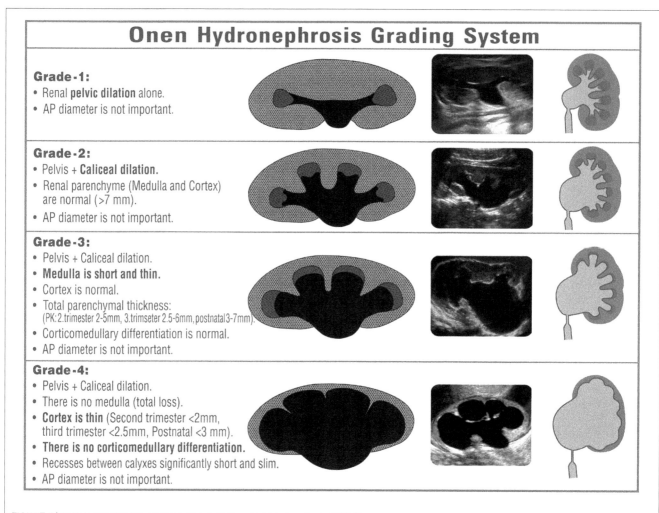

Onen Hydronephrosis Grading System

Grade-1:
- Renal **pelvic dilation** alone.
- AP diameter is not important.

Grade-2:
- Pelvis + **Caliceal dilation.**
- Renal parenchyme (Medulla and Cortex) are normal (>7 mm).
- AP diameter is not important.

Grade-3:
- Pelvis + Caliceal dilation.
- **Medulla is short and thin.**
- Cortex is normal.
- Total parenchymal thickness: (PK: 2.trimester 2–5mm, 3.trimeseter 2.5–6mm, postnatal 3–7mm).
- Corticomedullary differentiation is normal.
- AP diameter is not important.

Grade-4:
- Pelvis + Caliceal dilation.
- There is no medulla (total loss).
- **Cortex is thin** (Second trimester <2mm, third trimester <2.5mm, Postnatal <3 mm).
- **There is no corticomedullary differentiation.**
- Recesses between calyxes significantly short and slim.
- AP diameter is not important.

FIGURE 4 | Onen hydronephrosis grading system for both prenatal and post-natal UPJHN.

system. Because it determines clearly those infants who can be followed with ultrasound alone, who need renal scan, and who require surgery.

Our treatment and follow-up protocol for UPJHN based on the Onen grading system

- *Onen-1 UPJHN* cases neither need invasive evaluation nor need surgical treatment or antibiotic due to their benign nature; all they need is follow-up with ultrasound alone (**Figure 5**). A detailed urinary ultrasound at post-natal 1–3–6th months, 1 year, and 2 years of age is enough. If the Onen-1 does not increase or resolve, the follow-up can be ceased.
- *Onen-2 UPJHN* cases neither need invasive evaluation nor need antibiotic due to their benign nature; all they need is follow-up with ultrasound alone. However, about 10% of such infants will worsen and need pyeloplasty during follow-up. Therefore, they might be followed with ultrasound more closely comparing those of Onen-1 hydronephrosis. A detailed urinary ultrasound at post-natal 1–3–6th months and every 6 months until 3 years of age is enough. If Onen-2 decreases

to Onen-1 or resolve, the follow-up can be ceased. If Onen-2 persists, an ultrasound might be seen annually until 5 years of age and then the follow-up can be ceased with informing patients about such a symptom as pain or UTI.

- *Onen-3 UPJHN (medulla thin, PK = 3–7 mm)* patients need close follow-up including renal scan because about one-third of such children need pyeloplasty during follow-up. A detailed urinary ultrasound at post-natal 1st month, every 3 months until 2 years of age, and every 6 months until 3 years of age is reasonable. If the asymptomatic Onen-3 persists until 3 years of age with normal renal function, one of two ways might be discussed with the family; one is continuing invasive follow-up until adulthood, the other is performing a pyeloplasty with high success and thus preventing long-life invasive follow-up and prophylactic antibiotics (1, 5). If Onen-3 is diagnosed, we perform a renal scan. If the function and appearance (on ultrasound) of the ipsilateral kidney as well as contralateral kidney are normal, we follow them and see another ultrasound in 3 months. If Onen-3 decreases or stabilizes, we see the patient in the next 3 months; however, if Onen-3 gets worse,

Treatment and follow up protocol for UPJHN based on Onen grading system*									
	Ultrasound	Ultrasound interval	Renal scan	Renal scan interval	Prophylaxis	Treatment	Followup period	Surgical risk	Information
Onen-1	Yes	6 months	No	No	No	Conservative	2 years	1 %	Neither need invasive evaluation nor surgical treatment or antibiotic due to their benign atüre; they do not develop UTI or renal deterioration.
Onen-2	Yes	3-6 months	No	No	No	Conservative	3 years	10 %	Neither need invasive evaluation nor surgical treatment or antibiotic due to their benign atüre; they do not develop UTI or renal deterioration. They need more frequent ultrasound compared to Onen-1 hydronephrosis.
Onen-3	Yes	3 months	Yes	6 months	Yes (first year of life)	Conservative	3 years	30 %	Surgical indications: Onen-3 (thin medulla) (3-7mm) + • Presence of symptom (UTI, pain, stone) or • >20% compensatory growth in contralateral kidney • >10 units decrease in renal function or • Renal function <35% • Persistence until 3 years of age? (discuss with family)
Onen-4	Yes	2 weeks	Yes	1 month	Yes	Surgery	2 years	99%	Early intervention, after a short period (1-3 months) of follow up, is safer for preservation of renal function. Kidney function may not be measured accurately with this severity of hydronephrosis. This is particularly true for bilateral cases. Delay in prompt treatment may cause irreversible renal deterioration.

*Criteria for bad prognosis: Cortex less than half (<1,5mm), cyst-like kidney with no obvious recesses, cortical atrophy (marked reduction of kidney size), hyperechogenicity.

FIGURE 5 | Treatment and follow-up protocol for UPJHN based on the Onen grading system.

we perform a second renal scan to see renal function. If the function is under 35 or decrease by > 10 units, we perform pyeloplasty. If Onen-3 is diagnosed with renal function under 35, we look at the pictures of the scan in detail. If we believe that the decrease in renal function is correct and the reason of decrease in function is UPJHN, we decide to do surgery because we do not use the washout curve as a treatment criterion. On the other hand, if there is normal clearance of the pelvis and good washout, we look to ultrasound, renal scan, and sometimes VCUG to see if there is any other reason for the hydronephrosis such as a megaureter and reflux.

- *Onen-4 UPJHN (cortex thin, PK < 3 mm, no corticomedullary differentiation)* patients need surgical correction after a short period of follow-up (1–3 months). Renal function cannot objectively and accurately be assessed with this severity of hydronephrosis. It is particularly true for bilateral once (1, 4–6, 11, 30). Progressive permanent renal damage is inevitable when surgery is delayed in such cases (1, 4–6, 31). On the other hand, timely prompt surgical correction promises to improve decreased renal function in those severe cases (1, 4–6, 11, 30–32). When we see such a neonate with Onen-4, we perform an ultrasound in 1 week of life and then a second ultrasound with MAG3 1 month later. According to the results of these two tests, we decide to perform surgery or follow them conservatively for another month.

SURGICAL INDICATIONS FOR SEVERE HYDRONEPHROSIS ASSOCIATED WITH UPJ ANOMALIES BASED ON GRADING SYSTEMS

In the literature, a surgical decision for UPJHN has been made based on the increase in hydronephrosis on ultrasound in 70%

of cases, increase in hydronephrosis on ultrasound, decrease in renal function on scintigraphy in 15%, decrease in renal function on scintigraphy in 10%, and presence of symptom in 5% of UPJHN cases (1). Overall, a surgical decision has been made based on ultrasound findings in 85% of such cases. This rate will even increase if the false-positive findings and misleading (hydration, immobilization, catheterization, position, etc.) of renal scan is taken into account and if nobody uses drainage problems as a surgical indication. Therefore, correct determination of hydronephrosis severity is crucial for infants associated with UPJHN.

Surgical Indications for UPJHN Based on EAU and ESPU 2019 Guideline

Based on EAU and ESPU 2019 Guidelines on pediatric urology, surgical indications for UPJHN are impaired renal function (<40%), significant renal functional decrease (>10%) in control scans, poor drainage after furosemide injection, increased AP diameter, and SFU-III/IV (33). *All of these indications are problematic:*

- Impaired renal function (<40%) or a decrease in renal function of >10% can be a surgical indication with at least presence of Onen-3 or 4 (thin parenchyma) UPJHN. However, in children with calyceal dilation (Onen-2) alone, the reason of impaired function may be that either an etiology other than UPJHN or the impaired function may actually be false positive.
- Poor drainage function after administration of furosemide by itself should never be used as a surgical indication. This is because the drainage is poor even in UPJHN cases with only calyceal dilation (Onen-2).
- An increased AP diameter on ultrasound by itself should never be used as a surgical indication. It is very discussable. What degree is the increase in AP diameter? How many mm or

percent is the increase in AP diameter? At what location of renal pelvis is the AP diameter measured?

- SFU-3 represents only calyceal dilation with the normal renal parenchyma which should never be used as a surgical indication by itself.
- SFU-4 represents any degree of thinning in the renal parenchyma. The wide definition of SFU-4 fails to demonstrate accurately the severity of hydronephrosis and thus significantly misleads from prompt treatment. Those with cortical thinning definitely will need surgery while medullary thinning by itself (with normal renal function) does not need surgery.

Surgical Indications for UPJHN Based on the Hydronephrosis Severity Score (HSS)

It has been developed to determine the predictivity of pyeloplasty based on ultrasound and diuretic renogram findings (34). The crucial problem and disadvantage of HSS is that it relies on diuretic renogram and its curve. As we all know, renal scan is greatly affected from hydration, bladder catheterization, position, immobilization, function of the affected kidney, laterality (bilateral), diuretic timing, and operator experience (35–38).

Surgical Indications for UPJHN Based on the Pyeloplasty Prediction Score (PPS)

A recent study has suggested a pyeloplasty prediction score (PPS) using three ultrasound parameters to determine who need surgery and who do not in infants with UPJ-like hydronephrosis (39). They recommend a combination of SFU grade (A), transverse AP diameter (B), and the absolute percentage difference of ipsilateral and contralateral renal lengths at baseline (C) to predict a criterion for surgical need. This study suggests that any infant with UPJO-like hydronephrosis with a PPS of 8 or higher is 8 times more likely to undergo pyeloplasty (39). Unfortunately, none of these parameters is ideal to use due to many disadvantages and/or limitations as described in this review in details. We think that when we put problematic parameters together, it is difficult to get a correct beneficial result from them. Moreover, the laterality (normal right and left long length is different), contralateral or bilateral hydronephrosis, ipsilateral atrophy, or contralateral hypertrophy significantly changes the results of the pyeloplasty prediction score (A + B + C). The absolute percentage (C) would be low when there is a contralateral compensatory growth or an atrophy in ipsilateral kidney which will miss the severity of hydronephrosis. In addition, how would it be an objective criterion in bilateral cases? Any of these parameters can change the percentage (C) from 5 to 20%, which means the score may change from 0 to 4. We should use objective and reproducible criteria that are not affected by many parameters and are applicable for all patients.

Our Surgical Indications for UPJHN Based on the Onen Grading System

- Onen-4 (thin cortex) (<3 mm)
- Onen-3 (thin medulla) (3–7 mm) plus
- Presence of symptom (UTI, pain, stone) or

- >20% compensatory growth in contralateral kidney or
- >10 units decrease in renal function or
- Renal function <35%.

DISCUSSION

Although there are many studies in the literature, indications for invasive diagnostics, and surgery in infants with asymptomatic primary UPJHN are an ongoing challenge, and there is no consensus between different disciplines (1, 40). The surgical decision of such patients is done mostly based on ultrasound findings in the literature due to the invasiveness and high negative predictivity of renal scans in infants.

The crucial point for prompt diagnostics, ideal therapeutic approach, and follow-up of such patients is the severity of hydronephrosis. Such many hydronephrosis grading systems as AP diameter, SFU, radiology, UTD, and Onen have been developed to evaluate hydronephrosis severity in infants (1, 2, 4, 7, 9, 18, 23, 40–42) (Figure 6).

Though some authors have proposed cutoff values for the anterior posterior diameter of the renal pelvis, a simple threshold AP diameter value which separates non-obstructive dilation from obstructive dilatation of kidney does not exist (43). AP diameter is a very dynamic parameter and is affected by many factors (1, 10–12, 18, 19). Its measurement is very variable and misleading due to different renal pelvic configurations (1, 4, 10). Therefore, the use of AP diameters has certain disadvantages and limitations. It does not promptly demonstrate the degree of hydronephrosis (1, 2, 4–6, 11, 43). In the literature, there is no study determining intraobserver and interobserver reproducibility of the measurement of AP diameter. In addition, AP diameter does not consider calyceal dilation or the quality of the parenchyma, which may suggest severe cases of obstruction (1, 4, 12, 43).

The radiology grading system has the same grades 1, 2, and 3 as the SFU grading system with addition of the AP diameter for these 3 groups (7, 9). As we discussed above in detail, the AP diameter should not be a parameter in determining the severity of hydronephrosis for many significant reasons. This grading system divides parenchymal loss into two different grades, suggesting the importance of the renal parenchyma to determine the severity of hydronephrosis, which has somewhat a similar idea as that of the Onen hydronephrosis grading system (1, 4, 7). Radiology grade-4 hydronephrosis represents mild parenchymal loss while grade-5 represents severe parenchymal loss (7). However, it is operator dependent, is not decisive, and does not differentiate grades 4 and 5 clearly. Therefore, between- and intra-rater reliability is low.

The SFU grading system has many certain disadvantages and limitations. All grades are problematic and subjective. Both SFU-1 and SFU-2a represent different degrees of renal pelvic dilation. Therefore, it is confusing and is very difficult to differentiate each other (1, 2, 4). Moreover, follow-up, treatment, and prognosis of these two degree are similar; all of them resolve spontaneously without renal damage (1, 2, 4, 11, 20). They should be in

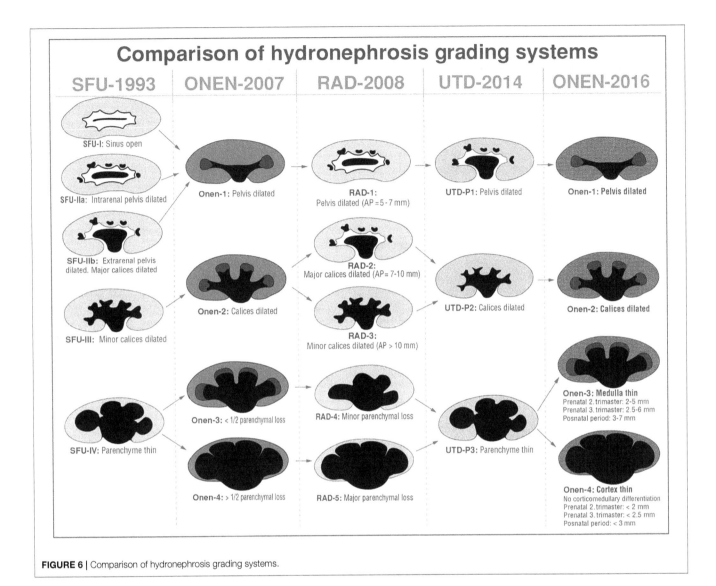

FIGURE 6 | Comparison of hydronephrosis grading systems.

the same degree of hydronephrosis. Both SFU-2b and SFU-3 represent different degrees of calyceal dilation (major vs. minor). Therefore, it is subjective, confusing, and very difficult to differentiate each other (1, 4). It can be influenced by the examiner (22). It has modest inter-rater reliability. Although SFU-3 represents only calyceal dilation, the pictures for SFU-3 show severe medullary thinning clearly. This causes significant confusion among the clinicians and radiologists (1, 4). High grades of SFU represent various features, making prognosis difficult to predict (1, 4, 8, 11, 28). It is subjective and can be influenced by the examiner (22). It has modest inter-rater reliability (43).

UTD-P classification appears to be modified partially from SFU and Onen grading system (4, 9). UTD-P1 and 2 have been modified from the Onen grading system (Onen-1 and 2) (4) while UTD-P3 has been modified from the SFU grading system (SFU-4) (9). This classification includes 3 different risk groups: low-risk (UTD-P1), intermediate-risk (UTD-P2), and high-risk (UTD-P3) groups (2, 29). None of these risk groups is the

gold standard for all patients. AP diameter >15 mm, peripheral calyceal dilation, and dilated ureter represent intermediate risk (UTD-P2). For example, bilateral grade-4 intra-renal reflux has exactly these findings. However, we all know that this does not represent intermediate risk. It should be in the high-risk group due to the fact that most of these patients develop significant renal damage and UTI breakthrough with fever. There are many similar examples suggesting that this risk scoring is not the standard for all such patients. Between- and within-rater reliability is moderate for this classification (26, 27).

Significant variability exists within and between raters in SFU, radiology grading, and UTD classification. This is because it is significantly operator dependent to differentiate the dilation of peripheral (minor) calices from those of central (major) calices due to a high discrepancy between raters for interpretation of the two types of calyceal dilation (26, 27). Therefore, the UTD score reliability has been found to be low (26, 27). It is exactly the same for SFU-2b and SFU-3 as well as radiology grades 2 and 3 (1, 4, 7, 9, 26, 27). Central (major) calices are somewhat like a neck between the renal pelvis and peripheral (minor) calices. In fact, the real calices are peripheral ones. Therefore, in our opinion, the exact calyceal dilation should be accepted as peripheral (minor) calyceal dilation. It is because it is significant dilation that is clearly different from renal pelvic dilation and is well-visualized and there is no high discrepancy between raters for interpretation (1, 4). Opposite to SFU, radiology, and UTD classification, the Onen grading system does not differ the central and peripheral calyceal dilation.

SFU-4 and UTD-P3 represent the same degree of hydronephrosis. Both represent any kind of renal parenchymal thinning (medulla or cortex), which is a considerable range of severity of hydronephrosis (2, 9). This wide definition of SFU-4 and UTD-P3 fails to demonstrate accurately the severity of hydronephrosis and thus significantly misleads from prompt treatment. They do not suggest who need surgical treatment and who can safely be followed non-operatively in infants with severe UPJHN (1, 2, 4–6, 11). In addition, these two grades make prognosis difficult to predict in UPJHN cases (1, 4, 8, 28).

The Onen hydronephrosis grading system which has been updated in 2016 determined specific detailed findings of significant renal damage, which clearly showed and suggested who can safely be treated conservatively from who will need surgical intervention for UPJHN (1). The intra-rater reliability of Onen grading is higher than that of SFU (2, 20). This grading system has been shown to have good inter- and intra-observer agreements in the diagnosis and follow-up of hydronephrosis in children (20). Intra-observer agreement for the diagnosis of hydronephrosis in prenatal ultrasound recently showed an almost perfect agreement in the Onen grading system (22).

Onen grading system has a sensitivity of 100%, specificity of 76%, and accuracy of 86.4% (21). In a recent study, all units that had Onen-1 and 2 were not obstructed and had renal function > 40% while Onen grade-4 had 100% specificity, meaning that it consistently predicts kidney damage due to obstruction when present (1, 21). Therefore, renal scan is required for only Onen-3 patients; thus, renal scan could be avoided in more than two-thirds of cases (1, 21).

The upgraded Onen grading system not only uses the quality of the renal parenchyma but also takes into account both affected and contralateral kidney size including longitudinal length and atrophy (1). Considering parenchymal loss, SFU and UTD are the same, differing from the Onen grading system that stratifies it in cortical and medullary loss, which was found clearly more precise (1, 21). Recent studies have shown that patients with Onen-3 had better renal function than Onen-4, proving that this difference is relevant to choosing this grading system for children (1, 4, 5, 11, 21). Bienias and Sikora have shown that 21/25 (84%) children with Onen grades 3 and 4 developed obstructive nephropathy with impaired relative function from 15 to 35% (44). If the study separated Onen-3 and 4, almost 100% of Onen-4 would have shown significant renal damage when they did not undergo surgery. Patients with Onen grade-4 had a 100% specificity while those with parenchymal loss not specified (SFU-4, UTD-3) had only 76% specificity regarding obstruction (21). Therefore, dividing SFU-4 or UTD-P3 into Onen grade-3 (medulla thin) and Onen-4 (cortex thin) provides

valuable important information in the follow-up and prognosis of high-grade hydronephrosis (1, 4, 8, 11, 21, 28).

DRF and SFU grade of hydronephrosis do not correctly reflect renal injury in bilateral UPJO; however, Onen hydronephrosis grade shows a significant relationship with renal histopathologic grade and can be an indicator for renal injury in UPJO (45). The Onen grading system is more relevant to post-natal prognosis of fetal hydronephrosis compared to SFU and UTD classification (1, 4, 5, 11). It has previously been shown that the Onen grading system determines the severity of UPJHN better and make follow-up more practical compared to SFU and UTD (1, 11). It is reliable and easily reproducible and plays a significant role in the diagnosis of obstruction in children (1, 21). Therefore, the use and popularity of this grading system are increasing around the world (20–22, 45).

In summary, neither AP diameter nor radiology or SFU or UTD is the gold standard in determining the severity of hydronephrosis. They have been shown to be unsuitable for standardizing due to evaluation criteria (1, 4, 21). All these grading systems are based on subjective parameters and are affected by many factors (1, 2, 4–7, 11, 25). They do not determine the exact severity of UPJHN and thus cause permanent renal damage due to delay in surgical decision in some infants while causing unnecessary surgery in others. In addition, they make prognosis difficult in UPJHN cases (1, 4, 8, 11, 28).

The 4 special structures of the kidney (pelvis, calices, medulla, cortex), each having different anatomophysiologic properties, should be taken into account in determining the severity of hydronephrosis. This is because each produces different risks of renal damage. The upgraded Onen hydronephrosis grading system has been developed based on this basic evidence. Therefore, it has resolved all disadvantages of other grading systems. It is an accurate and easily reproducible grading that has high sensitivity and specificity for diagnosis of obstruction, follow-up, prompt treatment (surgical requirement), and prognosis of infants with UPJHN (1, 4–6, 11, 21).

Regardless of the type of hydronephrosis grading systems, AP diameter and calyceal dilation by themselves are insufficient parameters in determining the severity of hydronephrosis. The quality of the renal parenchyma (thickness and appearance) which is the crucial parameter that parallels with renal function and damage should be taken into account in determining the severity of hydronephrosis. This is because it is an important parameter that significantly and objectively suggests who need invasive diagnostic and surgery while giving information about the clinical prognosis of infants associated with UPJHN.

AUTHOR CONTRIBUTIONS

The author confirms being the sole contributor of this work and has approved it for publication.

ACKNOWLEDGMENTS

The author would like to give his sincere thanks to Prof Steve Koff for improving my vision on hydronephrosis.

REFERENCES

1. Onen A. Üreteropelvik bileşke darligi. *Çocuk Cerrahisi Dergisi.* (2016) 30:55–79. doi: 10.5222/JTAPS.2016.055

2. Nguyen HT, Benson CB, Bromley B, Campbell JB Chow J, Coleman B, Cooper C, et al. Multidisciplinary consensus on the classification of prenatal and postnatal urinary tract dilation (UTD classification system). *J Pediatr Urol.* (2014) 10:982–99. doi: 10.1016/j.jpurol.2014.10.002

3. Passerotti CC, Kalish LA, Chow J, Passerotti AMS, Recabal P, Cendron M, et al. The predictive value of the first postnatal ultrasound in children with antenatal hydronephrosis. *J Pediatr Urol.* (2011) 7:128–36. doi: 10.1016/j.jpurol.2010.09.007

4. Onen A. An alternative hydronephrosis grading system to refine the criteria for exact severity of hydronephrosis and optimal treatment guidelines in neonates with primary UPJ-type hydronephrosis. *J Pediatr Urol.* (2007) 3:200–5. doi: 10.1016/j.jpurol.2006.08.002

5. Onen A. Treatment and outcome of prenatally detected newborn hydronephrosis. *J Pediatr Urol.* (2007) 3:469–76. doi: 10.1016/j.jpurol.2007.05.002

6. Onen A. Neonatal Hidronefrozlar. In: Onen A, editor. *Çocuk Cerrahisi ve Çocuk Ürolojisi Kitabi.* Istanbul: Nobel Tip Kitabevi. (2006). p. 345–66.

7. Riccabona M, Avni FE, Blickman JG, Dacher JN, Darge K, Lobo ML, et al. Imaging recommendations in paediatric uroradiology: minutes of the ESPR workgroup session on urinary tract ultrasonography and voiding cystourethrography. *Pediatr Radiol.* (2008) 38:138–45. doi: 10.1007/s00247-007-0695-7

8. Onen A. Üreteropelvik bileşke darliklari ve nadir üreter anomalileri. In: Onen A, editor. *Çocuk Cerrahisi ve Çocuk Ürolojisi Kitabi.* Istanbul: Nobel Tip Kitabevi (2006). p. 367–72.

9. Fernbach SK, Maizels M, Conway JJ. Ultrasound grading of hydronephrosis: introduction to the system used by the society for fetal urology. *Pediatr Radiol.* (1993) 23:478–80. doi: 10.1007/BF02012459

10. Kadioglu A. Renal measuruments, including lenght, parenchymal thicness, and medullary pyramid thickness, in healthy children: what are the normative ultrasound values? *Am J Roentgenol.* (2010) 194:509–15. doi: 10.2214/AJR.09.2986

11. Onen A, Yalinkaya A. *Possible Predictive Factors for A Safe Prenatal Follow-Up of Fetuses with Hydonephrosis. The 29th Congress of European Society of Pediatric Urology 11th – 14th April.* Helsinki: ESPU (2018).

12. Nguyen HT, Herndon ACD, Cooper C, Gatti J, Kirsch A, Kokorowski P, et al. The society for fetal urology consensus statement on the evaluation and management of antenatal hydronephrosis. *J Pediatr Urol.* (2010) 6:212–31. doi: 10.1016/j.jpurol.2010.02.205

13. Eze CU, Agwu KK, Ezeasor DN, Agwuna KK, Aronu AE, EI Mba El. Sonographic biometry of normal kidney dimensions among school-age children in Nsukka, Southeast Nigeria. *West Indian Med J.* (2014) 63:46–53. doi: 10.7727/wimj.2013.010

14. Konda R, Sakai K, Ota S, Abe Y, Hatakeyama T, Orikasa S. Ultrasound grade of hydronephrosis and severity of renal cortical damage on 99mtechnetium dimercaptosuccinic acid renal scan in infants with unilateral antenatal hydronephrosis during followup and after pyeloplasty. *J Urol.* (2002) 167:2159–63. doi: 10.1016/S0022-5347(05)65118-X

15. Moghazi S, Jones E, Schroepple J, Arya K, Mcclellan W, Hennigar RA, et al. Correlation of renal histopathology with sonographic findings. *Kidney Int.* (2005) 67:1515–20. doi: 10.1111/j.1523-1755.2005.00230.x

16. Stock JA, Krous HF, Heffernan J, Packer M, Kaplan GW. Correlation of renal biopsy and radionuclide renal scan differential function in patients with unilateral ureteropelvic junction obstruction. *J Urol.* (1995) 154:716–8. doi: 10.1016/S0022-5347(01)67142-8

17. Chevalier RL, Thornhill BA, Forbes MS, Kiley SC. Mechanism of renal injury and progression of renal disease in congenital obstructive nephropathy. *Pediatric Nephrol.* (2010) 25:687–97. doi: 10.1007/s00467-009-1316-5

18. Timberlake MD, Herndon CDA. Mild to moderate postnatal hydronephrosis grading systems and management. *Nat Rev Urol.* (2013) 10:649–56. doi: 10.1038/nrurol.2013.172

19. Pereira AK, Reis ZS, Bouzada MC, de Oliveira EA, Osanan G, Cabral AC. Antenatal ultrasonographic antero-posterior renal pelvis diameter measurement: is it a reliable way of defining fetal hydronephrosis? *Obstet Gynecol Int.* (2011) 2011:861–5. doi: 10.1155/2011/861865

20. Kim SY, Kim MJ, Yoon CS, Lee MS, Han KH, Lee MJ. Comparison of the reliability of two hydronephrosis grading systems: the society for fetal urology grading system vs. the Onen grading system. *Clin Radiol.* (2013) 68:484–90. doi: 10.1016/j.crad.2013.03.023

21. De Bessa Jr, Rodrigues CM, Chammas MC, Miranda EP, Gomes CM, Moscardi PR, et al. Diagnostic accuracy of Onen's alternative grading system combined with doppler evaluation of ureteral jets as an alternative in the diagnosis of obstructive hydronephrosis in children. *Peer J.* (2018) 6:e4791. doi: 10.7717/peerj.4791

22. Cho HY, Jung I, Kim YH, Kwon JY. Reliability of society of fetal urology and Onen grading system in fetal hydronephrosis. *Obstet Gynecol Sci.* (2019) 62:87–92. doi: 10.5468/ogs.2019.62.2.87

23. Dhillon HK. Prenatally diagnosed hydronephrosis: the great ormond street experience. *Br J Urol.* (1998) 81:39–44. doi: 10.1046/j.1464-410X.1998.0810s2039.x

24. Keays MA, Guerra LA, Mihill J, Raju G, Al-Asheeri N, Geier P, et al. Reliability assessment of society for fetal urology ultrasound grading system for hydronephrosis. *J Urol.* (2008) 180:1680–2. doi: 10.1016/j.juro.2008.03.107

25. Yamaçake KGR, Nguyen HT. Current management of antenatal hydronephrosis. *Pediatr Nephrol.* (2013) 28:237–43. doi: 10.1007/s00467-012-2240-7

26. Back SJ, Edgar JC, Weiss DA, Oliver ER, Bellah RD, Darge K. Rater reliability of postnatal urinary tract consensus classification. *Pediatric Radiol.* (2018) 48:1606–11. doi: 10.1007/s00247-018-4173-1

27. Rickard M, Easterbrook B, Kim S, DeMaria J, Lorenzo AJ, Braga LH, et al. Six of one, half a dozen of the other: a measure of multdicsiplinary inter/intra-rater reliability of the society for fetal urology and urinary tract dilation grading systems for hydronephrosis. *J Pediatr Urol.* (2017) 13:80.e81–5. doi: 10.1016/j.jpurol.2016.09.005

28. Sidhu G, Beyene J, Rosenblum ND. Outcome of isolated antenatal hydronephrosis. A systematic review and metanalysis. *Pediatr Nephrol.* (2006) 21:218–24. doi: 10.1007/s00467-005-2100-9

29. Pelliccia P, Papa SS, Cavallo F, Tagi VM, Serafino MD, Esposito F, et al. Prenatal and postnatal urinary tract dilation: advantages of a standardized ultrasound definition and classification. *J Ultrasound.* (2018) 22:5–12. doi: 10.1007/s40477-018-0340-3

30. Onen A, Jayanthi VR, Koff SA. Long-term follow-up of prenatally detected severe bilateral newborn hydronephrosis initially managed nonoperatively. *J Urol.* (2002) 168:1118e20. doi: 10.1016/S0022-5347(05)64604-6

31. Bansal R, Ansari MS, Srivastava A, Kapoor R. Longterm results of pyeloplasty in poorly functioning kidneys in the pediatric age group. *J Pediatr Urol.* (2012) 8:25–8. doi: 10.1016/j.jpurol.2010.12.012

32. Jindal B, Bal CS, Bhatnagar V. The role of renal function reserve estimation in children with hydronephrosis. *J Indian Assoc Paediatr Surg.* (2007) 12:196–201. doi: 10.4103/0971-9261.40834

33. Radmayr C, Bogaert G, Dogan HS, Kocvara R, Nijman JM, Stein R, et al. EAU guidelines on pediatric urology. In: *European Society for Paediatric Urology and European Association of Urology.* Arnhem: EAU Guidelines Office (2019). p. 55–9.

34. Babu R, Venkatachalapathy E, Sai V. Hydronephrosis severity score: an objective assessment of hydronephrosis severity in children-a preliminary report. *J Pediatr Urol.* (2019) 15:68.e6. doi: 10.1016/j.jpurol.2018.09.020

35. Shulkin BL, Mandell GA, Cooper JA, Leonard JC, Majd M, Parisi MT, et al. Procedure guideline for diuretic renography in children 3.0. *J Nucl Med Technol.* (2008) 36:162–8. doi: 10.2967/jnmt.108.056622

36. Piepsz A. Antenatal detection of pelviureteric junction stenosis: main controversies. *Semin Nucl Med.* (2011) 41:11–9. doi: 10.1053/j.semnuclmed.2010.07.008

37. Wong DC, Rossleigh MA, Farnsworth RH. Diuretic renography with the addition of quantitative gravity-assisted drainage in infants and children. *J Nucl Med.* (2000) 41:1030–6.

38. Turkolmez S, Atasever T, Turkolmez K, Gogus O. Comparison of three different diuretic renal scintigraphy protocols in patients with dilated upper urinary tracts. *Clin Nucl Med.* (2004) 29:154–60. doi: 10.1097/01.rlu.0000113852.57445.23

39. Li B, McGrath M, Farrokhyar F, Braga LH. Ultrasound-based scoring system for indication of pyeloplasty in patients with UPJO-like hydronephrosis. *Front Pediatr.* (2020) 8:353. doi: 10.3389/fped.2020.00353

40. Zanetta VC, Rosman BM, Bromley B, Shipp TD, Chow JS, Campbell JB, et al. Variations in management of mild prenatal hydronephrosis among maternal-fetal medicine obstetricians, pediatric urologists and radiologists. *J Urol.* (2012) 188:1935–9. doi: 10.1016/j.juro.2012.07.011

41. Carr MC. Ureteropelvic junction obstruction and multicystic dysplastic kidney: surgical management. In: Docimo SG, Canning DA, Khoury AE, editors. *The Kelalis-King-Belman Textbook of Clinical Pediatric Urology*, 5th ed. United Kingdom: Informa Healthcare UK Ltd. (2007). p. 479–86.

42. Carr MC, Ghoneimi AE. Anomalies and surgery of the ureteropelvic junction in children. In: Wein AJ, Kavoussi LR, Novick AC, Partin AW, Peters CA, editors. *Campbell-Walsh Urology*, 9th ed. Philadelphia: Saunders Elsevier (2007). p. 3359–82.

43. Sarin YK. Is it always necessary to treat an asymptomatic hydronephrosis due to ureteropelvic junction obstruction? *Indian J Pediatr.* (2017) 84:531–9. doi: 10.1007/s12098-017-2346-9

44. Bienias B Sikora P. Potential novel biomarkers of obstructive nephropathy in children with hydronephrosis. *Hindawi Dis.* (2018) 2018:105726. doi: 10.1155/2018/1015726

45. Lee YS, Jeong HJ, Im YJ, Kim MJ, Lee MJ, Yun M, et al. Factors indicating renal injury in pediatric bilateral ureteropelvic-junction obstruction. *Urology.* (2013) 81:873–9. doi: 10.1016/j.urology.2012.09.064

15

Redo Laparoscopic Pyeloplasty in Infants and Children: Feasible and Effective

Hamdan Al-Hazmi[1,2†], Matthieu Peycelon[1,3,4†], Elisabeth Carricaburu[1,3], Gianantonio Manzoni[1,5], Khalid Fouda Neel[1,2], Liza Ali[1,3], Christine Grapin[1,3,4], Annabel Paye-Jaouen[1,3] and Alaa El-Ghoneimi[1,3,4*]

[1] Department of Pediatric Urology, Robert-Debré University Hospital, Assistance Publique - Hôpitaux de Paris (APHP), Paris, France, [2] College of Medicine and King Saud University Medical City, King Saud University, Riyad, Saudi Arabia, [3] National Reference Center of Rare Urinary Tract Malformations (MARVU), Paris, France, [4] University of Paris, Paris, France, [5] Department of Pediatric Urology Fondazione Cà Granda Ospedale Maggiore Policlinico, Milan, Italy

*Correspondence:
Alaa El-Ghoneimi
alaa.elghoneimi@aphp.fr

Purpose: To determine the feasibility and effectiveness of redo laparoscopic pyeloplasty among patients with failed previous pyeloplasty, specifically examining rates of success and complications.

Materials and Methods: We retrospectively reviewed the charts of all patients, who underwent redo laparoscopic pyeloplasty from 2006 to 2017. This included patients who underwent primary pyeloplasty at our institution and those referred for failures. Analysis included demographics, operative time, complications, length of hospital stay, complications, and success. Success was defined as improvement of symptoms and hydronephrosis and/or improvement in drainage demonstrated by diuretic renogram, especially in those with persistent hydronephrosis. Descriptive statistics are presented.

Results: We identified 22 patients who underwent redo laparoscopic pyeloplasty. All had Anderson-Hynes technique except two cases in which ureterocalicostomy was performed. Median (IQR) follow-up was 29 (2–120) months, median time between primary pyeloplasty and redo laparoscopic pyeloplasty was 12 (7–49) months. The median operative time was 200 (50–250) min, and median length of hospital stay was 3 (2–10) days. The procedure was feasible in all cases without conversion. During follow-up, all but two patients demonstrated an improvement in the symptoms and the degree of hydronephrosis. Ninety-one percent of patients experienced success and no major complications were noted.

Conclusions: Redo laparoscopic pyeloplasty is feasible and effective with a high success rate and low complication rate.

Keywords: redo laparoscopic pyeloplasty, uretero-pelvic junction obstruction, open pyeloplasty, minimally invasive surgical procedures, children

INTRODUCTION

Secondary uretero-pelvic junction obstruction (UPJO) may occur following pyeloplasty in up to 11% of patients who may require redo surgical intervention (1). Redo surgical intervention (open, laparoscopic, or robotic) has been shown to be more effective than endourological procedures (JJ stent insertion, balloon dilatation, and endopyelotomy) (2, 3). Laparoscopic and robotic redo pyeloplasty are alternatives to redo open pyeloplasty (ROP), which have been reported with good success (2, 4, 5).

Redo laparoscopic pyeloplasty (RLP) offers a minimally invasive approach with the benefits of a shorter period of convalescence and decreased morbidity compared to open surgery; however, it requires advanced laparoscopic skills (6). Herein, we report our outcomes with redo laparoscopic pyeloplasty to determine the feasibility and effectiveness of this procedure in a relatively large case series. And our hypothesis was: do infants and children with persistent UPJO undergoing redo laparoscopic pyeloplasty have the same overall success rate in comparison to the ones reported in open redo pyeloplasty series?

MATERIALS AND METHODS

Patient Selection and Study Design

After obtaining ethical board approval for conduct of the study, we retrospectively reviewed the charts of all patients who underwent laparoscopic pyeloplasty for secondary UPJO at a single institution, University Hospital of Robert-Debré, Paris, France, from December 2006 to October 2017. Inclusion criteria were all patients with persistent UPJO undergoing redo transperitoneal laparoscopic pyeloplasty at our institution regardless of if their primary pyeloplasty was performed at our institution or elsewhere. Exclusion criteria were: primary UPJO repair or any redo pyeloplasty performed by an open, retroperitoneal laparoscopic or robot-assisted approach.

Variables and Outcome Measures

Variables collected from the reviewed charts included: patient sex, age at primary surgery and redo surgery; type of previous interventions and number of attempts to repair the UPJO; confirmation of persistent UPJO following initial surgery, both clinically and radiologically (renal ultrasound, dynamic renal scintigraphy (MAG-3) and/or magnetic resonance urography (MRU); indication for redo pyeloplasty; use of stents and drains; length of hospitalization; postoperative complications; need for readmission and subsequent procedures; and success rate.

Indications for redo laparoscopic pyeloplasty were persistent severe hydronephrosis (defined as (1) AP diameter > 30 mm or (2) AP diameter > 15 mm and flank pain or (3) AP diameter > 15 mm and other US criteria (calyceal dilation, thin parenchyma)] associated with at least one of the following:

repeated febrile urinary tract infection (UTI) documented by positive urine culture, flank pain, and persistence obstruction on retro or ante grade imaging (retrograde pyelography, renal scintigraphy, MRU). Surgical complications were classified according to the Clavien-Dindo classification (7). Febrile UTIs included both a fever and a urine cultures with >100,000 colony forming units.

Follow-up evaluation was performed using renal ultrasound and dynamic renal scintigraphy. Success defined as improvement of symptoms (neither UTI, nor flank pain) and decrease of hydronephrosis, determined by the measurement of post-operative anteroposterior diameter (APD, in millimeters) and/or the absence of calyceal dilation. In patients with persistent hydronephrosis, an absence of obstruction on the drainage curve on functional imaging (defined as a $t_{1/2}$ <20 min on nuclear scan) was used to define success. A single dedicated radiologist was not available to perform all follow-up imaging.

Surgical Details

The surgery was performed by staff pediatric urologists. A transperitoneal approach was used for all patients undergoing redo laparoscopic pyeloplasty. The patient was positioned in the supine position with an inflatable device under the flank of the operated side. The surgeon stood on the opposite side of the obstructed kidney (**Figure 1**), and all ports were inserted with the child in the supine position. Four ports were used for all patients (**Figure 2**), namely a 5-mm umbilical port by open access for the camera; and insufflation was maintained at 10 mm Hg. Then two 3-mm working ports were inserted under direct vision, one midway between the xiphoid process and umbilicus and the other midway between the symphysis pubis and the umbilicus, and the fourth accessory trocar, 3-mm, in the ipsilateral iliac fossa. The fourth was used to help to reduce the operative time for suction and exposition. There was some modification in the placing of trocars between young and older children (**Figures 2A,B**). A 45° lateral position was obtained by inflating the device. The

Abbreviations: APD, Anteroposterior diameter; IQR, Interquartile; Kg, kilogram; MCUG, Micturating cysto-urethrogram; MRU, Magnetic resonance urography; OP, Open pyeloplasty; PP, Primary pyeloplasty; RLP, Redo laparoscopic pyeloplasty; ROP, Redo open pyeloplasty; UPJ, Uretero-pelvic junction; UPJO, Uretero-pelvic junction obstruction; UTI, Urinary tract infection.

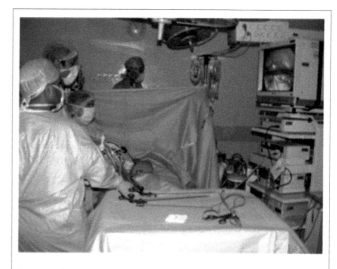

FIGURE 1 | Position of the surgeon and all assistants.

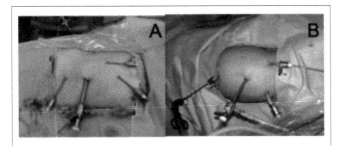

FIGURE 2 | (A) Placement of the four trocars in older children: all in the midline; **(B)** Placement of the four trocars in young children.

TABLE 1 | Previous surgical details (N = 22).

	Patients (%)
Initial surgeries	
Retroperitoneal laparoscopic pyeloplasty	3 (13.6)
Open dorsal lumbotomy	15 (68.1)
Open anterior subcostal incision	4 (18.2)
Temporizing interventions	
Nephrostomy tube	8 (36.4)
JJ stent	5 (22.7)
Endoscopic balloon dilatation	2 (9.1)
None	7 (31.2)

TABLE 2 | Demographic and clinical data (N = 22).

	Minimum	Maximum	Median
Age at redo (months)	4.5	183	22
Weight (kg)	6	50	10
Operative time (min)	50	250	200
Hospital stay (days)	2	10	3
Follow-up duration (months)	2	120	29

colon was mobilized to expose the renal pelvis after removing all the adhesions until the UPJ was identified. The reason for the failure of previous surgery was identified. All patients underwent Anderson-Hynes dismembered pyeloplasty except two cases in which ureterocalicostomy was performed because the renal pelvis was intrarenal and difficult to identify due to severe fibrosis from the prior surgery, one of them had already failed redo robotic pyeloplasty elsewhere. Continuous suture was used for the anastomosis in all patients except one in whom interrupted suturing was required due to a thick-walled renal pelvis and signs of inflammation. We used a 5-0 Polyglactin suture for all patients. A JJ stent was placed in an antegrade fashion in all cases except one who had trouble in passing the JJ stent through the ureterovesical junction, so an externalized stent was placed instead (Multipurpose stent, BARD®, Salt Lake City, UT). A Foley catheter was placed and left until day 1 postoperatively.

All patients were followed-up clinically for pain or UTI, and radiologically by renal ultrasound (four times the 1st year, then twice the next year and finally once a year for 5 years). An isotopic renal scan or MRU was obtained in the setting of persistent severe hydronephrosis. The choice to use either an isotopic renal scan or a MRU was done on the functional imaging studies used for the preoperative evaluation.

Descriptive statistics were performed with SPSSV20 software (IBM SPSS Statistics, IBM Corp, Armonk, NY).

RESULTS

Twenty-two patients (four girls and 18 boys) underwent laparoscopic pyeloplasty for persistent UPJO during the study period. Thirteen patients (59.1%) were referred from an outside hospital after failed pyeloplasty. Median age at initial surgery was 8 months (IQR: 3–48). Surgery was performed on the right side in 10 patients and the left in 12 patients. Pre-operative micturating cysto-urethrogram (MCUG) was ordered in case of UTI after the first pyeloplasty (N = 4) and was normal in these selected patients except one patient with contralateral grade I vesicoureteral reflux that was observed. Previous surgical details are listed in **Table 1**.

Median age at redo pyeloplasty was 22 months (IQR: 11–84 months), median weight at surgery was 10 kg (8–15 kg), and median time between primary and redo repair was 12 months (7–49 months). Patient details at time of redo laparoscopic

pyeloplasty are shown in **Table 2**. Cause of failure of the primary repair was identified during laparoscopy as follows: adhesions around the UPJ area causing the obstruction (10 patients, 45.4%), stenotic UPJ area (seven patients, 31.8%), high anastomosis (anastomosis was not in the dependent area) (two patients, 9.1%), crossing vessels (one patient, post primary open repair, 4.5%), long segment stricture (one patient, 4.5%), and one patient had a twist of the anastomosis (4.5%) (**Table 3**). Preoperative and postoperative imaging features are reported in **Table 4**.

A JJ stent was used for all patients for a median duration of 2.5 months (IQR: 2–3 months). There was a single exception to this in the case of a patient in whom there was difficulty passing the JJ stent beyond the uretero-vesical junction, so an externalized ureteral catheter was used for 10 days.

Median operative time was calculated from the start of insufflation until exsufflation and was 200 min (IQR: 180–225 minutes). Median length of hospital stay was 3 days (IQR: 3–4.25 days). Two patients had a prolonged hospital stay: the first one kept admitted 10 days to await resolution of a urine leak from the anastomosis site. The other was readmitted on day 11 after surgery for pyelonephritis Intravenous antibiotics were injected at hospital for 6 days.

The procedure was feasible in all cases without conversion to open surgery. No major complications (Clavien ≥ III) were recorded.

Median follow-up duration was 29 months (IQR: 15–62 months). All patients were asymptomatic except one patient who presented with post-operative pain and pyelonephritis 11 days after surgery. Nineteen patients demonstrated an improvement in hydronephrosis. Three showed severe hydronephrosis with an obstructed curve on nuclear study. One patient had a wide dependent draining anastomosis on retrograde pyelography

TABLE 3 | Side, intraoperative finding, procedure, and outcome ($N = 22$).

	Number	Percentage (%)
Symptoms	10	45.5
UTI	7	31.8
Pain	4	18.2
Asymptomatic	12	54.5
Obstruction side: Right/Left	10/12	45.5/54.5
Intraoperative Cause of Failure		
1. Adhesions causing obstruction	10	45.5
2. UPJ obstruction	7	31.8
3. Highly inserted ureter	2	9
4. Crossing vessels	1	4.5
5. Long segment stricture	1	4.5
6. Twist of the anastomosis	1	4.5
Intraoperative Procedure:		
1. Anderson-Hynes technique	20	90.9
2. Ureterocalicostomy	2	9.1
Readmission		
Yes	2	9.1
No	20	90.9
Outcome		
Success	20	90.9
Failure	2	9.1

TABLE 4 | Preoperative and postoperative imaging features (N=22).

	Preoperative evaluation	Postoperative evaluation	p-value
Anteroposterior diameter on renal ultrasound (mm) (median and IQR)	36 (34–50)	15 (9–45)	0.04
Functional imaging (N, %)			0.99
Renal scintigraphy	3 (13.6)	2 (9)	
MRU	19 (86.4)	10 (45.5)	
$t_{1/2}$ (median and IQR)	40 (35–50)	14 (13.5–14.5)	
Split renal function on functional studies (%) (median and IQR)	32 (24–46)	33 (21–39)	0.79
Pyelography (N, %)			0.52
Antegrade	5 (22.7)	0 (0)	
Retrograde	8 (36.4)	2 (9)	

without obstruction and therefore was not considered a failure. The other two patients had obstruction confirmed on retrograde pyelography (RPG). In these patients, the kidney was palpable and on ultrasound exhibited worsening of hydronephrosis with the average APD increased from 33 mm to 51 mm and decreased renal function by renography from 25 to 7%. One underwent endoscopic balloon dilatation after the RPG and the second underwent a redo laparoscopic pyeloplasty. Both are doing well after their repeat intervention.

Overall success of redo laparoscopic pyeloplasty was 90.9%.

DISCUSSION

The first attempt of laparoscopic pyeloplasty for primary ureteropelvic junction obstruction was described for adults at the end of twentieth century in 1993 followed by reports for children in 1995 (8–10). Only one of these cases had secondary ureteropelvic junction obstruction after failure of open pyeloplasty (8). Since that time, the role of laparoscopic and robotic assisted pyeloplasty has evolved to take a more primary role in the management of primary UPJO, regardless of age or trans peritoneal vs. retroperitoneal approach (11–15). However, the gold standard for redo cases has general been considered an open pyeloplasty and thus redo laparoscopic pyeloplasty in children has not been widely applied. With the advent of improving minimally invasive techniques and increasing familiarity with these approaches, many have advocated using minimally invasive techniques in the redo setting. In a prospective, case–control study of open vs. laparoscopic pyeloplasty, 30 patients with UPJO were compared. This showed comparable results with the laparoscopic approach

being associated with a decrease in hospital stay and complication rates when compared to children in the open cohort (16, 17).

Management options in failed pyeloplasty include JJ stent placement, balloon dilatation endopyelotomy, and redo surgery (2, 3). Lower success rates have been reported endoscopic procedures as compared to redo pyeloplasty, which is not surprising (2, 3, 18). However, Dy et al. reported that at least one endoscopic procedure was performed prior to definitive redo-pyeloplasty in 11% of children with failed pyeloplasty (1).

Performing a redo-UPJO is a challenging surgery. Despite encouraging outcomes achieved with both laparoscopy and robotics, success rates are likely to be lower than those obtained in the primary setting (19).

Redo laparoscopic pyeloplasty has well-established merits, including reduced morbidity, reduced hospital stays, and reduced pain compared to open pyeloplasty (19). However, this challenging technique must be performed by experienced surgeons due to the extensive scarring and fibrosis noted from the previous procedure (4). Basiri et al. evaluated the feasibility and effectiveness of RLP and found that 100% of children showed improved renal function after undergoing secondary UPJO treated by RLP, lending credence to its value over immediately attempting an open repair (20).

In our previously reported experience, primary laparoscopic pyeloplasty has a 98% success rate, which is higher than the 90.9% reported in the current study of redo laparoscopic pyeloplasties (21). Our current findings are similar to those reported by Abdel-Karim et al. (22). Similarly, Moscardi et al. had a 90% success rate of 11 redo laparoscopic pyeloplasty, and they showed no difference in the outcome between primary laparoscopic pyeloplasty and redo laparoscopic pyeloplasty in terms of operative time, complications, and success rate (23).

Redo laparoscopic pyeloplasty has been reported in adults and children usually using the transperitoneal approach but occasionally through a retroperitoneal approach (4, 24). Although the retroperitoneal approach is still our preference for primary cases, we have chosen the transperitoneal approach for secondary cases (21). This choice has been made to avoid dissecting through secondary adhesions in the retroperitoneal space, and to limit the dissection to the UPJ and proximal ureter.

Interestingly, most of the cases that we report in the current study were performed in an open fashion for the primary surgery, and not all initially underwent a retroperitoneal approach for their initial surgery. It raises the question of whether a better option would be a retroperitoneal laparoscopic approach for a redo pyeloplasty if the patient originally underwent a transperitoneal approach.

Factors, such as young age at initial surgery (<6 months), missed anatomic findings at the first intervention (long ureteral segment narrowing or crossing vessels) and dry anastomosis (prolonged urinary diversion) have been associated with pyeloplasty failure (13, 25). The degree of adhesion and fibrosis is highly variable, which may be secondary to healing factors of the patients as well as the technical difficulty in the primary surgery, such as an incomplete or unfavorable position of the anastomosis between the renal pelvis and ureter or urinoma (26). Additionally, peri pelvic fibrosis, excessive scarring, and thermal energy, which can cause more tissue reactions and fibrosis can be associated with failures (27). These reasons support the findings we report in our cohort.

The long median time between primary and redo surgeries in our series is explained by the large (13 out of 22) number of patients referred to us from outside, which is the same observation noticed by Moscardi et al. (23). It would have been pertinent to examine factors associated with primary pyeloplasty failure, given the fact that over half of the patients were referrals, we did not feel that we could justify such an analysis using our data.

In our experience, two factors have been identified for the success of this procedure. First, the use of MRU as an anatomical and functional imaging studies during the preoperative management is a useful tool to assess the anatomy of the kidney and the renal pelvis, to measure the thickness of the parenchyma and to evaluate the split renal function. The first study from Perez-Brayfield et al. in 2003 concluded that dynamic contrast enhanced MRI provided equivalent information about renal function but superior information regarding morphology in a single study without ionizing radiation (28). A multi-institutional study in 2014 including 369 patients reported an equivalence of MRU to renal scintigraphy making substitution of MRU for RS acceptable (29). In our study, 19 (86.4%) patients were evaluated with a MRU. We strongly believe this imaging is better than a renal scintigraphy as it provides a better evaluation of the pelvis anatomy. Median split renal function of the operated kidney was 32 and 33% preoperatively and postoperatively, respectively ($p > 0.05$). However, functional studies were not unfortunately performed routinely after the redo surgery either in cases of preoperative evaluation showed asymmetrical function or remaining hydronephrosis. Secondly, the experience of our team in using minimally invasive surgery in our daily practice helps the laparoscopic approach to provide easily a global exposure of the pelvis and the ureter without the need to extensively dissect or mobilize the kidney (12, 21, 30–34). In selected cases with an extensive fibrosis of multi-operated renal pelvis, an alternative approach by ureterocalicostomy was deemed most appropriate.

There are multiple limitations worth discussing in the present study. First and foremost is the retrospective nature and small number of included patients. Furthermore, the fact that over half of the patients were referred to our institution makes it challenging to comment at all on how the initial surgical approach could have impacted the redo procedure that we report upon herein. The minority of patients underwent a laparoscopic pyeloplasty for their primary repair. However, as the primary goal of the study was to examine the feasibility and effectiveness of performing laparoscopic pyeloplasty in the redo setting, particularly in the setting of such a high proportion of prior open repairs, we feel that the limitations are acceptable so long as the reader is aware of them.

CONCLUSION

Redo laparoscopic pyeloplasty is both a feasible and effective procedure for the management of failed primary pyeloplasty, regardless of whether the initial surgery was performed open or laparoscopic. Given the benefits of shorter hospitalization and reduced pain following any minimally invasive procedure, it should be strongly considered as an option for any pediatric patient presenting with a recurrent UPJ obstruction.

AUTHOR CONTRIBUTIONS

HA-H, MP, EC, GM, CG, AP-J, and AE-G contributed conception and design of the study. HA-H, MP, EC, KN, LA, and AE-G organized the database. HA-H, LA, and MP performed the statistical analysis. HA-H wrote the first draft of the manuscript. MP, GM, AP-J, LA, and AE-G wrote sections of the manuscript. All authors contributed to manuscript revision, read, and approved the submitted version.

ACKNOWLEDGMENTS

The authors thank M. Francesca MONN, Department of Urology, Eastern Virginia Medical School, VA (USA) for valuable comments on the study and for assistance with language editing and proofreading.

REFERENCES

1. Dy GW, Hsi RS, Holt SK, Lendvay TS, Gore JL, Harper JD. National trends in secondary procedures following pediatric pyeloplasty. *J Urol.* (2016) 195:1209–14. doi: 10.1016/j.juro.2015.11.010

2. Romao RLP, Koyle MA, Pippi Salle JL, Alotay A, Figueroa VH, Lorenzo AJ, et al. Failed pyeloplasty in children: revisiting the unknown. *Urology.* (2013) 82:1145–7. doi: 10.1016/j.urology.2013.06.049

3. Thomas JC, de Marco RT, Donohoe JM, Adams MC, Pope JC, Brock JW. Management of the failed pyeloplasty: a contemporary review. *J Urol.* (2005) 174:2363–6. doi: 10.1097/01.ju.0000180420.11915.31

4. Piaggio LA, Noh PH, González R. Reoperative laparoscopic pyeloplasty

in children: comparison with open surgery. *J Urol.* (2007) 177:1878–82. doi: 10.1016/j.juro.2007.01.053

5. Lindgren BW, Hagerty J, Meyer T, Cheng EY. Robot-assisted laparoscopic reoperative repair for failed pyeloplasty in children: a safe and highly effective treatment option. *J Urol.* (2012) 188:932–7. doi: 10.1016/j.juro.2012.04.118

6. Knoedler J, Han L, Granberg C, Kramer S, Chow G, Gettman M, et al. Population-based comparison of laparoscopic and open pyeloplasty in paediatric pelvi-ureteric junction obstruction. *BJU Int.* (2013) 111:1141–7. doi: 10.1111/bju.12039

7. Clavien PA, Barkun J, de Oliveira ML, Vauthey JN, Dindo D, Schulick RD, et al. The clavien-Dindo classification of surgical complications: five-year experience. *Ann Surg.* (2009) 250:187–96. doi: 10.1097/SLA.0b013e3181b13ca2

8. Schuessler WW, Grune MT, Tecuanhuey LV, Preminger GM. Laparoscopic dismembered pyeloplasty. *J Urol.* (1993) 150:1795–9. doi: 10.1016/S0022-5347(17)35898-6

9. Kavoussi LR, Peters CA. Laparoscopic pyeloplasty. *J Urol.* (1993) 150:1891–4. doi: 10.1016/S0022-5347(17)35926-8

10. Peters CA, Schlussel RN, Retik AB. Pediatric laparoscopic dismembered pyeloplasty. *J Urol.* (1995) 153:1962–5. doi: 10.1016/S0022-5347(01)67378-6

11. Yeung CK, Tam YH, Sihoe JD, Lee KH, Liu KW. Retroperitoneoscopic dismembered pyeloplasty for pelvi-ureteric junction obstruction in infants and children. *BJU Int.* (2001) 87:509–13. doi: 10.1046/j.1464-410X.2001.00129.x

12. El-Ghoneimi A, Farhat W, Bolduc S, Bagli D, McLorie G, Aigrain Y, et al. Laparoscopic dismembered pyeloplasty by a retroperitoneal approach in children. *BJU Int.* (2003) 92:104–8. doi: 10.1046/j.1464-410X.2003.04266.x

13. Metzelder ML, Schier F, Petersen C, Truss M, Ure BM. Laparoscopic transabdominal pyeloplasty in children is feasible irrespective of age. *J Urol.* (2006) 175:688–91. doi: 10.1016/S0022-5347(05)00179-5

14. Atug F, Burgess SV, Castle EP, Thomas R. Role of robotics in the management of secondary ureteropelvic junction obstruction. *Int J Clin Pract.* (2006) 60:9–11. doi: 10.1111/j.1368-5031.2006.00701.x

15. Reddy M, Nerli RB, Bashetty R, Ravish IR. Laparoscopic dismembered pyeloplasty in children. *J Urol.* (2005) 174:700–2. doi: 10.1097/01.ju.0000164738.78606.78

16. Piaggio LA, Corbetta JP, Weller S, Dingevan RA, Duran V, Ruiz J, et al. Comparative, prospective, case-control study of open versus laparoscopic pyeloplasty in children with ureteropelvic junction obstruction: long-term results. *Front Pediatr.* (2017) 5:10. doi: 10.3389/fped.2017.00010

17 Bansal P, Gupta A, Mongha R, Narayan S, Das RK, Bera M, et al. Laparoscopic versus open pyeloplasty: comparison of two surgical approaches- a single centre experience of three years. *Indian J Surg.* (2011) 73:264–7. doi: 10.1007/s12262-011-0237-2

18. Braga LHP, Lorenzo AJ, Skeldon S, Dave S, Bagli DJ, Khoury AE, et al. Failed pyeloplasty in children: comparative analysis of retrograde endopyelotomy versus redo pyeloplasty. *J Urol.* (2007) 178:2571–5. doi: 10.1016/j.juro.2007.08.050

19. Autorino R, Eden C, El-Ghoneimi A, Guazzoni G, Buffi N, Peters CA, et al. Robot-assisted and laparoscopic repair of ureteropelvic junction obstruction: a systematic review and meta-analysis. *Eur Urol.* (2014) 65:430–52. doi: 10.1016/j.eururo.2013.06.053

20. Basiri A, Behjati S, Zand S, Moghaddam SMH. Laparoscopic pyeloplasty in secondary ureteropelvic junction obstruction after failed open surgery. *J Endourol.* (2007) 21:1045–51. doi: 10.1089/end.2006.0414

21. Blanc T, Muller C, Abdoul H, Peev S, Paye-Jaouen A, Peycelon M, et al. Retroperitoneal laparoscopic pyeloplasty in children: long-term outcome and critical analysis of 10-year experience in a teaching center. *Eur Urol.* (2013) 63:565–72. doi: 10.1016/j.eururo.2012.07.051

22. Abdel-Karim AM, Fahmy A, Moussa A, Rashad H, Elbadry M, Badawy H, et al. Laparoscopic pyeloplasty versus open pyeloplasty for recurrent ureteropelvic junction obstruction in children. *J Pediatr Urol.* (2016) 12:401.e1–6. doi: 10.1016/j.jpurol.2016.06.010

23. Moscardi PRM, Barbosa JABA, Andrade HS, Mello MF, Cezarino BN, Oliveira LM, et al. Reoperative laparoscopic ureteropelvic junction obstruction repair in children: safety and efficacy of the technique. *J Urol.* (2017) 197:798–804. doi: 10.1016/j.juro.2016.10.062

24. Eden C, Gianduzzo T, Chang C, Thiruchelvam N, Jones A. Extraperitoneal laparoscopic pyeloplasty for primary and secondary ureteropelvic junction obstruction. *J Urol.* (2004) 172:2308–11. doi: 10.1097/01.ju.0000143904.17666.0b

25. Kapoor A, Allard CB. Laparoscopic pyeloplasty: the standard of care for ureteropelvic junction obstruction. *Can Urol Assoc J.* (2011) 5:136–8. doi: 10.5489/cuaj.11036

26. Kojima Y, Sasaki S, Mizuno K, Tozawa K, Hayashi Y, Kohri K. Laparoscopic dismembered pyeloplasty for ureteropelvic junction obstruction in children. *Int J Urol.* (2009) 16:472–6. doi: 10.1111/j.1442-2042.2009.02282.x

27. Song SH, Lee C, Jung J, Kim SJ, Park S, Park H, et al. A comparative study of pediatric open pyeloplasty, laparoscopy-assisted extracorporeal pyeloplasty, and robot-assisted laparoscopic pyeloplasty. *PLoS ONE.* (2017) 12:e0175026. doi: 10.1371/journal.pone.0175026

28. Perez-Brayfield MR, Kirsch AJ, Jones RA, Grattan-Smith JD. A prospective study comparing ultrasound, nuclear scintigraphy and dynamic contrast enhanced magnetic resonance imaging in the evaluation of hydronephrosis. *J Urol.* (2003) 170:1330–4. doi: 10.1097/01.ju.0000086775.66329.00

29. Claudon M, Durand E, Grenier N, Prigent A, Balvay D, Chaumet-Riffaud P, et al. Chronic urinary obstruction: evaluation of dynamic contrast-enhanced MR urography for measurement of split renal function. *Radiology.* (2014) 273:801–12. doi: 10.1148/radiol.14131819

30. El-Ghoneimi A, Sauty L, Maintenant J, Macher MA, Lottmann H, Aigrain Y. Laparoscopic retroperitoneal nephrectomy in high risk children. *J Urol.* (2000) 164:1076–9. doi: 10.1097/00005392-200009020-00039

31. Bonnard A, Fouquet V, Carricaburu E, Aigrain Y, El-Ghoneimi A. Retroperitoneal laparoscopic versus open pyeloplasty in children. *J Urol.* (2005) 173:1710–3. doi: 10.1097/01.ju.0000154169.74458.32

32. Blanc T, Koulouris E, Botto N, Paye-Jaouen A, El-Ghoneimi A. Laparoscopic pyeloplasty in children with horseshoe kidney. *J Urol.* (2014) 191:1097–103. doi: 10.1016/j.juro.2013.10.059

33. Blanc T, Muller C, Pons M, Pashootan P, Paye-Jaouen A, El Ghoneimi A. Laparoscopic mitrofanoff procedure in children: critical analysis of difficulties and benefits. *J Pediatr Urol.* (2015) 11:28.e1–8. doi: 10.1016/j.jpurol.2014.07.013

34. Peycelon M, Rembeyo G, Tanase A, Muller CO, Blanc T, Alhazmi H, et al. Laparoscopic retroperitoneal approach for retrocaval ureter in children. *World J Urol.* (2019) 38:2055–62. doi: 10.1007/s00345-019-02849-w

16

Ultrasound-Based Scoring System for Indication of Pyeloplasty in Patients with UPJO-Like Hydronephrosis

Bruce Li[1], Melissa McGrath[2,3,4], Forough Farrokhyar[4,5] and Luis H. Braga[2,3,4,5]*

[1] Michael G. DeGroote School of Medicine, McMaster University, Hamilton, ON, Canada, [2] McMaster Pediatric Surgical Research Collaborative, McMaster University, Hamilton, ON, Canada, [3] Division of Urology, McMaster University, Hamilton, ON, Canada, [4] McMaster Children's Hospital Foundation, Hamilton, ON, Canada, [5] Department of Health Research, Methods, Evidence & Impact, McMaster University, Hamilton, ON, Canada

Correspondence:
Luis H. Braga
lhbraga@gmail.com

Background: Previous scoring systems have used renal scan parameters to assess severity of ureteropelvic junction obstruction-like hydronephrosis (UPJO-like HN), however this information is not always reliable due to protocol variation across centers and renogram limitations. Therefore, we sought to evaluate the Pyeloplasty Prediction Score (PPS), which utilizes only baseline ultrasound measurements to predict the likelihood of pyeloplasty in infants with UPJO-like.

Methods: PPS was developed using three ultrasound parameters, Society of Fetal Urology (SFU) grade, transverse anteroposterior (APD), and the absolute percentage difference of ipsilateral and contralateral renal lengths at baseline. PPS was evaluated using prospectively collected prenatal hydronephrosis data ($n = 928$) of patients with UPJO-HN. Children with vesicoureteral reflux. primary megaureter, other associated anomalies, bilateral HN and <3 months of follow-up were excluded. Scores were analyzed regarding its usefulness in predicting which patients would be more likely to undergo pyeloplasty. Sensitivity, specificity, likelihood ratios (LR) and receiver operating characteristic (ROC) curve were determined.

Results: Of 353 patients, 275 (78%) were male, 268 (76%) had left UPJO-like HN, and 81 (23%) had a pyeloplasty. The median age at baseline was 3 months (IQR 1–5). The PPS system was highly accurate in distinguishing patients who underwent pyeloplasty using baseline ultrasound measurements (AUC: 0.902). PPS of 7 and 8 were found to have a sensitivity of 85 and 78%, and specificity of 81 and 90%, respectively. PPS of 8 was associated with a LR of 7.8, indicating that these patients were eight times more likely to undergo pyeloplasty.

Conclusion: Overall, PPS could detect patients more likely to undergo pyeloplasty using baseline ultrasound measurements. Those with a PPS of eight or higher were eight times more likely to undergo pyeloplasty.

Keywords: ureteropelvic junction obstruction, prenatal hydronephrosis, pyeloplasty, classification, ultrasonography

INTRODUCTION

Prenatal hydronephrosis is one of the most commonly detected ultrasound findings, affecting 1–5% of pregnancies, and is usually detected during the third trimester as an incidental finding (1). Ureteropelvic junction obstruction-like hydronephrosis (UPJO-like HN) is one of the most common congenital causes of prenatal hydronephrosis (1). If left untreated, the severe hydronephrosis (HN) due to obstruction can lead to a clinical symptoms such as urinary tract infections, hematuria, progressive deterioration of renal function, and permanent kidney damage (1–3). Thus, early detection and surgical intervention of UPJO cases provides benefits by reducing the length of time the kidney is obstructed. However, a large proportion of UPJO-like [isolated hydronephrosis (pelvic distension) with or without dilated calyces] cases are benign in nature and spontaneously resolve. Therefore, the challenge with UPJO-like patients is identifying those that warrant further testing and would benefit from intervention in a timely manner to reduce associated morbidities.

Scoring systems have been developed to be utilized as an adjunctive tool to help predict those patients in need of pyeloplasty. Many of these scoring systems rely on ultrasound measurements of the afflicted kidney and on diuretic renogram findings. Nevertheless, nuclear studies pose an issue to the external validity of these scoring systems, as their protocols vary significantly across different centers (4). Consequently, interpretation of the drainage patterns, renogram curves and T1/2 times can be subjective and unreliable.

The primary objective of this study was to create a scoring system, the pyeloplasty prediction score (PPS), based on baseline ultrasound findings only, and evaluate its utility in predicting pyeloplasty in infants with UPJO-like. We hypothesized that the proposed scoring system could discriminate those who will resolve spontaneously from those who will end up having surgical intervention.

MATERIALS AND METHODS

After obtaining Research Ethics Board approval (13-62D), we reviewed our prospectively collected prenatal hydronephrosis database ($n = 928$) from a tertiary pediatric hospital and identified those who were diagnosed with UPJO-like hydronephrosis between 2008 and 2019. We excluded infants with vesicoureteral reflux, primary megaureter (hydroureteronephrosis), duplication anomalies, bilateral cases, other genitourinary anomalies (Prune-Belly, posterior urethral valves, horseshoe kidneys, neurogenic bladder, multicystic dysplastic kidney), and those with <3 months of follow-up.

Calculation of the Pyeloplasty Prediction Score

For each case, characteristics were collected, and only baseline (initial visit) ultrasound measurements were analyzed. The PPS scoring system was then retrospectively applied to each included case. Ultrasound measurements were conducted following institutional protocol, such as no pretest patient hydration to minimize measurement bias, with the patient in supine position, measurement pre- and post-void to confirm an empty bladder, using the same two ultrasound machines, by two technicians specialized in pediatric renal bladder ultrasound, who were specifically assigned to the Pediatric Urology Service.

The clinical outcome was resolution of HN or surgical intervention with a pyeloplasty. HN resolution was defined as two consecutive ultrasounds showing either Society for Fetal Urology (SFU) grade 1 or less, or renal pelvis anteroposterior diameter (APD) of 10 mm or less (5). Indications for pyeloplasty were based on the following protocol: 1-Worsening of hydronephrosis, characterized by increase in the transverse APD of the renal pelvis with or without change (increase) of SFU grade on repeat ultrasounds; or 2-Deterioration of differential renal function (DRF) >10% on repeated renal scans; or 3-Initial renal function <40% associated with an obstructive (ascending) curve on renogram; or 4-Worsening of hydronephrosis associated with a T1/2 time >30 min, or 5-Development of symptoms (sepsis, febrile urinary tract infections, stones).

PPS was based on three widely used ultrasound variables at baseline: SFU grade, transverse APD, and absolute percentage difference in renal length. APD was calculated in the transverse view, by measuring the distance between the parenchymal lips at the renal hilum in the mid-section. The extra-renal and intra-renal measurements for APD were taken and the larger of the two was recorded in the prospective database to be used in the PPS calculation. Renal length was measured in ipsilateral and contralateral kidneys in the longitudinal view, such that the distance between the most distant points of the upper and lower poles was captured. **Figures 1A,B** demonstrate the technique for measuring renal length and APD using electronic calipers, respectively. Each of these variables were assigned a value out of four, with zero being normal variant or least severe and four being the most severe; thus, making the PPS score total range from 0 to 12.

The SFU grading system ranges from normal, 1, 2, 3, 4 which corresponded to a score of 0, 1, 2, 3, 4, respectively (6).

The APD measurement was grouped as <5, 5–10, 11–15, 16–19, ≥20 mm corresponding to scores of 0, 1, 2, 3, 4, respectively. The APD category values were established based on current evidence that generally, the larger the APD, the greater the risk of obstructive uropathy (7–9), and thus a greater likelihood of surgical intervention (8, 10–12). An APD <5 mm is not considered as HN, which is why a score of 0 was assigned. A post-natal APD value <10 mm is considered as physiologic HN and APD values from 10 to 15 mm are associated with low risk of obstructive uropathy, which both correspond to the Urinary Tract Dilation (UTD) Classification System's P1 designation (13). The P1 designation is the lowest risk stratum in the UTD

Abbreviations: UPJO-like, Ureteropelvic junction obstruction-like (isolated hydronephrosis); PPS, Pyeloplasty Prediction Score; HN, Hydronephrosis; SFU, Society of Fetal Urology; APD, Anteroposterior diameter; IQR, Interquartile range; CI, Confidence interval; ROC, Receiver operating characteristic curve; LR, Likelihood ratio; PPV, Positive predictive value; HSS, Hydronephrosis Severity Score; DMSA, Dimercaptosuccinic acid; DRF, Differential renal function; SNDRF, Supra-normal differential renal function.

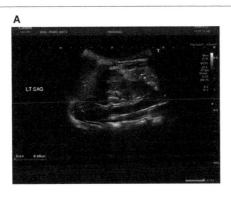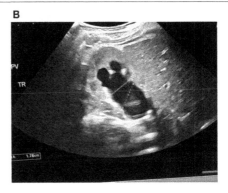

FIGURE 1 | Example measurements of ultrasound renal parameters for the Pyeloplasty Prediction Score in **(A)** longitudinal view of the left kidney with electronic calipers measuring renal length as the maximal distance between the upper and lower poles and **(B)** transverse view of the right kidney with green electronic calipers measuring true anteroposterior diameter (APD) as the distance between the parenchymal lips at the renal hilum in the mid-section. Blue electronic calipers represent the incorrect method of measuring APD as the calipers are not aligned to the parenchymal lips.

post-natal classification, which is why those two APD categories been assigned lower severity scores as 1 and 2, respectively. An APD value of 16 or greater was found by Dias et al. to have the best diagnostic odds ratio to identify infants who had pyeloplasty performed, which corresponds to the category of 16–19 mm (10). Multiple literature sources vary in terms of what APD cutoff value has the greatest likelihood of surgery, but are generally consistent in that an APD of at least 20 mm or greater is associated with the highest likelihood of pyeloplasty, which is why it was designated the greatest score of 4 (14, 15).

Absolute percentage difference between renal lengths was grouped as <5% (error variation), 5–10, 11–15, 16–19, ≥20% corresponding to scores of 0, 1, 2, 3, 4, respectively. The absolute percentage difference was taken by the following equation:

$$\left[100\% \times \frac{\left(\dfrac{Ipsilateral\ Renal}{Length} - \dfrac{Contralateral\ Renal}{Length} \right)}{Ipsilateral\ Renal\ Length} \right].$$

The three scores were then summed for a total score out of 12. The details of scoring criteria are described in **Table 1**.

The PPS system was analyzed for its usefulness in predicting which patients were more likely to undergo pyeloplasty. A trial of various cut-points was done to establish an optimal threshold that would maximize sensitivity and specificity of the scoring system. Sensitivity, specificity, likelihood ratios (LR) with their corresponding 95% confidence intervals (CI) and a receiver-operating characteristic (ROC) curve were determined. A p-value equal to or <0.05 was considered statistically significant. SPSS version 26 (www.ibm.com) were used for analysis.

RESULTS

Overall, from 928 prenatal HN patients in our database, a total of 353 with UPJO-like (isolated HN) qualified for analysis based on inclusion and exclusion criteria. Of the 353 included infants, 275 (78%) were male and 268 had HN on the left side (76%). The

median age of the cohort at baseline (initial visit) was 3 months (IQR 1–5 months). In 81 of the 353 patients (23%), kidneys were considered obstructed based on our criteria (previously stated in the methods section), and a pyeloplasty was performed.

The area under the ROC curve (AUC) was 0.902, demonstrating the accuracy of the PPS score in identifying patients more likely to undergo a pyeloplasty (**Figure 2A**). The PPS could result in a score of 1 to 12, through testing of various modeling scenarios, a score of 7–8 was found to be the optimal cut-off point, with the highest levels of sensitivity and specificity for discriminating patients that would likely be candidates for a pyeloplasty. The sensitivities of a PPS score of 7 and 8 were found to be 85 and 78%, respectively (**Figure 2B**). The specificities of a PPS score of 7 and 8 were found to be 81 and 90%, respectively (**Figure 2B**).

The LRs of the PPS score range (1–12) increased progressively as the score increased, as expected. The optimal cut-point score of 8 was found to have a LR of 7.8 (**Figure 3**). Based on LR values, we stratified the patients into three risk categories, according to the likelihood of undergoing pyeloplasty (**Figure 3**).

DISCUSSION

The present study involved the development and analysis of a prediction scoring system for pyeloplasty in UPJO-like HN using only baseline ultrasound characteristics. Our findings show that PPS was highly accurate in distinguishing patients who ended up having a pyeloplasty from those managed non-surgically. Based on our findings, the optimal cut-off point where pediatric urologists could consider indicating a pyeloplasty should be a PPS ≥8, provided they followed the same pyeloplasty indications, as outline in our protocol. Only two patients were recorded as false negatives, such that the PPS score was below eight at baseline, yet eventually had pyeloplasty. These two cases initially presented to office with very mild hydronephrosis but over repeated follow-up found worsening of the condition. As previously described, one of the indications for pyeloplasty at our institution is worsening of hydronephrosis by APD or SFU grade, which is why these two

TABLE 1 | The Pyeloplasty Prediction Score is based on three parameters: society of fetal urology (SFU) grade of the ultrasound, transverse anteroposterior diameter (APD) measurement, and the absolute percentage difference between the lengths of the ipsilateral and contralateral kidneys.

A.	SFU grading of affected kidney on ultrasound
0	Normal
1	SFU Grade 1
2	SFU Grade 2
3	SFU Grade 3
4	SFU Grade 4

B.	APD measurement of affected kidney on ultrasound
0	<5 mm
1	5–10 mm
2	11–15 mm
3	16–19 mm
4	≥20 mm

C.	Absolute percentage difference between the ipsilateral and contralateral renal lengths |[100% * (Ipsilateral Renal Length- Contralateral Renal Length)/Ipsilateral Renal Length]|
0	<5%
1	5%–10%
2	11%–15%
3	16%–19%
4	≥20%

PPS = A + B + C

Each parameter is assigned a score from 0 to 4, 0 being least severe and 4 being most.

patients qualified for surgical intervention. With respect to false positives, there were no patients that scored above 8 and did not have surgical intervention. Based on the sensitivity and specificity calculations, clinicians can expect a 90% probability that those with a score ≥ 8 will end up having a pyeloplasty in the future. The LR indicated that patients with a PPS ≥ 8 were eight times more likely to have surgery vs. no surgery.

Indications for Pyeloplasty

The indications for pyeloplasty at our center are consistent with what has been previously published in the literature. Within the entire prenatal hydronephrosis database of 928 patients, there were 353 cases of UPJO-like HN which were followed prospectively. Of those 353 patients, only 81 had surgical intervention, which translates into a pyeloplasty rate of 23%. Dhillon et al., one of the first groups to introduce the concept of non-surgical management for UPJO-like HN, had highlighted that approximately one-third of the infants in their series ended up having surgical intervention, which is similar to our figures (15).

Pyeloplasty indications have been well-established in the main urological textbooks. According to Campbell-Walsh 12th edition textbook, widely accepted indications for pyeloplasty include

"increasing APD on ultrasonography, low or decreasing DRF, breakthrough infections while on prophylactic antibiotics, or symptomatic hydronephrosis in older infants and children" (16).

Nevertheless, controversy surrounding some of these indications due to inherent subjectivity still exists. Low or decreasing differential renal function does not specify an actual value for decreased function or decreasing function, thus how low or how much has decreased to indicate need for pyeloplasty is subjective to some degree. Some authors may consider < 40% DRF as a cut-off (17) while others may push it even lower to <35% (18). Similarly, this subjectivity issue arises with increase in the APD of renal pelvis. At what APD value and at what rate of increase does pyeloplasty outweigh non-surgical management? Again, these values vary from surgeon-to-surgeon and are the subject of many debates within pediatric urology.

Historically, decreased or decreasing renal function as an indication for pyeloplasty had been controversial (17). Waiting until function has dropped and then performing surgery with the hopes to regain what has already been lost seems to be contradictory to the philosophy in pediatrics of maximizing a child's potential (19). While this view does not convey the thought that surgery should be performed on every child, this does highlight the need for a more advanced measure for screening patients that would benefit significantly from early surgical intervention rather than observation.

Early Intervention Compared to Non-surgical Management

Argument against early intervention of UPJO-like HN consists of evidence demonstrating that most cases of UPJO-like HN are clinically benign and will self-resolve. Koff followed neonates with suspected UPJO-like HN (regardless of degree of HN, shape of diuretic renogram curve, or initial degree of functional impairment) and showed that only 7% eventually had pyeloplasty performed for obstruction, suggesting that due to diagnostic inaccuracy and low risk of developing obstructive injury, many newborn kidneys with HN may rapidly improve without intervention (20, 21). This was further validated by Onen et al. who followed 19 newborns (38 kidneys) with primary SFU grade 3 to 4 bilateral HN for a mean of 54 months. Overall, 25 hydronephrotic kidneys (65%) resolved spontaneously, with renal dilatation and function improving over time in most kidneys (22). Furthermore, Braga et al. analyzed a cohort of 501 UPJO-like HN patients with all SFU grades and observed that 68% of those with grades 3 and 4 HN resolved with non-surgical management over 48 months of follow-up (23). This rate compares well to a recent study from a center known for its conservative approach regarding pyeloplasty indications. They reported a pyeloplasty rate of 38% in 64 patients with grades 3/4 UPJO-like HN at a median age of 21 months (24).

In contrast, benefit of early pyeloplasty in UPJO-like HN has been vastly reported in the literature. With respect to renal function, Babu et al. compared children with UPJO-like HN and SFU grade 3 or 4 who had pyeloplasty done at a mean age of 2.8 vs. 12.5 months. They found that at 1 year follow-up, the

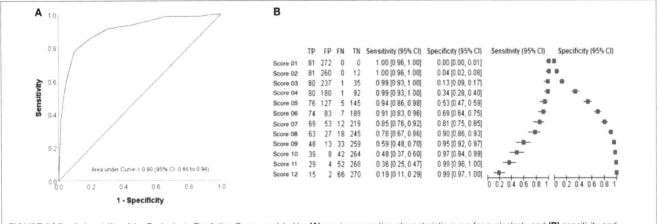

	TP	FP	FN	TN	Sensitivity (95% CI)	Specificity (95% CI)
Score 01	81	272	0	0	1.00 [0.96, 1.00]	0.00 [0.00, 0.01]
Score 02	81	260	0	12	1.00 [0.96, 1.00]	0.04 [0.02, 0.08]
Score 03	80	237	1	35	0.99 [0.93, 1.00]	0.13 [0.09, 0.17]
Score 04	80	180	1	92	0.99 [0.93, 1.00]	0.34 [0.28, 0.40]
Score 05	76	127	5	145	0.94 [0.86, 0.98]	0.53 [0.47, 0.59]
Score 06	74	83	7	189	0.91 [0.83, 0.96]	0.69 [0.64, 0.75]
Score 07	69	53	12	219	0.85 [0.76, 0.92]	0.81 [0.75, 0.85]
Score 08	63	27	18	245	0.78 [0.67, 0.86]	0.90 [0.86, 0.93]
Score 09	48	13	33	259	0.59 [0.48, 0.70]	0.95 [0.92, 0.97]
Score 10	39	8	42	264	0.48 [0.37, 0.60]	0.97 [0.94, 0.99]
Score 11	29	4	52	268	0.36 [0.25, 0.47]	0.99 [0.96, 1.00]
Score 12	15	2	66	270	0.19 [0.11, 0.29]	0.99 [0.97, 1.00]

FIGURE 2 | Predictive ability of the Pyeloplasty Prediction Score modeled by **(A)** receiver operating characteristic curve for pyeloplasty and **(B)** sensitivity and specificity at various score cut-points.

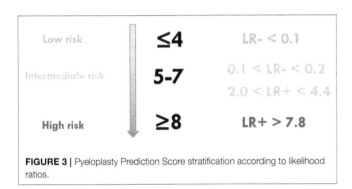

FIGURE 3 | Pyeloplasty Prediction Score stratification according to likelihood ratios.

early group had a significant improvement of split DRF while the delayed group generally had a marginal loss in function (25). Tabari et al. analyzed functional and anatomic indices (cortical thickness, polar length, SFU grade) in patients with early surgical pyeloplasty compared to those with non-surgical management. The early surgical group noted a faster return to anatomical and functional baseline parameters, whereas the non-surgical group had a significant deterioration in function compared to baseline (26). Thus, it is clinically essential to be able to identify those patients with UPJO-like HN that would benefit most from early pyeloplasty, which is exactly what the PPS was intended to do.

Limitations of Other Scoring Systems

Other scoring systems, such as the Hydronephrosis Severity Score (HSS) developed by Babu et al. attempted to predict pyeloplasty using ultrasound and diuretic renogram results (27). The main limitation of the HSS is that it relies greatly on the diuretic renogram and the interpretation of its curve, all factors which are heavily exam and operator dependent. Confounders such as time of furosemide dose (F + 20, F – 15, F – 0), bladder catheterization or no catherization, oral or intravenous hydration, DRF of the affected kidney, and conjugate views, all may influence the results of the scan (4, 28–31).

Bladder distension and elevated bladder pressures can restrict the upper urinary tract's ability to drain and can prolong the excretory phase, which is difficult to control without bladder catheterization. Patient position has also been demonstrated to affect urine flow, such that when the patient is supine the urine flow can resemble obstruction whereas upright gravity-assisted position can increase flow significantly (29). Timing of furosemide administration is controversial. Earlier furosemide administration (F + 0, F – 15) urine flow is dramatically increased and can increase the specificity by decreasing the false-positive rate but also results in underestimation of renal function due to acceleration of renal transit (30, 32). Later administration of furosemide (F + 20) allows the examiner to compare the drainage curve before and after furosemide to directly observe the modifications to excretion by diuretic. However, prolongation of the excretory phase does run the increased risk of false-positive findings of obstruction (28). It is not difficult to imagine that even with just the variability of one of these three factors, how many protocol variations can be expected across different centers. This will lead to inconsistencies when interpreting study results involving different protocols and radiotracers.

Pyeloplasty Prediction Score Parameters

Therefore, the concept of creating a score relying exclusively on ultrasound parameters was attractive because of its reproducibility. SFU grade, APD and renal length discrepancy measurements were chosen as the components of the PPS system because each one of them has been shown to be significantly associated with obstruction/pyeloplasty, as previously reported. Increasing severity of SFU grade, specifically SFU grades 3 and 4 of post-natal UPJO-like HN, were shown to be independent risk factors for surgery (6, 23, 33, 34). In a prospective study including 501 UPJO-like HN patients, Braga et al. showed that the pyeloplasty rate in patients with SFU grades 3 and 4 was significantly higher than that in those with SFU grades I and II (2% vs. 32%) (23). In a meta-analysis, Lee et al. had demonstrated that severe hydronephrosis (antenatal APD >

15 mm) found during the third trimester had an 88% chance of post-natal pathology (35). Dias et al. had also established that with a prenatal APD > 18 mm in the third trimester and >16 mm in the postnatal period, the sensitivity and specificity of eventually needing pyeloplasty for UPJO-like HN were 100 and 86% (10). Renal length discrepancy on ultrasound has already been shown to be a significantly reliable predictor of abnormal DMSA scans, representing function, and SFU grade, representing obstructive severity. Khazaei et al. showed in children of all ages with a left kidney longer than the right by ≥10 mm or right longer than the left by ≥7 mm corresponded with a positive predictive value (PPV) of 79 and 100% of abnormal DMSA scan (36). Kelley et al. had found that an increase in renal length was significantly associated with SFU 3 and 4 as compared to SFU 1 and 2 (37). The three parameters chosen for the PPS have thus been shown to capture significant anatomical and functional measures independently, so the next logical step was to combine them into a single scoring system.

Though drop in differential renal function (DRF) is commonly listed as an indication for pyeloplasty, it has been omitted from the PPS formula. DRF can occasionally be misleading with the supra-normal differential renal function (SNDRF) phenomenon. A finding of SNDRF is generally defined as when the hydronephrotic kidney is found to have higher than normal DRF (>55%) (38, 39). It is hypothesized that this finding does not reflect true elevated function but reflects hyper-filtration in the setting of obstruction (38). SNDRF has been found in studies to be associated with significant post-operative decrease in DRF (38, 40). Pippi Salle et al. suggested that SNDRF observed during renography is a true phenomenon and that parenchymal proximity and distribution in relation to the pelvis are critical determinants, thus recommending the conjugate view technique for HN renography (41). There is intrinsic measurement error in renal scans of hydronephrotic kidneys making DRF measurement unreliable, due to variation in technique and the presence of the SNDRF phenomenon. Thus, DRF measurements do not have a consistent unidirectional relationship with disease severity that can be effectively utilized in a prediction model such as with the PPS.

Limitations

The main limitation of this study is that despite including widely accepted parameters that vary according to the severity of UPJO-like HN as components of the PPS, surgery indications are operator-dependent. A surgeon can determine his or her own criteria for pyeloplasty with some degree of flexibility from guidelines. Thus, the PPS system should be adopted for research at other

centers for evaluation of the external validity of its predictive abilities.

Another limitation of the present study is that there have been debates regarding using pyeloplasty as an outcome in single-center studies involving UPJO-like HN. Those that are against using surgery as an outcome argue that pyeloplasty is inherently a surgeon's threshold for surgery rather than an objective point of need for surgery. However, pyeloplasty is one of the few concrete outcomes that is available in the UPJO-like HN natural history. If pyeloplasty cannot be considered as an outcome, no other concrete objective outcomes are currently available, with the exception of renal function loss and symptoms. As previously discussed, waiting for renal function to deteriorate to indicate surgery with the hopes to regain what has already been lost seems counter-intuitive, especially when nephron preservation is the goal. Using an objective criterion for surgery such as DRF deterioration has its own problems. A recent study, which utilized DRF <40% as the main indication for pyeloplasty, regardless of HN grade and APD, showed a much higher febrile UTI rate of 12.5% for patients followed non-surgically, when compared to previous studies (24). This abnormally higher UTI rate seen, which can be considered as a true outlier, was most likely secondary to waiting too long for renal function loss to occur to intervene.

The PPS system was tested with a dataset from a single tertiary pediatric hospital. In order to further assess its external validity, it should be verified at other centers with prospectively collected data and larger sample sizes.

Despite these limitations, we propose that there is value in attempting to predict which UPJO-like HN patients will undergo pyeloplasty, using the PPS. We encourage that this scoring system be adopted at other centers to verify its findings, and to possibly establish an objective, simple, standard measure to quantitively compare thresholds for surgery between various pediatric urologists.

AUTHOR CONTRIBUTIONS

LB theorized the presented idea. MM and BL developed the theory and performed the computations. LB and FF verified the analytical methods. BL, MM, FF, and LB contributed to interpretation of the results. BL wrote the manuscript in consultation with MM, FF, and LB. LB supervised the project. All authors provided critical feedback and helped design the research, analysis, manuscript, and figures.

REFERENCES

1. Capolicchio J-P, Braga LH, Szymanski KM. Canadian urological association/pediatric urologists of Canada guideline on the investigation and management of antenatally detected hydronephrosis. *Can Urol Assoc J.* (2018) 12:85–92. doi: 10.5489/cuaj.5094

2. Thorup J, Jokela R, Cortes D, Nielsen OH. The results of 15 years of consistent strategy in treating antenatally suspected pelvi-ureteric junction obstruction. *BJU Int.* (2003) 91:850–2. doi: 10.1046/j.1464-410x.2003.04228.x

3. de Waard D, Dik P, Lilien MR, Kok ET, de Jong TPVM. Hypertension is an

indication for surgery in children with ureteropelvic junction obstruction. *J Urol.* (2008) 179:1976–9. doi: 10.1016/j.juro.2008.01.058

4. Shulkin BL, Mandell GA, Cooper JA, Leonard JC, Majd M, Parisi MT, et al. Procedure guideline for diuretic renography in children 3.0. *J Nucl Med Technol.* (2008) 36:162–8. doi: 10.2967/jnmt.108.056622

5. Braga LH, McGrath M, Farrokhyar F, Jegatheeswaran K, Lorenzo AJ. Society for fetal urology classification vs urinary tract dilation grading system for prognostication in prenatal hydronephrosis: a time to resolution analysis. *J Urol.* (2018) 199:1615–21. doi: 10.1016/j.juro.2017.11.077

6. Fernbach SK, Maizels M, Conway JJ. Ultrasound grading of hydronephrosis: introduction to the system used by the society for fetal urology. *Pediatr Radiol.* (1993) 23:478–80. doi: 10.1007/bf02012459

7. Coplen DE, Austin PF, Yan Y, Blanco VM, Dicke JM. The magnitude of fetal renal pelvic dilatation can identify obstructive postnatal hydronephrosis, and direct postnatal evaluation and management. *J Urol.* (2006) 176:724–7. doi: 10.1016/j.juro.2006.03.079

8. Duin LK, Willekes C, Koster-Kamphuis L, Offermans J, Nijhuis JG. Fetal hydronephrosis: does adding an extra parameter improve detection of neonatal uropathies? *J Matern Fetal Neonatal Med.* (2012) 25:920–3. doi: 10.3109/14767058.2011.600365

9. Psooy K, Pike J. Investigation and management of antenatally detected hydronephrosis. *Can Urol Assoc J.* (2009) 3:69–72. doi: 10.5489/cuaj.1027

10. Dias CS, Silva JMP, Pereira AK, Marino VS, Silva LA, Coelho AM, et al. Diagnostic accuracy of renal pelvic dilatation for detecting surgically managed ureteropelvic junction obstruction. *J Urol.* (2013) 190:661–6. doi: 10.1016/j.juro.2013.02.014

11. Barbosa JABA, Chow JS, Benson CB, Yorioka MA, Bull AS, Retik AB, et al. Postnatal longitudinal evaluation of children diagnosed with prenatal hydronephrosis: insights in natural history and referral pattern. *Prenat Diagn.* (2012) 32:1242–9. doi: 10.1002/pd.3989

12. Dicke JM, Blanco VM, Yan Y, Coplen DE. The type and frequency of fetal renal disorders and management of renal pelvis dilatation. *J Ultrasound Med.* (2006) 25:973–7. doi: 10.7863/jum.2006.25.8.973

13. Nguyen HT, Benson CB, Bromley B, Campbell JB, Chow J, Coleman B, et al. Multidisciplinary consensus on the classification of prenatal and postnatal urinary tract dilation (UTD classification system). *J Pediatr Urol.* (2014) 10:982–98. doi: 10.1016/j.jpurol.2014.10.002

14. Arora S, Yadav P, Kumar M, Singh SK, Sureka SK, Mittal V, et al. Predictors for the need of surgery in antenatally detected hydronephrosis due to UPJ obstruction–a prospective multivariate analysis. *J Pediatr Urol.* (2015) 11:248.e1–5. doi: 10.1016/j.jpurol.2015.02.008

15. Dhillon HK. Prenatally diagnosed hydronephrosis: the great ormond street experience. *Br J Urol.* (1998) 81(Suppl 2):39–44. doi: 10.1046/j.1464-410x.1998.0810s2039.x

16. Partin A, Peters C, Kavoussi L, Dmochowski R, Wein A. *Campbell-Walsh-Wein Urology, 12th Edition.* Philadelphia, PA: Elsevier. (2020).

17. Castagnetti M, Novara G, Beniamin F, Vezzu B, Rigamonti W, Artibani W. Scintigraphic renal function after unilateral pyeloplasty in children: a systematic review. *BJU Int.* (2008) 102:862–8. doi: 10.1111/j.1464-410X.2008.07597.x

18. Xu G, Xu M, Ma J, Chen Z, Jiang D, Hong Z, et al. An initial differential renal function between 35% and 40% has greater probability of leading to normal after pyeloplasty in patients with unilateral pelvic-ureteric junction obstruction. *Int Urol Nephrol.* (2017) 49:1701–6. doi: 10.1007/s11255-017-1665-0

19. Peters CA. Urinary tract obstruction in children. *J Urol.* (1995) 154:1874. doi: 10.1016/s0022-5347(01)66815-0

20. Koff SA, Campbell KD. The nonoperative management of unilateral neonatal hydronephrosis: natural history of poorly functioning kidneys. *J Urol.* (1994) 152:593–5. doi: 10.1016/s0022-5347(17)32658-7

21. Koff SA. Neonatal management of unilateral hydronephrosis. Role for delayed intervention. *Urol Clin North Am.* (1998) 25:181–6. doi: 10.1016/s0094-0143(05)70006-9

22. Onen A, Jayanthi VR, Koff SA. Long-term followup of prenatally detected severe bilateral newborn hydronephrosis initially managed nonoperatively. *J Urol.* (2002) 168:1118–20. doi: 10.1097/01.ju.0000024449.19337.8d

23. Braga LH, McGrath M, Farrokhyar F, Jegatheeswaran K, Lorenzo AJ. Associations of initial society for fetal urology grades and urinary tract dilatation risk groups with clinical outcomes in patients with isolated prenatal hydronephrosis. *J Urol.* (2017) 197:831–7. doi: 10.1016/j.juro.2016.08.099

24. Alsabban A, Romao R, Dow T, Anderson P, MacLellan D. Severe ureteropelvic junction obstruction (UPJO)-like hydronephrosis in asymptomatic infants: to operate or not? In: *SPU 68th Annual Meeting* (2020).

25. Babu R, Rathish VR, Sai V. Functional outcomes of early versus delayed pyeloplasty in prenatally diagnosed pelvi-ureteric junction obstruction. *J Pediatr Urol.* (2015) 11:63.e1–5. doi: 10.1016/j.jpurol.2014.10.007

26. Tabari AK, Atqiaee K, Mohajerzadeh L, Rouzrokh M, Ghoroubi J, Alam A, et al. Early pyeloplasty versus conservative management of severe ureteropelvic junction obstruction in asymptomatic infants. *J Pediatr Surg.* (2020) S0022-3468:30513–5. doi: 10.1016/j.jpedsurg.2019.08.006

27. Babu R, Venkatachalapathy E, Sai V. Hydronephrosis severity score: an objective assessment of hydronephrosis severity in children-a preliminary report. *J Pediatr Urol.* (2019) 15:68.e1–e6. doi: 10.1016/j.jpurol.2018.09.020

28. Piepsz A. Antenatal detection of pelviureteric junction stenosis: main controversies. *Semin Nucl Med.* (2011) 41:11–19. doi: 10.1053/j.semnuclmed.2010.07.008

29. Wong DC, Rossleigh MA, Farnsworth RH. Diuretic renography with the addition of quantitative gravity-assisted drainage in infants and children. *J Nucl Med.* (2000) 41:1030–6.

30. Turkolmez S, Atasever T, Turkolmez K, Gogus O. Comparison of three different diuretic renal scintigraphy protocols in patients with dilated upper urinary tracts. *Clin Nucl Med.* (2004) 29:154–60. doi: 10.1097/01.rlu.0000113852.57445.23

31. Kumar MT, Hanuwant S. Comparison of the F+20 and F-15 diuresis technetium-99m diethylenetriaminepentacetate renography protocols for diagnosis of ureteropelvic junction obstruction in adult patients with hydronephrosis. *Indian J Nucl Med.* (2018) 33:39–42. doi: 10.4103/ijnm.IJNM_113_17

32. Donoso G, Ham H, Tondeur M, Piepsz A. Influence of early furosemide injection on the split renal function. *Nucl Med Commun.* (2003) 24:791–5. doi: 10.1097/01.mnm.0000080253.50447.94

33. Chertin B, Pollack A, Koulikov D, Rabinowitz R, Hain D, Hadas-Halpren I, et al. Conservative treatment of ureteropelvic junction obstruction in children with antenatal diagnosis of hydronephrosis: lessons learned after 16 years of follow-up. *Eur Urol.* (2006) 49:734–8. doi: 10.1016/j.eururo.2006.01.046

34. Ross SS, Kardos S, Krill A, Bourland J, Sprague B, Majd M, et al. Observation of infants with SFU grades 3-4 hydronephrosis: worsening drainage with serial diuresis renography indicates surgical intervention and helps prevent loss of renal function. *J Pediatr Urol.* (2011) 7:266–71. doi: 10.1016/j.jpurol.2011.03.001

35. Lee RS, Cendron M, Kinnamon DD, Nguyen HT. Antenatal hydronephrosis as a predictor of postnatal outcome: a meta-analysis. *Pediatrics.* (2006) 118:586–93. doi: 10.1542/peds.2006-0120

36. Khazaei MR, Mackie F, Rosenberg AR, Kainer G. Renal length discrepancy by ultrasound is a reliable predictor of an abnormal DMSA scan in children. *Pediatr Nephrol.* (2008) 23:99–105. doi: 10.1007/s00467-007-0637-5

37. Kelley JC, White JT, Goetz JT, Romero E, Leslie JA, Prieto JC. Sonographic renal parenchymal measurements for the evaluation and management of ureteropelvic junction obstruction in children. *Front Pediatr.* (2016) 4:42. doi: 10.3389/fped.2016.00042

38. Rickard M, Braga LH, Gandhi S, Oliveria J-P, Demaria J, Lorenzo AJ. Comparative outcome analysis of children who underwent pyeloplasty for ureteropelvic junction obstruction associated with or without supranormal differential renal function. *Urology.* (2017) 99:210–4. doi: 10.1016/j.urology.2016.07.016

39. Inanir S, Biyikli N, Noshari O, Caliskan B, Tugtepe H, Erdil TY, et al. Contradictory supranormal function in hydronephrotic kidneys: fact or artifact on pediatric MAG-3 renal scans? *Clin Nucl Med.* (2005) 30:91–6. doi: 10.1097/00003072-200502000-00004

40. Cho SY, Kim IS, Lee S-B, Choi H, Park K. Nature and fate of supranormal differential renal function: lessons from long-term follow-up after pyeloplasty. *Urology.* (2013) 81:163–7. doi: 10.1016/j.urology.2012.09.017

41. Pippi Salle JL, Cook A, Papanikolaou F, Bagli D, Breen SL, Charron M, et al. The importance of obtaining conjugate views on renographic evaluation of large hydronephrotic kidneys: an *in vitro* and ex vivo analysis. *J Urol.* (2008) 180:1559–65. doi: 10.1016/j.juro.2008.06.010

17

Construction and Analysis of Immune Infiltration-Related ceRNA Network for Kidney Stones

Yuqi Xia[†], Xiangjun Zhou[†], Zehua Ye, Weimin Yu, Jinzhuo Ning, Yuan Ruan, Run Yuan, Fangyou Lin, Peng Ye, Di Zheng, Ting Rao* and Fan Cheng*

Department of Urology, Renmin Hospital of Wuhan University, Wuhan, China

*Correspondence:
Ting Rao
tinart@126.com
Fan Cheng
Urology1969@aliyun.com

[†]These authors have contributed equally to this work

Purpose: Kidney stones is a common medical issue that mediates kidney injury and even kidney function loss. However, the exact pathogenesis still remains unclear. This study aimed to explore the potential competing endogenous RNA (ceRNA)-related pathogenesis of kidney stones and identify the corresponding immune infiltration signature.

Methods: One mRNA and one long non-coding RNA (lncRNA) microarray dataset was obtained from the GEO database. Subsequently, we compared differentially expressed mRNAs (DE-mRNAs) and lncRNAs between Randall's plaques in patients with calcium oxalate (CaOx) stones and controls with normal papillary tissues. lncRNA-targeted miRNAs and miRNA–mRNA pairs were predicted using the online databases. lncRNA-related DE-mRNAs were identified using the Venn method, and GO and KEGG enrichment analyses were subsequently performed. The immune-related lncRNA–miRNA–mRNA ceRNA network was developed. The CIBERSORT algorithm was used to estimate the rate of immune cell infiltration in Randall's plaques. The ceRNA network and immune infiltration were validated in the glyoxylate-induced hyperoxaluric mouse model and oxalate-treated HK-2 cells.

Results: We identified 2,340 DE-mRNAs and 929 DE-lncRNAs between Randall's plaques in patients with CaOx stones and controls with normal papillary tissues. lncRNA-related DE-mRNAs were significantly enriched in extracellular matrix organization and collagen-containing extracellular matrix, which were associated with kidney interstitial fibrosis. The immune-related ceRNA network included 10 lncRNAs, 23 miRNAs, and 20 mRNAs. Moreover, we found that M2 macrophages and resting mast cells were differentially expressed between Randall's plaques and normal tissues. Throughout kidney stone development, kidney tubular injury, crystal deposition, collagen fiber deposition, TGF-β expression, infiltration of M1 macrophages, and activation of mast cells were more frequent in glyoxylate-induced hyperoxaluric mice compared with control mice. Nevertheless, M2 macrophage infiltration increased in early stages (day 6) and decreased as kidney stones progressed (day 12). Furthermore, treatment with 0.25 and 0.5 mM of oxalate for 48 h significantly upregulated NEAT1, PVT1, CCL7, and ROBO2 expression levels and downregulated hsa-miR-23b-3p, hsa-miR-429, and hsa-miR-139-5p expression levels in the HK-2 cell line in a dose-dependent manner.

Conclusion: We found that significant expressions of ceRNAs (NEAT1, PVT1, hsa-miR-23b-3p, hsa-miR-429, hsa-miR-139-5p, CCL7, and ROBO2) and infiltrating immune cells (macrophages and mast cells) may be involved in kidney stone pathogenesis. These findings provide novel potential therapeutic targets for kidney stones.

Keywords: kidney stones, ceRNA, immune cell infiltration, calcium oxalate, glyoxylate

INTRODUCTION

Kidney stones are common and have high incidence and recurrence rates. Kidney stone prevalence in China is 6.4% and increases annually worldwide (Zeng et al., 2017; Kittanamongkolchai et al., 2018), inducing a heavy burden on the healthcare system. Calcium oxalate (CaOx) kidney stones, the most common type of kidney stone, can induce urinary tract obstruction, renal tubular injury, interstitium inflammation and fibrosis, and even chronic renal disease (Rule et al., 2011). However, the process of kidney stone formation is complex, and the exact mechanism remains unclear. Currently, Randall's plaque (RP), the calcium phosphate crystal deposition at the tip of the renal papillae, is considered to be the origin of kidney stones (Daudon et al., 2015). Crystals in supersaturated urine nucleates deposit in the renal papillae and grow gradually, eventually forming kidney stones (Khan and Canales, 2015). Evidence from endoscopic images demonstrated that stones attach to RP, which appeared in approximately half of patients with kidney stones (Pless et al., 2019). Moreover, renal papillae biopsies have shown that RP formation was associated with high urinary calcium levels, acidic urine, and metabolic diseases (Marien and Miller, 2016). Thus, studying RP to explore the potential pathogenesis of kidney stones and effective therapeutic targets is essential.

Non-coding RNAs (ncRNAs) include long non-coding RNAs (lncRNAs), microRNAs (miRNAs), and circular RNAs, which regulate gene expression at transcriptional and post-transcriptional levels without coding proteins (Beermann et al., 2016). Accumulating evidence has shown that the regulation of mRNAs and ncRNAs is essential for kidney stone-induced renal injury, including apoptosis, oxidative stress, inflammation, and interstitial fibrosis (Liu et al., 2019; Li et al., 2020; Zhu et al., 2020). In recent years, a competing endogenous RNAs (ceRNAs) network hypothesis has been proposed. This hypothesis states that RNAs communicate with each other using miRNA response elements (MREs). LncRNAs regulate the function of mRNAs by competitively binding to the corresponding miRNAs through MREs (Salmena et al., 2011). Given their complexity, the dysregulation of lncRNA–miRNA–mRNA networks is closely related to the pathogenesis of acute and chronic kidney injuries, including ischemia-reperfusion injury and unilateral ureteral obstruction (Cheng et al., 2019; Ren et al., 2019). Nevertheless, few studies have concentrated on the ceRNA regulatory network in patients with kidney stones.

Conventionally, the immune system plays a crucial role in the formation and pathogenesis of kidney stones. Throughout kidney stone development, CaOx crystals promote the secretion of inflammatory cytokines and chemokines, possibly recruiting various immune cells to renal interstitium, including neutrophils, macrophages, and T cells (Zhu et al., 2019; Taguchi et al., 2021). The dysfunction of the immune microenvironment in the kidney could not only initiate adverse factors, but also further exacerbate kidney stone formation (Khan et al., 2021). Previous studies have revealed that M2 macrophages can phagocytize and degrade crystals to suppress stone formation and prevent CaOx inflammatory damage (Taguchi et al., 2021). However, the polarization of M1 macrophages induces cell damage and increases stone burden (Taguchi et al., 2021). In this context, another study has shown that aberrant $\gamma\delta$T cells were activated and accumulated in CaOx kidney stones in a mouse model (Zhu et al., 2019). Despite the importance of maintaining immune microenvironmental homeostasis, in patients with kidney stones, the landscape of immune cell infiltration has not been fully clarified.

In this study, we compared differentially expressed (DE) mRNAs and lncRNAs between RPs in patients with CaOx stones and controls with normal papillary tissues based on the Gene Expression Omnibus (GEO) database and constructed an immune-related ceRNA network. Subsequently, to the best of our knowledge, we were the first to estimate the rate of immune cell infiltration in RPs. Moreover, we validated the ceRNA network and immune infiltration in vivo and in vitro. This study aimed to explore the potential ceRNA-related pathogenesis of kidney stones and identify its corresponding immune infiltration signature.

MATERIALS AND METHODS

Data Acquisition and Differential Expression Analysis

The mRNA microarray dataset GSE73680 (Taguchi et al., 2017) and lncRNA microarray dataset GSE117518 (Zhu et al., 2021) were obtained from the GEO database (https://www.ncbi.nlm.nih.gov/geo/). The GSE73680 dataset included 24 RPs from patients with CaOx stones and six controls with normal papillary tissues. The GSE117518 dataset included three RPs from patients with CaOx stones and three controls with normal papillary tissues. The details of both datasets are presented in **Table 1**. Probe names were transformed into gene symbols according to platform annotation information. Moreover, immune-related genes were obtained from the Immunology Database and Analysis Portal (IMMPORT) database (http://www.immport.org/) (Bhattacharya et al., 2014).

Subsequently, DE-mRNAs and lncRNAs were analyzed and compared between RPs and normal–papillary tissue controls

TABLE 1 | Details of lncRNA and mRNA datasets of patients with calcium oxalate kidney stones.

Type	GEO accession	Platform	Sample organism	Samples (kidney tissues), *n*		Contributors. (Year)
				Randall's plaque	Normal papillary	
mRNA	GSE73680	GPL17077	*Homo sapiens*	24	6	Taguchi et al. (2015)
lncRNA	GSE117518	GPL21827	*Homo sapiens*	3	3	Cui et al. (2016)

using the "limma" package (Ritchie et al., 2015) in the R software (http://www.r-project.org). mRNAs that met the criteria of | log$_2$FC|>1 and $p < 0.01$ were considered as DE-mRNAs, and lncRNAs that met the criteria of |log$_2$FC|>0.58 and $p < 0.01$ were considered as DE-lncRNA. The "ggplot2" package was used to draw heatmaps and volcano plots for data visualization.

Prediction of lncRNA–miRNA and miRNA–mRNA Interactions

Potential DE-lncRNA-targeted miRNAs were predicted using the miRcode database (http://mircode.org/) (Jeggari et al., 2012). Subsequently, miRNA–mRNA pairs were analyzed using TargetScan (http://www.targetscan.org/vert_72/) (Agarwal et al., 2015), miRTarBase (https://mirtarbase.cuhk.edu.cn/php/index.php) (Huang et al., 2020), and miRDB (http://mirdb.org/) (Chen and Wang, 2020) databases. mRNAs that were found in at least two databases were considered as candidate targets of miRNAs.

Venn Method

The Venn method was used to analyze overlapping genes. Intersections between DE-mRNA and DE-lncRNA-targeted mRNAs, as well as lncRNA-related DE-mRNAs and immune-related genes were identified using the Venny version 2.1 online tool (https://bioinfogp.cnb.csic.es/tools/venny/index.html).

Functional Enrichment and Protein–Protein Interaction Analysis

To explore the functions of lncRNA-related DE-mRNAs, gene ontology (GO) and Kyoto Encyclopedia of Genes and Genomes (KEGG) enrichment analyses were conducted using the "org.Hs.eg.db" and "ClusterProfiler" packages (Yu et al., 2012) in the R software. An adjusted $p < 0.05$ was considered statistically significant. Subsequently, the STRING database (https://string-db.org/) (Szklarczyk et al., 2019) was used to determine the relationship between the DE-mRNAs, and Cytoscape software (https://cytoscape.org) was used to develop the PPI network.

Construction of the Immune-Related ceRNA Network

After identifying immune-related and lncRNA-related DE-mRNAs, the interaction between lncRNAs, miRNAs, and mRNAs was confirmed as described in item 3.2. Subsequently, the immune-related lncRNA–miRNA–mRNA ceRNA network was developed using the R software. The "ggalluvial" package was used to draw a sankey diagram for data visualization.

Analysis of Immune Cell Infiltration

To estimate the abundance of 22 types of immune cell types in Randall's plaques and normal–papillary tissue controls, the mRNA microarray dataset GSE73680 was uploaded to the platform of CIBERSORT (http://cibersort.stanford.edu/) (Newman et al., 2015). Only samples that had a CIBERSORT algorithm output of $p < 0.05$ were considered for further analysis. Histograms and heatmaps were drawn to show the rate of immune cell infiltration in different samples. Co-expression patterns in immune-related DE-mRNAs and infiltrating immune cells were analyzed using Pearson's correlation coefficient. Subsequently, the Wilcoxon rank-sum test was performed to compare differentially infiltrating immune cells between RPs in patients with CaOx stones and controls with normal papillary tissues. The relationship between DE-mRNA expression and the fractions of macrophages and mast cells was also investigated using the Wilcoxon test. Results were visualized using the "heatmap" and "vioplot" packages in the R software.

Animal Experiments

Thirty male C57BL/6J mice weighing 22–25 g and aging 6–8 weeks were acquired from the Center of Experimental Animals at the Renmin hospital of Wuhan University, Hubei, China. The mice were acclimatized in the animal house of our institution at a steady temperature of 22 ± 2°C and humidity of 40–70% on a 12/12-h light–dark cycle and with free access to water and feed. The animal experiments were conducted according to the Guide for the Care and Use of Laboratory Animals, and the study protocol was approved by the Laboratory Animal Welfare and Ethics Committee of the Renmin hospital of Wuhan University (approval number: WDRM-20200604).

According to previous publications (Okada et al., 2007; Usami et al., 2018), the mice were intraperitoneally injected with 80 or 120 mg/kg of glyoxylate (Sigma–Aldrich; St. Louis, MO, United States) daily for 6 or 12 days to establish a CaOx kidney stone model. Mice were randomly assigned to the five following dosage groups ($n = 6$): control, 80 mg/kg of glyoxylate for 6 days, 120 of mg/kg glyoxylate for 6 days, 80 mg/kg of glyoxylate for 12 days, and 120 mg/kg of glyoxylate for 12 days groups. After 6 or 12 days, the mice were sacrificed, and kidneys were removed for analyses.

Cell Culture and Treatment

Human renal tubular epithelial cell line (HK-2) cells were provided by Stem Cell Bank, Chinese Academy of Sciences, Shanghai, China. HK-2 cells were cultured in an MEM medium supplemented with 10% fetal bovine serum (Gibco, Waltham, MA, United States) and 1% antibiotics (penicillin/streptomycin). The cells were maintained at 37°C under a humidified atmosphere with 5% CO_2. Oxalate was purchased from Sigma–Aldrich and dissolved in the culture medium. Subsequently, the cells were cultured in six-well plates, and 0.25 mM or 0.5 mM of oxalate were added for 48 h.

Hematoxylin and Eosin, Von Kossal, and Masson Staining

After fixation in 4% paraformaldehyde, kidneys were imbedded in paraffin and were cut into 5-μm slices. HE staining was performed to assess the histopathological kidney tubular injuries as previously described (Dong et al., 2019). Injuries were scored as follows: 0, no tubular injury; 1, <10% tubular damage; 2, 10–25% tubular damage; 3, 25–50% tubular damage; 4, 50–74% tubular damage; and 5, >75% tubular damage. Subsequently, crystals were detected using Von Kossal staining, as previously described (Wang et al., 2019). The crystal deposition area was quantified using Image J software. Renal fibrosis was verified using Masson trichrome staining, and the collagen fiber deposition area on kidney sections was quantified using Image J software.

Immunohistochemistry and Immunofluorescence Staining

The protein expression levels of TGF-β, iNOS, and CD206 were analyzed using immunohistochemical and immunofluorescence staining. Antibodies (i.e., TGF-β [21898-1-AP], iNOS [18985-1-AP], and CD206 [60143-1-Ig]) were purchased from Proteintech (Chicago, IL, United States). All procedures were conducted according to the recommendations of the manufacturer. By comparing the positive area between groups using microscopy, figures were analyzed using Image J software.

Toluidine Blue Staining

Mast cells were detected using Toluidine blue staining as previously described (Zhang et al., 2017). Mast cells were identified using purple granules, and activated mast cells were characterized by disgorged and loosely packed granules. Activated mast cells per field were counted at a magnification of 400 ×.

Quantitative Real-Time PCR

Total RNA was extracted from HK-2 cells using TRIzol reagent (Invitrogen Life Technologies, Carlsbad, CA, United States), and RNA purity was measured using spectrophotometry. RNAs were reverse transcribed into cDNAs using the Takara RNA PCR kit (Takara Biotechnology, Shiga, Japan) according to the instructions of the manufacturer. Subsequently, cDNA was amplified by RT-qPCR using an Applied Biosystems SYBR Green mix kit (Applied Biosystems, Foster City, CA, United States). GAPDH was used as an internal reference for lncRNAs and mRNAs, while U6 was used as a reference for miRNA. The primers used for these reactions are shown in **Supplementary Table S1**. The reactions were measured on the ABI 7900 Real-Time PCR system (Applied Biosystems Life Technologies), and the $2^{-\Delta\Delta CT}$ method was used for analysis.

Statistical Analysis

All data are presented as the mean ± SD. Statistical analysis was conducted using SPSS version 19.0 (SPSS Inc., Chicago, IL, United States). Student's t-test was used to compare differences between groups. A p-value of <0.05 was considered statistically significant. All experiments were performed at least three times.

RESULTS

Identification of DE mRNAs and lncRNAs

To clarify the process of this research, a schematic representation is presented in **Figure 1**. Original data were downloaded from the GSE73680 and GSE117518 datasets in the GEO database. In the GSE73680 dataset, RNA-seq data of 24 RPs from patients with CaOx stones and from six controls with normal papillary tissues were analyzed using criteria of $|\log_2 FC|>1$ and $p < 0.01$. A total of 2,340 DE-mRNAs (2,098 upregulated and 242 downregulated) were compared between RPs and normal papillary tissues. In the GSE117518 dataset, the RNA-seq data of three RPs from patients with CaOx stones and three normal papillary tissues were analyzed using criteria of $|\log_2 FC|>0.58$ and $p < 0.01$. A total of 929 DE-lncRNAs (587 upregulated and 342 downregulated) were identified. Corresponding heatmaps and volcano plots are shown in **Figure 2**. Details of datasets are presented in **Table 1**.

Function Enrichment Analysis of lncRNA-Related DE-mRNAs

To establish the ceRNA network, DE-lncRNAs were further analyzed. Potential DE-lncRNA-targeted miRNAs were predicted using the miRcode database. Subsequently, miRNA–mRNA pairs were analyzed using the TargetScan, miRTarBase, and miRDB databases. A total of 197 miRNAs and 8,457 mRNAs were predicted. Subsequently, the Venn method was used to analyze the intersection between DE-mRNA and DE-lncRNA-targeted mRNAs (**Figure 3A**). Consequently, 278 overlapping lncRNA-related DE-mRNAs were identified. To determine the functions of lncRNA-related DE-mRNAs, GO and KEGG enrichment analyses were conducted (**Figures 3B,C**). A biological process analysis showed that lncRNA-related DE-mRNAs were significantly enriched in extracellular matrix organization, cellular calcium ion homeostasis, and regulation of cellular response to growth factor stimulus. A cellular component analysis showed that lncRNA-related DE-mRNAs were mostly enriched in collagen-containing extracellular matrix and endoplasmic reticulum lumen. A molecular function (MF) analysis showed that lncRNA-related DE-mRNAs were mostly enriched in channel activity and extracellular matrix structural constituent. The KEGG pathway enrichment analysis showed that lncRNA-related DE-mRNAs were significantly enriched in PI3K-Akt

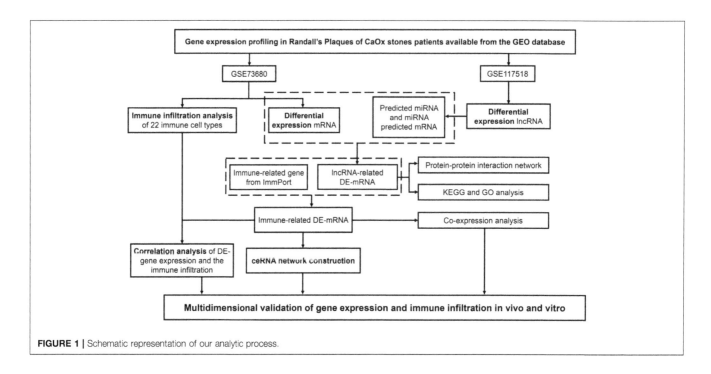

FIGURE 1 | Schematic representation of our analytic process.

signaling pathway, focal adhesion, and extracellular matrix-receptor interaction. Details of GO and KEGG enrichment analyses are presented in **Tables 2**, **3**. The PPI network of lncRNA-related DE-mRNAs is shown in **Supplementary Figure S1**.

Construction of the Immune-Related ceRNA Network

To construct the immune-related ceRNA network, the Venn method was used to analyze the intersection between lncRNA-related DE-mRNAs and immune-related genes obtained from the IMMPORT database. Consequently, 20 overlapping immune-related DE-mRNAs (12 upregulated and eight downregulated) were identified (**Figure 4A**). A co-expression analysis of immune-related DE-mRNAs was performed (**Figure 4B**). Subsequently, immune-related DE-mRNAs and their paired miRNAs and lncRNAs were chosen to develop the ceRNA regulatory network (**Figure 4C**). In total, the immune-related ceRNA network contained 10 lncRNAs, 23 miRNAs, and 20 mRNAs.

Composition of Infiltrating Immune Cells

The composition of 22 infiltrating immune cells in RPs in patients with CaOx stones and controls with normal papillary tissues were estimated using the CIBERSORT algorithm (**Figures 5A,B**). The relationships among these 22 immune cells are presented in **Figure 5C**. M1 macrophages were positively correlated with resting dendritic cells ($R = 0.70$). M2 macrophages were positively correlated with eosinophils ($R = 0.52$). Activated mast cells activated were positively correlated with neutrophils ($R = 0.59$). Resting mast cells were positively correlated with activated NK cells ($R = 0.55$) and negatively correlated with

resting dendritic cells ($R = -0.45$). The differential proportion of infiltrating immune cells between RPs in patients with CaOx stones and in controls with normal papillary tissues was analyzed. As shown in **Figure 5D**, compared with the RPs in controls, M2 macrophages ($p = 0.038$) and resting mast cells ($p = 0.019$) were significantly downregulated and M1 macrophages ($p = 0.49$) and activated mast cells ($p = 0.296$) were significantly upregulated in the RPs in patients with kidney stones.

Co-Expression Patterns of Infiltrating Immune Cells and DE-mRNAs

For further analysis, DE-mRNAs were divided to the high expression and low expression groups. The correlation between infiltrating immune cells and DE-mRNAs expression was estimated using the Wilcoxon test, and significantly correlated pairs with $p < 0.05$ are shown in **Figure 6**. Results indicated that the expression of IL-13, OGN, and VEGFC was significantly negatively correlated with the proportion of M1 macrophages ($p = 0.011$, $p = 0.002$, and $p = 0.05$, respectively), whereas the expression of VAV2 was significantly positively correlated with proportion of M1 macrophages ($p = 0.038$). The expression of ADM2, CCL7, FGF18, FGF21, CCR9, LEP, ROBO2, and VAV2 was significantly negatively correlated with the proportion of resting mast cells ($p = 0.011$, $p = 0.049$, $p = 0.001$, $p = 0.002$, $p < 0.001$, $p = 0.016$, $p = 0.007$, $p = 0.02$, and $p = 0.002$, respectively).

Validation in a Glyoxylate-Induced Hyperoxaluric Mouse Model

To validate the aforementioned pathway and differentially infiltrating immune cells, kidney tubular injury, crystal

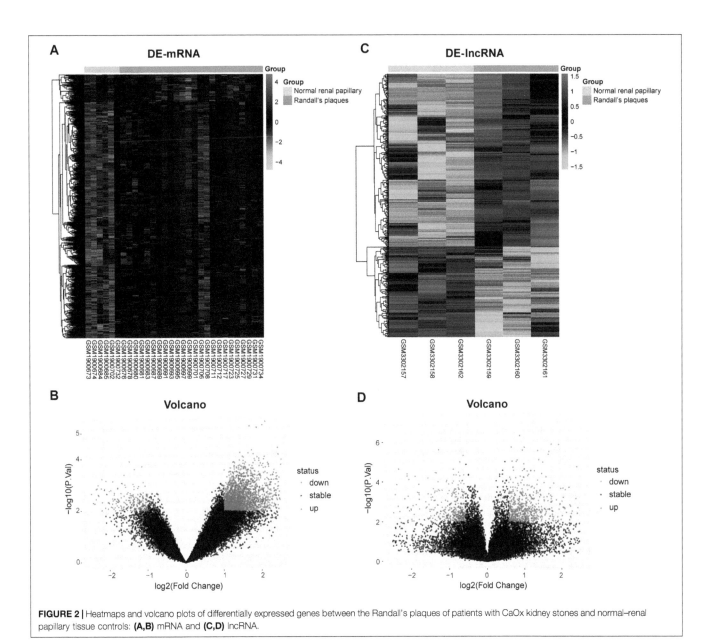

FIGURE 2 | Heatmaps and volcano plots of differentially expressed genes between the Randall's plaques of patients with CaOx kidney stones and normal–renal papillary tissue controls: **(A,B)** mRNA and **(C,D)** lncRNA.

deposition, fibrosis level, and macrophage and mast cell infiltration were evaluated in a glyoxylate (Gly)-induced hyperoxaluric mouse model. As shown in **Figure 7**, kidney tubular injury and crystal deposition were aggravated as treatment concentration and time of glyoxylate increased. Tubular injury and crystals were markedly worse in the day–12 Gly-treated groups than in the day–6 Gly-treated groups. Moreover, tubular injury and crystals were markedly worse in the 120–mg/kg Gly-treated mice than in the 80–mg/kg Gly-treated mice in both day-6 and day-12 groups. Fibrosis and collagen fiber deposition were evaluated using Masson staining and immunohistochemical staining of TGF-β. Results have shown that collagen fiber depositions

and TGF-β-positive areas were significantly more frequent in the Gly-treated groups than in the control group in a dose- and time-dependent manner; these results are consistent with those shown in **Figure 3B**.

Subsequently, the immunofluorescence staining of macrophage-related molecules iNOS (M1) and CD206 (M2) showed that M1 macrophage infiltration significantly increased as kidney stones aggravated, whereas M2 macrophage infiltration increased in the early stages (day 6) and decreased as kidney stones progressed (day 12). Toluidine blue staining showed that activated mast cell infiltration significantly increased in the kidneys of mice with stone formation. As treatment concentration and time of Gly increased, activated mast cells

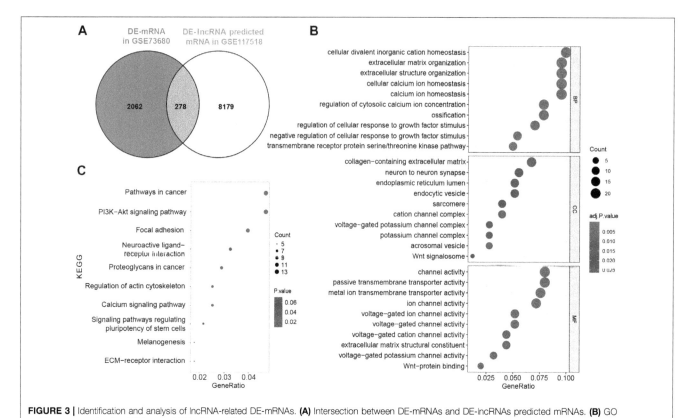

FIGURE 3 | Identification and analysis of lncRNA-related DE-mRNAs. **(A)** Intersection between DE-mRNAs and DE-lncRNAs predicted mRNAs. **(B)** GO enrichment analysis of lncRNA-related DE-mRNAs. **(C)** KEGG enrichment analysis of lncRNA-related DE-mRNAs. DE-mRNAs, differentially expressed mRNAs; DE-lncRNAs, differentially expressed lncRNAs; GO, gene ontology; and KEGG, Kyoto Encyclopedia of Genes and Genomes.

concomitantly increased. These immune cell infiltration results are consistent with our findings shown in **Figure 5**.

Construction of Immune-Related hub ceRNA Network and Validation in HK-2 Cells Stimulated With Oxalate

Through literature review and co-expression analysis of infiltrating immune cells, we established the immune-related hub ceRNA network, comprising 2 lncRNAs, 3 miRNAs, and 2 mRNAs (**Figure 8A**). Details of the immune-related hub ceRNA network developed from the GSE73680 and GSE117518 datasets are presented in **Table 4**. To validate the immune-related hub ceRNA network in kidney stones, RT-qPCR was used to detect the expression levels of the hub genes. As shown in **Figure 8B**, treatment with 0.25 and 0.5 mM oxalate for 48 h significantly upregulated the expression levels of NEAT1, PVT1, CCL7, and ROBO2 but downregulated the expression levels of hsa-miR-23b-3p, hsa-miR-429, and hsa-miR-139-5p in the HK-2 cell line in a dose-dependent manner. These results are consistent with the findings of GEO datasets.

DISCUSSION

Kidney stones are among the most common urological diseases and have a high recurrence rate. In the GEO database, several datasets assessed gene expression profiling by RNA-sequencing in kidney

stones. However, most experiments were based on animal models (GSE72135, GSE36446, and GSE75543 datasets) or cell lines (GSE110509, GSE75111, and GSE56934 datasets), rather than patient samples. RPs are considered as the origin of kidney stones (Daudon et al., 2015). Thus, analysis based on the gene expression profiling of RPs may provide more convincing results to reveal kidney stone pathogenesis. In this study, for the first time, an immune-related ceRNA network was constructed and the composition of infiltrating immune cells was estimated based on gene expression profiling in RPs from patients with CaOx kidney stones.

Kidney stones mediate kidney injury and even kidney function loss (Rule et al., 2011). A recent study has found that symptomatic patients with kidney stones have an increased risk off chronic kidney disease compared with the risk of normal individuals (Rule et al., 2009). A retrospective clinical study has demonstrated that 6.01% of patients with kidney stones experience renal atrophy 2 years after percutaneous nephrolithotomy; kidney stones lasting more than 12 months and multiple calyces stone are independent risk factors (Xiangrui et al., 2020), indicating the serious outcomes of kidney stones. The underlying mechanisms may be associated with urinary tract obstruction, infection, and crystal-induced injury and fibrosis (Uribarri, 2020). Convento et al. (2017) demonstrated that the expression levels of TGF-β and epithelial-mesenchymal transition-associated proteins increased in hyperoxaluric mice and HK-2 cells treated with oxalate and CaOx, accompanied by progressive renal failure. In this study, we found that lncRNA-related DE-mRNAs are significantly enriched

TABLE 2 | Top 10 GO enrichment terms of differential expression genes.

GO term ID	Term description	GeneRatio	adj.p.val
Biological process			
GO:0072503	Cellular divalent inorganic cation homeostasis	24/243	2.30E-05
GO:0030198	Extracellular matrix organization	23/243	3.25E-06
GO:0043062	Extracellular structure organization	23/243	3.25E-06
GO:0006874	Cellular calcium ion homeostasis	23/243	2.30E-05
GO:0055074	Calcium ion homeostasis	23/243	2.96E-05
GO:0051480	Regulation of cytosolic calcium ion concentration	19/243	9.83E-05
GO:0001503	Ossification	19/243	0.00055
GO:0090287	Regulation of cellular response to growth factor stimulus	17/243	0.00025
GO:0090288	Negative regulation of cellular response to growth factor stimulus	13/243	0.00026
GO:0090101	Negative regulation of transmembrane receptor protein serine/threonine kinase signaling pathway	12/243	8.63E-05
Cellular component			
GO:0062023	Collagen-containing extracellular matrix	17/254	0.01691
GO:0098984	Neuron to neuron synapse	14/254	0.01987
GO:0005788	Endoplasmic reticulum lumen	13/254	0.01863
GO:0030139	Endocytic vesicle	13/254	0.01863
GO:0030017	Sarcomere	10/254	0.01987
GO:0034703	Cation channel complex	10/254	0.02633
GO:0008076	Voltage-gated potassium channel complex	7/254	0.01863
GO:0034705	Potassium channel complex	7/254	0.01863
GO:0001669	Acrosomal vesicle	7/254	0.02647
GO:1990909	Wnt signalosome	3/254	0.01987
Molecular function			
GO:0015267	Channel activity	20/251	0.00085
GO:0022803	Passive transmembrane transporter activity	20/251	0.00085
GO:0046873	Metal ion transmembrane transporter activity	19/251	0.00085
GO:0005216	Ion channel activity	18/251	0.00153
GO:0005244	Voltage-gated ion channel activity	13/251	0.00057
GO:0022832	Voltage-gated channel activity	13/251	0.00057
GO:0022843	Voltage-gated cation channel activity	11/251	0.00057
GO:0005201	Extracellular matrix structural constituent	11/251	0.00148
GO:0005249	Voltage-gated potassium channel activity	8/251	0.00153
GO:0017147	Wnt-protein binding	5/251	0.00236

TABLE 3 | KEGG pathway enrichment analysis of differentially expressed genes.

KEGG term ID	Term description	Count	p.val
hsa05200	Pathways in cancer	13	0.00692
hsa04151	PI3K-Akt signaling pathway	13	0.00243
hsa04510	Focal adhesion	11	4.70E-04
hsa04080	Neuroactive ligand-receptor interaction	9	0.03502
hsa05205	Proteoglycans in cancer	8	0.01920
hsa04810	Regulation of actin cytoskeleton	7	0.06697
hsa04020	Calcium signaling pathway	7	0.03532
hsa04550	Signaling pathways regulating pluripotency of stem cells	6	0.04222
hsa04916	Melanogenesis	5	0.04751
hsa04512	Extracellular matrix-receptor interaction	5	0.03078

in extracellular matrix organization, regulation of cellular response to growth factor stimulus, and collagen-containing extracellular matrix, which were associated with kidney interstitial fibrosis. Moreover, we revealed that, throughout kidney stone development, collagen fiber deposition and TGF-β expression were significantly increased in glyoxylate-induced hyperoxaluric mice in a dose- and time-dependent manner. Hence, we speculated that more attention should be paid to kidney stone-induced fibrosis and that lncRNAs may play a crucial role on the corresponding process.

miRNAs, as transcription regulators, are essential in various physiological and pathological processes, including kidney stone-induced renal injury (Jiang et al., 2020; Su et al., 2020). Su et al. (2020) indicated that miR-21 expression increased in hyperoxaluric mice, which promoted CaOx-induced renal tubular injury by PPARA. Jiang demonstrated that miR-155-5p upregulated and promoted oxalate and that CaOx induced oxidative stress injury in HK-2 cells (Jiang et al., 2020). In recent years, the lncRNA–miRNA–mRNA ceRNA network has been proved to be involved in various kidney diseases, including

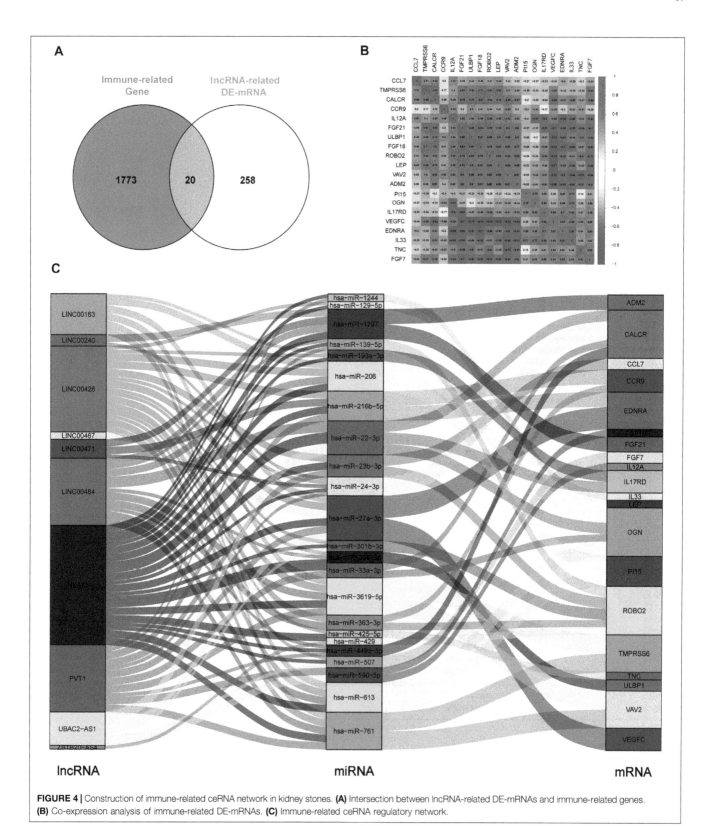

FIGURE 4 | Construction of immune-related ceRNA network in kidney stones. **(A)** Intersection between lncRNA-related DE-mRNAs and immune-related genes. **(B)** Co-expression analysis of immune-related DE-mRNAs. **(C)** Immune-related ceRNA regulatory network.

kidney stones (Liang et al., 2019; Liu et al., 2019; Ren et al., 2019). Liu et al. (2019) determined that the interaction between lncRNA H19 and miR-216b facilitated CaOx-induced kidney injury *via* the HMGB1/TLR4/NF-κB pathway. Moreover, Liang et al. (2019)

identified the lncRNA–miRNA–mRNA expression variation profile in the urine of patients with CaOx stones. In this study, we constructed an immune-related ceRNA network based on gene expression profiling in RPs, including 10

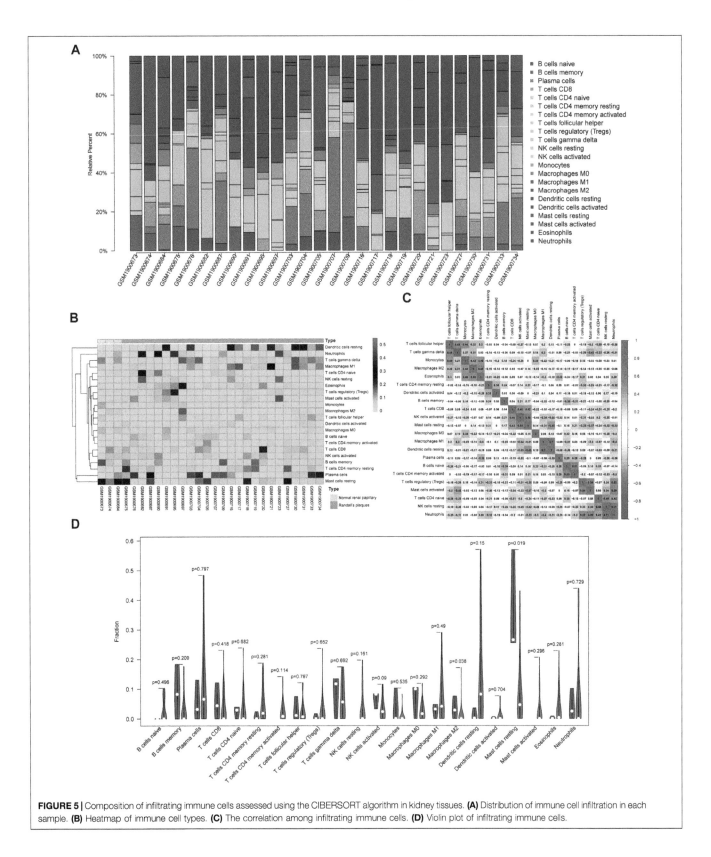

FIGURE 5 | Composition of infiltrating immune cells assessed using the CIBERSORT algorithm in kidney tissues. **(A)** Distribution of immune cell infiltration in each sample. **(B)** Heatmap of immune cell types. **(C)** The correlation among infiltrating immune cells. **(D)** Violin plot of infiltrating immune cells.

lncRNAs, 23 miRNAs, and 20 mRNAs, which are potential therapeutic targets. Subsequently, the immune-related hub ceRNA network was established and validated *in vitro*.

Treatment with 0.25 and 0.5 mM of oxalate significantly upregulated NEAT1 and PVT1 expression levels and downregulated hsa-miR-23b-3p, hsa-miR-429, and hsa-miR-

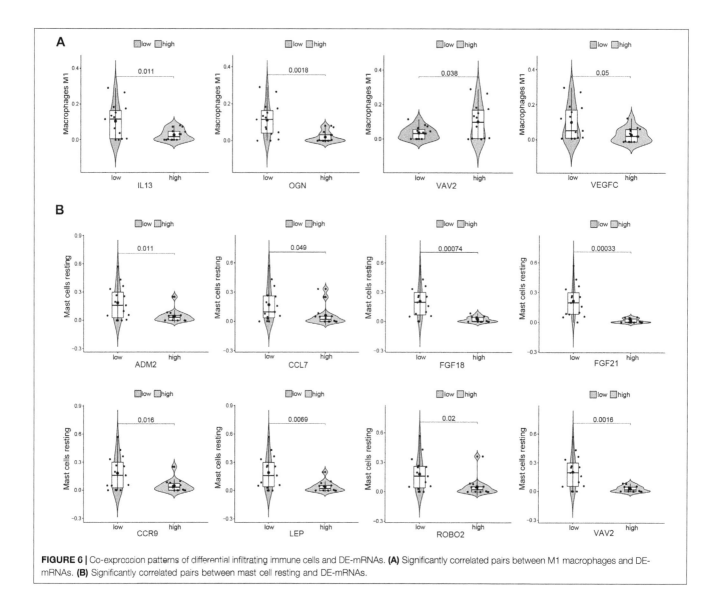

FIGURE 6 | Co-expression patterns of differential infiltrating immune cells and DE-mRNAs. **(A)** Significantly correlated pairs between M1 macrophages and DE-mRNAs. **(B)** Significantly correlated pairs between mast cell resting and DE-mRNAs.

139-5p expression levels in the HK-2 cell line in a dose-dependent manner. The interaction between NEAT1, PVT1, miR-429, miR-139-5p, and miR-23b-3p may regulate CaOx-induced kidney injury via CCL7 and ROBO2.

The CCL7 gene encodes C-C motif chemokine 7, which can attract monocytes to mediate inflammation and fibrosis (Klein et al., 2009). Inaba et al. (2020) demonstrated that CCL7 increased in a murine model of folic acid-induced acute kidney injury and that the blockade of CCL7 expression reduced monocyte recruitment and ameliorated injury. Sun et al. (2018) reported that CCL7 expression increased in the papillary and urine of patients with nephrolithiasis. The ROBO2 gene encodes the roundabout homolog 2, which is a receptor of slit homolog proteins (SLITs) and is associated with cellular migration guidance (Daehn and Duffield, 2021). ROBO2 dysfunction has been considered to cause congenital kidney and urinary tract abnormalities (Daehn and Duffield, 2021). Moreover, the SLITs/ROBO2 pathway was found to mediate inflammation and acute kidney injury (Chaturvedi and Robinson,

2015). In this study, treatment with 0.25 and 0.5 mM of oxalate significantly upregulated the expression levels of CCL7 and ROBO2 in the HK-2 cell line in a dose-dependent manner, yet the underlying mechanism still needed further investigation.

The polarization of macrophages has been recognized to be involved in the pathogenesis of kidney stones (Taguchi et al., 2021). Taguchi et al. (2016) found that M1-macrophage transfusion promoted kidney stone formation in hyperoxaluric mice and that M2-macrophage transfusion suppressed stone formation. Moreover, Xi et al. (2019) demonstrated that Sirtuin 3-overexpression suppressed crystal deposition through the promotion of the polarization of M2 macrophages. Mast cells have been considered as important components in kidney disease development (Vibhushan et al., 2020). Summers et al. (2012) demonstrated that mast cell activation and degranulation promoted renal fibrosis in mice with unilateral ureteric obstruction, while mast cell-deficient mice showed decreased collagen deposition. Moreover, it has been reported that mast cells can mediate cisplastin-induced acute kidney injury through

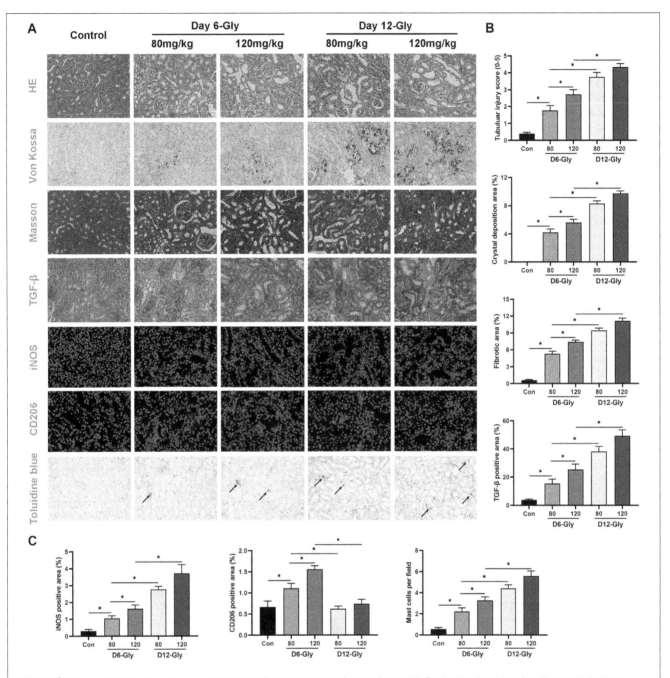

FIGURE 7 | Evaluation of kidney tubular injury, crystal deposition, fibrosis level, macrophage, and mast cell infiltration in a glyoxylate-induced hyperoxaluric mouse model. **(A)** Representative pictures of HE staining, Von Kossal staining, Masson staining, immunohistochemical staining, immunofluorescence staining, and Toluidine blue staining (magnification, 400×). **(B)** Quantification of kidney tubular injury score, CaOx crystal deposition area, collagen fiber deposition area, and TGF-β positive area. **(C)** Quantification of macrophage-related molecules in the iNOS (M1) and CD206 (M2) positive areas, and quantification of activated mast cell per field. Gly, glyoxylate. The arrow indicates activated mast cells. *$p < 0.05$.

the recruitment of leukocytes and secretion of TNF (Summers et al., 2011). However, the role of mast cells in the development of kidney stones has not been reported. Consistent with the aforementioned studies, we found that the proportion of M2 macrophages and resting mast cells decreased in the RPs of patients with CaOx stones. Furthermore, throughout kidney stone development, the infiltration of M1 macrophages and activated mast cells increased in mice with

glyoxylate-induced hyperoxaluria. M2-macrophage infiltration increased in the early stage and decreased as kidney stones progressed. Together, these results indicate that the polarization of macrophages and recruitment of mast cells may play crucial roles in the development of kidney stones.

This study has several limitations. First, although we analyzed two microarray datasets of kidney stones, the sample size was still

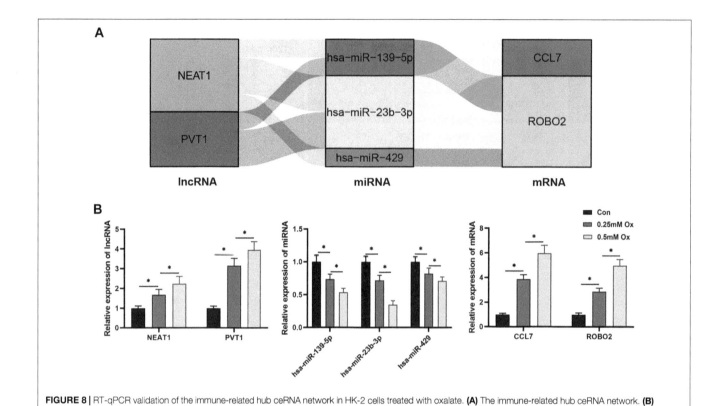

FIGURE 8 | RT-qPCR validation of the immune-related hub ceRNA network in HK-2 cells treated with oxalate. **(A)** The immune-related hub ceRNA network. **(B)** Quantification of the relative expression levels of NEAT1, PVT1, hsa-miR-23b-3p, hsa-miR-429, hsa-miR-139-5p, CCL7, and ROBO2 using RT-qPCR. *p < 0.05.

TABLE 4 | The details of hub ceRNA network from GEO datasets.

	LncRNA			microRNA	mRNA			
Name	Fold change	p.val	Status	Name	Name	Fold change	p.val	Status
NEAT1	1.58	0.00053	up	hsa-miR-23b-3p	CCL7	2.96	0.00013	up
					ROBO2	2.27	0.00607	up
				hsa-miR-429	ROBO2	2.27	0.00607	up
PVT1	2.70	0.00043	up	hsa-miR-23b-3p	CCL7	2.96	0.00013	up
					ROBO2	2.27	0.00607	up
				hsa-miR-139-5p	ROBO2	2.27	0.00607	up

limited; this was partly due to the low biopsy rate and low morbidity of kidney stones. Second, no miRNA microarray dataset of patients with kidney stones was available from an open database, thus potential target miRNAs were predicted by online tools. Third, the analysis of infiltrating immune cells only included 22 types; accordingly, the subtypes of macrophages and mast cells require further investigation. Fourth, HK-2 cell line was the only cell line for *in vitro* validation, other renal tubular epithelial cell lines should be studied in the further research. Finally, further functional experiments are needed to demonstrate the mechanisms of the immune-related ceRNA network and their relationship with immune cell infiltration.

In conclusion, in this comprehensive study, we construct an immune-related ceRNA regulatory network and estimate the composition of immune cell infiltration in the RPs of patients with kidney stones. Based on one mRNA and one lncRNA microarray datasets, we identified the DE-mRNA and DE-lncRNA present in RPs and normal papillary tissues and used them for the construction of the ceRNA network. Subsequently, we estimated DE infiltrating immune cells between RPs and normal papillary tissues and their correlation with immune-related DE-mRNAs. Among these cells, macrophages and mast cells were considered to be important immune cells associated with kidney stone formation. Moreover, we validated the ceRNA network and immune infiltration *in vivo* and *in vitro*. These findings provide new insights on the pathogenesis of kidney stones and novel potential therapeutic targets.

AUTHOR CONTRIBUTIONS

FC, TR, and YX designed the study. YX, TR, XZ, ZY, WY, and JN performed the experiments and collected the data. YR, RY, FL, PY, and DZ analyzed the data. YX, XZ, and ZY wrote the manuscript.

ACKNOWLEDGMENTS

We would like to thank the staffs of the central laboratory, Renmin Hospital of Wuhan University, for their full support.

SUPPLEMENTARY MATERIAL

Supplementary Figure 1 | PPI network of lncRNA-related differentially expressed mRNAs.

Supplementary Table S1 | Sequence of primers used for RT-qPCR.

REFERENCES

1. Agarwal, V., Bell, G. W., Nam, J.-W., and Bartel, D. P. (2015). Predicting Effective microRNA Target Sites in Mammalian mRNAs. *Elife* 4, e05005. doi:10.7554/eLife.05005

2. Beermann, J., Piccoli, M.-T., Viereck, J., and Thum, T. (2016). Non-coding RNAs in Development and Disease: Background, Mechanisms, and Therapeutic Approaches. *Physiol. Rev.* 96 (4), 1297–1325. doi:10.1152/physrev.00041.2015

3. Bhattacharya, S., Andorf, S., Gomes, L., Dunn, P., Schaefer, H., Pontius, J., et al. (2014). ImmPort: Disseminating Data to the Public for the Future of Immunology. *Immunol. Res.* 58 (2-3), 234–239. doi:10.1007/s12026-014- 8516-1

4. Chaturvedi, S., and Robinson, L. A. (2015). Slit2-Robo Signaling in Inflammation and Kidney Injury. *Pediatr. Nephrol.* 30 (4), 561–566. doi:10.1007/s00467-014- 2825-4

5. Chen, Y., and Wang, X. (2020). miRDB: an Online Database for Prediction of Functional microRNA Targets. *Nucleic Acids Res.* 48 (D1), D127–D131. doi:10.1093/nar/gkz757

6. Cheng, W., Li, X.-W., Xiao, Y.-Q., and Duan, S.-B. (2019). Non-coding RNA-Associated ceRNA Networks in a New Contrast-Induced Acute Kidney Injury Rat Model. *Mol. Ther. - Nucleic Acids* 17, 102–112. doi:10.1016/j.omtn.2019.05.011

7. Convento, M. B., Pessoa, E. A., Cruz, E., da Glória, M. A., Schor, N., and Borges, F. T. (2017). Calcium Oxalate Crystals and Oxalate Induce an Epithelial-To- Mesenchymal Transition in the Proximal Tubular Epithelial Cells: Contribution to Oxalate Kidney Injury. *Sci. Rep.* 7, 45740. doi:10.1038/srep45740

8. Daehn, I. S., and Duffield, J. S. (2021). The Glomerular Filtration Barrier: a Structural Target for Novel Kidney Therapies. *Nat. Rev. Drug Discov.* 20, 770–788. doi:10.1038/s41573-021-00242-0

9. Daudon, M., Bazin, D., and Letavernier, E. (2015). Randall's Plaque as the Origin of Calcium Oxalate Kidney Stones. *Urolithiasis* 43 (Suppl. 1), 5–11. doi:10.1007/ s00240-014-0703-y

10. Dong, Y., Zhang, Q., Wen, J., Chen, T., He, L., Wang, Y., et al. (2019). Ischemic Duration and Frequency Determines AKI-To-CKD Progression Monitored by Dynamic Changes of Tubular Biomarkers in IRI Mice. *Front. Physiol.* 10, 153. doi:10.3389/fphys.2019.00153

11. Huang, H.-Y., Lin, Y.-C. -D., Li, J., Huang, K.-Y., Shrestha, S., Hong, H.-C., et al. (2020). miRTarBase 2020: Updates to the Experimentally Validated microRNA-Target Interaction Database. *Nucleic Acids Res.* 48 (D1), D148–D154. doi:10.1093/nar/gkz896

12. Inaba, A., Tuong, Z. K., Riding, A. M., Mathews, R. J., Martin, J. L., Saeb-Parsy, K., et al. (2020). B Lymphocyte-Derived CCL7 Augments Neutrophil and Monocyte Recruitment, Exacerbating Acute Kidney Injury. *J.I.* 205 (5), 1376–1384. doi:10.4049/jimmunol.2000454

13. Jeggari, A., Marks, D. S., and Larsson, E. (2012). miRcode: a Map of Putative microRNA Target Sites in the Long Non-coding Transcriptome. *Bioinformatics* 28 (15), 2062–2063. doi:10.1093/bioinformatics/bts344

14. Jiang, K., Hu, J., Luo, G., Song, D., Zhang, P., Zhu, J., et al. (2020). Promotes Oxalate- and Calcium-Induced Kidney Oxidative Stress Injury by Suppressing MGP Expression. *Oxidative Med. Cell Longevity* 2020 (5863617), 1–14. doi:10.1155/2020/5863617

15. Khan, S. R., Canales, B. K., and Dominguez-Gutierrez, P. R. (2021). Randall's Plaque and Calcium Oxalate Stone Formation: Role for Immunity and Inflammation. *Nat. Rev. Nephrol.* 17 (6), 417–433. doi:10.1038/s41581-020- 00392-1

16. Khan, S. R., and Canales, B. K. (2015). Unified Theory on the Pathogenesis of Randall's Plaques and Plugs. *Urolithiasis* 43 (Suppl. 10 1), 109–123. doi:10.1007/s00240-014-0705-9

17. Kittanamongkolchai, W., Vaughan, L. E., Enders, F. T., Dhondup, T., Mehta, R. A., Krambeck, A. E., et al. (2018). The Changing Incidence and Presentation of Urinary Stones over 3 Decades. *Mayo Clinic Proc.* 93 (3), 291–299. doi:10.1016/j.mayocp.2017.11.018

18. Klein, J., Gonzalez, J., Duchene, J., Esposito, L., Pradere, J. P., Neau, E., et al. (2009). Delayed Blockade of the Kinin B1 Receptor Reduces Renal Inflammation and Fibrosis in Obstructive Nephropathy. *FASEB j.* 23 (1), 134–142. doi:10.1096/ fj.08-115600

19. Li, Y., Yan, G., Zhang, J., Chen, W., Ding, T., Yin, Y., et al. (2020). LncRNA HOXA11-AS Regulates Calcium Oxalate crystal-induced Renal Inflammation via miR-124-3p/MCP-1. *J. Cel Mol Med.* 24 (1), 238–249. doi:10.1111/ jcmm.14706

20. Liang, X., Lai, Y., Wu, W., Chen, D., Zhong, F., Huang, J., et al. (2019). LncRNA-miRNA-mRNA Expression Variation Profile in the Urine of Calcium Oxalate Stone Patients. *BMC Med. Genomics* 12 (1), 57. doi:10.1186/s12920-019-0502-y

21. Liu, H., Ye, T., Yang, X., Liu, J., Jiang, K., Lu, H., et al. (2019). H19 Promote Calcium Oxalate Nephrocalcinosis-Induced Renal Tubular Epithelial Cell Injury via a ceRNA Pathway. *EBioMedicine* 50, 366–378. doi:10.1016/j.ebiom.2019.10.059

22. Marien, T. P., and Miller, N. L. (2016). Characteristics of Renal Papillae in Kidney Stone Formers. *Minerva Urol. Nefrol* 68 (6), 496–515.

23. Newman, A. M., Liu, C. L., Green, M. R., Gentles, A. J., Feng, W., Xu, Y., et al. (2015). Robust Enumeration of Cell Subsets from Tissue Expression Profiles. *Nat. Methods* 12 (5), 453–457. doi:10.1038/nmeth.3337

24. Okada, A., Nomura, S., Higashibata, Y., Hirose, M., Gao, B., Yoshimura, M., et al.(2007). Successful Formation of Calcium Oxalate crystal Deposition in Mouse Kidney by Intraabdominal Glyoxylate Injection. *Urol. Res.* 35 (2), 89–99. doi:10.1007/s00240-007-0082-8

25. Pless, M. S., Williams, J. C., Jr, Andreassen, K. H., Jung, H. U., Osther, S. S., Christensen, D. R., et al. (2019). Endoscopic Observations as a Tool to Define Underlying Pathology in Kidney Stone Formers. *World J. Urol.* 37 (10), 2207–2215. doi:10.1007/s00345-018-02616-3

26. Ren, G. L., Zhu, J., Li, J., and Meng, X. M. (2019). Noncoding RNAs in Acute Kidney Injury. *J. Cel Physiol* 234 (3), 2266–2276. doi:10.1002/jcp.27203

27. Ritchie, M. E., Phipson, B., Wu, D., Hu, Y., Law, C. W., Shi, W., et al. (2015). Limma powers Differential Expression Analyses for RNA-Sequencing and Microarray Studies. Nucleic Acids Res. 43 (7), e47. doi:10.1093/nar/gkv007

28. Rule, A. D., Bergstralh, E. J., Melton, L. J., 3rd, Li, X., Weaver, A. L., and Lieske, J. C. (2009). Kidney Stones and the Risk for Chronic Kidney Disease. Cjasn 4 (4), 804–811. doi:10.2215/CJN.05811108

29. Rule, A. D., Krambeck, A. E., and Lieske, J. C. (2011). Chronic Kidney Disease in Kidney Stone Formers. Cjasn 6 (8), 2069–2075. doi:10.2215/CJN.10651110 Salmena, L., Poliseno, L., Tay, Y., Kats, L., and Pandolfi, P. P. (2011). A ceRNA Hypothesis: the Rosetta Stone of a Hidden RNA Language? Cell 146 (3), 353–358. doi:10.1016/j.cell.2011.07.014 Nucleic Acids Res. 43 (7), e47. doi:10.1093/nar/gkv007

30. Su, B., Han, H., Ji, C., Hu, W., Yao, J., Yang, J., et al. (2020). MiR-21 Promotes Calcium Oxalate-Induced Renal Tubular Cell Injury by Targeting PPARA. Am.

31. J. Physiology-Renal Physiol. 319 (2), F202–F214. doi:10.1152/ajprenal.00132.2020

32. Summers, S. A., Chan, J., Gan, P.-Y., Dewage, L., Nozaki, Y., Steinmetz, O. M., et al. (2011). Mast Cells Mediate Acute Kidney Injury through the Production of TNF. Jasn 22 (12), 2226–2236. doi:10.1681/ASN.2011020182

33. Summers, S. A., Gan, P.-y., Dewage, L., Ma, F. T., Ooi, J. D., O'Sullivan, K. M., et al. (2012). Mast Cell Activation and Degranulation Promotes Renal Fibrosis in Experimental Unilateral Ureteric Obstruction. Kidney Int. 82 (6), 676–685. doi:10.1038/ki.2012.211

34. Sun, A. Y., Hinck, B., Cohen, B. R., Keslar, K., Fairchild, R. L., and Monga, M. (2018). Inflammatory Cytokines in the Papillary Tips and Urine of Nephrolithiasis Patients. J. Endourology 32 (3), 236–244. doi:10.1089/end.2017.0699

35. Szklarczyk, D., Gable, A. L., Lyon, D., Junge, A., Wyder, S., Huerta-Cepas, J., et al. (2019). STRING V11: Protein-Protein Association Networks with Increased Coverage, Supporting Functional Discovery in Genome-wide Experimental Datasets. Nucleic Acids Res. 47 (D1), D607–D613. doi:10.1093/nar/gky1131

36. Taguchi, K., Hamamoto, S., Okada, A., Unno, R., Kamisawa, H., Naiki, T., et al. (2017). Genome-Wide Gene Expression Profiling of Randall's Plaques in Calcium Oxalate Stone Formers. Jasn 28 (1), 333–347. doi:10.1681/ASN.2015111271

37. Taguchi, K., Okada, A., Hamamoto, S., Unno, R., Moritoki, Y., Ando, R., et al. (2016). M1/M2-macrophage Phenotypes Regulate Renal Calcium Oxalate crystal Development. Sci. Rep. 6, 35167. doi:10.1038/srep35167

38. Taguchi, K., Okada, A., Unno, R., Hamamoto, S., and Yasui, T. (2021). Macrophage Function in Calcium Oxalate Kidney Stone Formation: A

39. Systematic Review of Literature. Front. Immunol. 12, 673690. doi:10.3389/fimmu.2021.673690

40. Uribarri, J. (2020). Chronic Kidney Disease and Kidney Stones. Curr. Opin. Nephrol. Hypertens. 29 (2), 237–242. doi:10.1097/mnh.0000000000000582 Usami, M., Okada, A., Taguchi, K., Hamamoto, S., Kohri, K., and Yasui, T. (2018).

41. Genetic Differences in C57BL/6 Mouse Substrains Affect Kidney crystal Deposition. Urolithiasis 46 (6), 515–522. doi:10.1007/s00240-018-1040-3

42. Vibhushan, S., Bratti, M., Montero-Hernández, J. E., El Ghoneimi, A., Benhamou, M., Charles, N., et al. (2020). Mast Cell Chymase and Kidney Disease. Ijms 22 (1), 302. doi:10.3390/ijms22010302

43. Wang, X. F., Zhang, B. H., Lu, X. Q., and Wang, R. Q. (2019). Gastrin-releasing Peptide Receptor Gene Silencing Inhibits the Development of the Epithelial- Mesenchymal Transition and Formation of a Calcium Oxalate crystal in Renal Tubular Epithelial Cells in Mice with Kidney Stones via the PI3K/Akt Signaling Pathway. J. Cel Physiol 234 (2), 1567–1577. doi:10.1002/jcp.27023

44. Xi, J., Chen, Y., Jing, J., Zhang, Y., Liang, C., Hao, Z., et al. (2019). Sirtuin 3 Suppresses the Formation of Renal Calcium Oxalate Crystals through Promoting M2 Polarization of Macrophages. J. Cel Physiol 234 (7), 11463–11473. doi:10.1002/jcp.27803

45. Xiangrui, Y., Xiong, W., Xi, W., Yuanbing, J., Shenqiang, Q., and Yu, G. (2020). Clinical Assessment of Risk Factors for Renal Atrophy after Percutaneous Nephrolithotomy. Med. Sci. Monit. 26, e919970. doi:10.12659/MSM.919970

46. Yu, G., Wang, L.-G., Han, Y., and He, Q.-Y. (2012). clusterProfiler: an R Package for Comparing Biological Themes Among Gene Clusters. OMICS: A J. Integr. Biol. 16 (5), 284 –287. doi:10.1089/omi.2011.0118

47. Zeng, G., Mai, Z., Xia, S., Wang, Z., Zhang, K., Wang, L., et al. (2017). Prevalence of Kidney Stones in China: an Ultrasonography Based Cross-Sectional Study. BJU Int. 120 (1), 109–116. doi:10.1111/bju.13828

48. Zhang, L., Wu, J.-H., Otto, J. C., Gurley, S. B., Hauser, E. R., Shenoy, S. K., et al. (2017). Interleukin-9 Mediates Chronic Kidney Disease-dependent Vein Graft Disease: a Role for Mast Cells. Cardiovasc. Res. 113 (13), 1551–1559. doi:10.1093/cvr/cvx177

49. Zhu, C., Liang, Q., Liu, Y., Kong, D., Zhang, J., Wang, H., et al. (2019). Kidney Injury in Response to Crystallization of Calcium Oxalate Leads to Rearrangement of the Intrarenal T Cell Receptor delta Immune Repertoire. J. Transl Med. 17 (1), 278. doi:10.1186/s12967-019-2022-0

50. Zhu, Z., Cui, Y., Huang, F., Zeng, H., Xia, W., Zeng, F., et al. (2020). Long Non-coding RNA H19 Promotes Osteogenic Differentiation of Renal Interstitial Fibroblasts through Wnt-β-Catenin Pathway. Mol. Cel Biochem 470 (1-2), 145–155. doi:10.1007/s11010-020-03753-3

51. Zhu, Z., Huang, F., Xia, W., Zeng, H., Gao, M., Li, Y., et al. (2021). Osteogenic Differentiation of Renal Interstitial Fibroblasts Promoted by lncRNA MALAT1 May Partially Contribute to Randall's Plaque Formation. Front. Cel Dev. Biol. 8, 596363. doi:10.3389/fcell.2020.596363

18

Urinary Extracellular Vesicles for Renal Tubular Transporters Expression in Patients with Gitelman Syndrome

Chih-Chien Sung [1], Min-Hsiu Chen [1], Yi-Chang Lin [2], Yu-Chun Lin [3], Yi-Jia Lin [3], Sung-Sen Yang [1] and Shih-Hua Lin [1]*

[1] Division of Nephrology, Department of Medicine, National Defense Medical Center, Tri-Service General Hospital, Taipei, Taiwan, [2] Division of Cardiovascular Surgery, Department of Surgery, National Defense Medical Center, Tri-Service General Hospital, Taipei, Taiwan, [3] Deparment of Pathology, National Defense Medical Center, Tri-Service General Hospital, Taipei, Taiwan

*Correspondence:
Shih-Hua Lin
l521116@ndmctsgh.edu.tw

Background: The utility of urinary extracellular vesicles (uEVs) to faithfully represent the changes of renal tubular protein expression remains unclear. We aimed to evaluate renal tubular sodium (Na^+) or potassium (K^+) associated transporters expression from uEVs and kidney tissues in patients with Gitelman syndrome (GS) caused by inactivating mutations in *SLC12A3*.

Methods: uEVs were isolated by ultracentrifugation from 10 genetically-confirmed GS patients. Membrane transporters including Na^+-hydrogen exchanger 3 (NHE3), $Na^+/K^+/2Cl^-$ cotransporter (NKCC2), NaCl cotransporter (NCC), phosphorylated NCC (p-NCC), epithelial Na^+ channel β (ENaCβ), pendrin, renal outer medullary K1 channel (ROMK), and large-conductance, voltage-activated and Ca^{2+}-sensitive K^+ channel (Maxi-K) were examined by immunoblotting of uEVs and immunofluorescence of biopsied kidney tissues. Healthy and disease (bulimic patients) controls were also enrolled.

Results: Characterization of uEVs was confirmed by nanoparticle tracking analysis, transmission electron microscopy, and immunoblotting. Compared with healthy controls, uEVs from GS patients showed NCC and p-NCC abundance were markedly attenuated but NHE3, ENaCβ, and pendrin abundance significantly increased. ROMK and Maxi-K abundance were also significantly accentuated. Immunofluorescence of the representative kidney tissues from GS patients also demonstrated the similar findings to uEVs. uEVs from bulimic patients showed an increased abundance of NCC and p-NCC as well as NHE3, NKCC2, ENaCβ, pendrin, ROMK and Maxi-K, akin to that in immunofluorescence of their kidney tissues.

Conclusion: uEVs could be a non-invasive tool to diagnose and evaluate renal tubular transporter adaptation in patients with GS and may be applied to other renal tubular diseases.

Keywords: Gitelman syndrome, renal tubular transporters, hypokalemia, renal tubular disease, urinary extracellular vesicles (exosomes)

INTRODUCTION

Gitelman syndrome (GS) is one of the most common inherited tubulopathy with a prevalence ranging from 0.25 to 4/10,000 per population. It is caused by biallelic inactivating mutations in the *SLC12A3* gene encoding thiazide-sensitive sodium-chloride cotransporter (NCC) expressed in the apical membrane of distal convoluted tubules (DCT) (1, 2). To date, more than 450 different mutations scattered throughout *SLC12A3* have been identified in GS (1, 3, 4). Clinical characteristics include renal sodium (Na^+) wasting with secondary hyperreninemia and hyperaldosteronism, renal potassium (K^+) wasting with chronic hypokalemia and metabolic alkalosis, and renal magnesium wasting with hypomagnesemia, but hypocalciuria (5). The defective NCC function caused by different classes of *SLC12A3* mutations leads to the reduced sodium chloride (NaCl) reabsorption in DCT with increased luminal NaCl delivery to downstream collecting ducts (CD) responsible for NaCl reabsorption via epithelial Na^+ channel (ENaC) and K^+ secretion via renal outer medullary K1 channel (ROMK) and large-conductance, voltage-activated and Ca^{2+}-sensitive K^+ channel (Maxi-K). Although the expression of ENaCβ, ROMK and Maxi-K in mouse GS model has been reported to be significantly increased in both immunoblotting and immunofluorescence of mouse kidney (6), the adaptive response of upstream and downstream Na^+ and K^+ associated transporters in response to renal Na^+ and K^+ wasting in GS patients remains unknown.

Urinary extracellular vesicles (uEVs) containing membrane and cytosolic proteins, mRNAs, miRNA and signaling molecules from each renal epithelial cell type may reflect the physiological state of their cells of origin (7, 8). The isolation of uEVs had the potential to shed much insight on the health status of the kidney and expression of urinary proteins (9–11). Knepper et al. has identified more than one thousand proteins including solute and water transporters, vacuolar H^+-ATPase subunits, and disease related proteins (12). It has been also reported that the isolated uEVs had an increased NCC abundance in patients with primary aldosteronism (13, 14) and Cushing syndrome (15) as well as a rapid increase in abundance of NCC and p-NCC in healthy subjects following the mineralocorticoid administration (16). In the inherited renal tubular disorders, uEVs have been used as a non-invasive tool to detect the defect of mutated renal tubular transporter such as NCC and $Na^+/K^+/2Cl^-$ cotransporter (NKCC2) expression in patients with GS and Bartter syndrome, respectively (17, 18). Nevertheless, uEVs for other renal Na^+ and K^+ associated transporters expression has not been also investigated in GS.

The aim of this study was to evaluate the changed expression of NCC, phosphorylated NCC (p-NCC), upstream DCT such as Na^+-hydrogen exchanger 3 (NHE3), NKCC2, downstream DCT such as ENaCβ, pendrin, as well as K^+-secreting channels such as ROMK and Maxi-K from uEVs and representative kidney tissues in patients with GS. Results to be reported indicated that a marked attenuation of NCC and p-NCC expression from uEVs could be used as a non-invasive diagnostic biomarker for GS. Both upstream NHE3 and downstream ENaCβ and pendrin from uEVs were increased in response to salt-losing and an enhanced

ROMK and Maxi-K expression were associated with renal K^+ wasting in GS patients. These findings from uEVs were similar to those obtained from renal biopsied tissues in GS patients.

MATERIALS AND METHODS
Study Design

The study protocol was approved by the Ethics Committee on Human Studies at Tri-Service General Hospital (TSGHIRB No.2-103-05-160 and TSGHIRB No.2-105-05-062). We prospectively collected 10 genetically confirmed GS patients. Their mutations included homozygous intronic mutation ($n = 2$), compound heterozygous mutati on ($n = 8$) in the *SLC12A3* gene encoding NCC (**Table 1**). Five healthy controls and three bulimic patients as hypokalemic disease controls were also enrolled. The diagnosis of bulimia was based on the American Psychiatric Association's Diagnostic and Statistical Manual, Fifth Edition (19). Clinical characteristics and laboratory examination were collected and determined. Renal biopsied tissues were collected from three different GS patients with definite *SLC12A3* mutations (compound heterozygous mutation of intronic c1670-191/p.I888_H916del, p.T60M/p.R959fs, and p.T60M/splicing c.965-1G>A+c965-977gcggacatttttgt>accgaaaatttt) and one bulimic patient. All of them had long-standing, severe hypokalemia refractory to aggressive K^+ supplementation and significant proteinuria. Control kidney tissue was obtained from normal part of kidney in one patient with renal cell carcinoma undergoing total nephrectomy.

uEVs Studies
Urine Collection and uEVs Isolation

Secondary morning spot urine with forty milliliters with protease inhibitors were collected for uEVs isolation by ultracentrifugation-based protocol. The urine sample was centrifuged at 17,000 × g for 10 min at 37°C. Supernatant was then ultracentrifuged at 200,000 × g for 2 h at 4°C. The pellet was resuspended in PBS or laemmli buffer with dithiothreitol.

Nanoparticle Tracking Analysis

Nanoparticles from isolated uEVs were analyzed using the NanoSight NS300 instrument (NanoSight Ltd, Amesbury, UK). Following published method (20), all experiments were carried out at a 1:1,000 dilution, yielding particle concentrations in the region of 1×10^8 particles ml^{-1} in accordance with the manufacturer's recommendations.

Transmission Electron Microscopy

uEVs pellet was carefully fixed the with enough volume of 2.5% glutaraldehyde (G5882, Sigma-Aldrich) in 0.1 M sodium cacodylate, pH 7.4 and 4% paraformaldehyde mix buffer (1:1) for 1 h at 4°C and then washed with PBS. Pre-fix the sample with 1 ml of 1% Osmium tetroxide (in ddH_2O) for 50 min at 4°C in dark. Post-fix the sample with 5% uranyl acetate (UA) blocking overnight at 4°C. Incubate for 10 min with a graded EtOH series (50, 70, 90, 95, 100%) and followed by EPON (Resin 20 ml, DDSA 7 ml, NMA 14 ml, DMP-30 0.8 ml). The uEVs samples

TABLE 1 | Characteristics of *SLC12A3* mutation among 10 patients with Gitelman syndrome.

Patients	Genotypes	Nucleotide change (NM_000339.3)	AA change (NP_000330.3)	Topological localization
1	Compound heterozygous	c.1924C>T + c.2548+253	p.R642C + Intronic	Transmembrane + C-terminal
2	Homozygous	c.1670-191C>T + c.1670-C>T	Intronic + Intronic	Transmembrane + Transmembrane
3	Compound heterozygous	c.2875_76delAG + c.2548+253	p.R959fs + Intronic	C-terminal + C-terminal
4	Compound heterozygous	c.2129C>A + c.2875-76delAG	p.S710X + p.R959fs	C-terminal + C-terminal
5	Compound heterozygous	c.488C>T+c.2660+1G>A	p.T163M + splicing	Transmembrane + C-terminal
6	Compound heterozygous	c.1000C>T+c.1326C>G	p.R334W + p.N442K	Transmembrane + Transmembrane
7	Homozygous	c.1670-191C>T + c.1670-C>T	Intronic+ Intronic	Transmembrane + Transmembrane
8	Compound heterozygous	c.2129C>A + c.2875_76delAG	p.S710X + p.R959fs	C-terminal + C-terminal
9	Compound heterozygous	c.911C>T/c.2875_76delAG	p.T304M + p.R959fs	Transmembrane + C-terminal
10	Compound heterozygous	c.2532G>A+c.805-06insTTGGCGTGGTCTCGG	p.W844X + p.T269delinsIGVVSA	C-terminal + Transmembrane

were analyzed with a Hitachi TEM HT7700 electron microscope operated at 60 kV.

Immunoblotting

For immunoblotting, the loading volume of each uEVs sample was adjusted so that the loaded amount of creatinine was constant (21, 22). SDS/PAGE was carried out on an 8% polyacrylamide gel, and proteins were transferred to Immobilon®-P membranes (Millipore, Amsterdam, The Netherlands). The primary antibodies were as follows: NSE (ab254088, Abcam, Cambridge, UK), TSG101 (ab125011, Abcam, Cambridge, UK), CD9 (GTX55564, Genetex, HsinChu City), AQP2 (sc-515770, Santa Cruz Biotechnology, Santa Cruz, CA), NHE3 (NHE31-A, Alpha Diagnostic Intl Inc., San Antonio, TX) (6), NKCC2 (AB2281, Millipore, Temecula, CA), NCC (AB3553, Millipore, Temecula, CA) (23), ENaCβ (ASC-019, Alomone labs, Jerusalem, Israel) (23), p-NCC (17T, in-house antibody) (23), Maxi-K (APC-021, Alomone labs, Jerusalem, Israel) (6), ROMK (APC-001, Alomone labs, Jerusalem, Israel) (6), and pendrin (ARP41739_P050, Aviva system biology, San Diego, CA). The membranes were incubated with the secondary antibody. Immunoreactive proteins were detected by the enhanced chemiluminescence method (Pierce, Rockford, IL, USA). The immunopositive bands from immunoblotting were quantified using pixel density scanning and calculated using Image J and the relative band intensity was normalized to the healthy controls.

Immunofluorescence of Kidney Tissue

After paraffin removal and rehydration, the slides were heated in 1× citrate buffer (ThermoFisher) and exposed to 3% H_2O_2 (ThermoFisher) at room temperature and then the blocking solution. After washing with PBS plus 0.1% Tween 20 (J.T. Baker), the tissue was incubated with primary antibodies at 4°C overnight. The primary antibodies of AQP2, NHE3, NKCC2, NCC, p-NCC, ENaCβ, Maxi-K, ROMK, and

pendrin were used. The tissues were exposed to species-specific secondary antibodies conjugated to Alexa Fluor fluorophores (ThermoFisher). Immunofluorescence images were obtained by Zeiss LSM880 confocal microscope.

Statistical Analyses

Serum and urine biochemistry data were expressed as mean ± standard deviation. Correlation between uEVs particles and urine creatinine were calculated by Pearson's correlation coefficient statistic in Excel. Data analyses were performed with the Prism (v5) software (GraphPad Software). Group comparisons of renal transporters from uEVs between GS patients and healthy controls were made using a two-tailed unpaired Student's *t*-test. Statistical significance was defined as *p*-values <0.05.

RESULTS

Clinical Characteristics in GS

As shown in **Table 2**, all GS patients (Male/Female = 9/1, age 33.4 ± 7.8 years old) were normotensive with renal Na^+ and Cl^- wasting and secondary hyperreninemia (plasma renin activity, PRA 28.9 ± 14.4 ng/mL/h) but normal to high plasma aldosterone concentration (PAC) (229.4 ± 69.6 pg/mL), chronic hypokalemia (K^+, 2.34 ± 0.45 mmol/L) with higher urinary K^+ excretion (transtubular potassium gradient, 13.46 ± 10.91), metabolic alkalosis ($HCO3^-$, 28.7 ± 3.9 mmol/L), hypomagnesemia (Mg^{2+} 0.63 ± 0.07 mmol/L), and hypocalciuria (Ca^{2+}/Creatinine 0.07 ± 0.06 mmol/mmol).

Characterization of uEVs

Characterization of the uEVs in healthy controls was validated by nanoparticle tracking analysis (NTA), transmission electron microscopy (TEM), and immunoblotting of uEVs makers. NTA identified size distribution of particles in the expected uEVs size range of 20–120 nm shown in **Figures 1A,B**. The mean particle size and concentration were 132.9 ± 65.8 nm and 6.6 × 10^{14}/ml,

TABLE 2 | Clinical characteristics and biochemistries in patients with Gitelman syndrome.

Patients		1	2	3	4	5	6	7	8	9	10	Mean ± SD
SBP/DBP (mmHg)		123/65	111/68	120/80	114/78	128/70	120/64	126/64	120/70	105/84	115/68	116.2 ± 7.5/69.7 ± 7.4
Serum	Reference											
BUN (mmol/L)	2.50–8.93	5.71	5.36	7.85	4.64	6.07	5.36	7.14	4.64	4.28	5.71	5.68 ± 1.12
Creatinine (μmol/L)	61.9–106.1	79.6	88.4	114.9	53 0	106.1	106.1	88.4	97.2	70.7	97.2	90.17.0 ± 18.54
Sodium (mmol/L)	136–145	135	135	138	132	140	142	138	137	134	134	137.1 ± 3.1
Potassium (mmol/L)	3.5–5.1	2.6	1.9	2.4	2.9	2.8	2.3	2.1	2.1	1.5	2.8	2.34 ± 0.45
Chloride (mmol/L)	98–107	97	100	98	94	97	99	97	98	96	96	97.2 ± 1.7
Total Calcium (mmol/L)	2.15–2.55	2.33	2.20	2.33	2.35	2.53	2.45	2.50	2.23	2.45	2.45	2.38 ± 0.11
Magnesium (mmol/L)	0.7–1.05	0.53	0.66	0.62	0.62	0.70	0.66	0.74	0.58	0.62	0.53	0.63 ± 0.67
Hematocrit (%)	38.0–47.0	45.7	49.0	46.3	39.9	53.9	54.0	48.3	46.8	44.4	45.6	47.4 ± 4.3
Albumin (g/L)	35–57	43	37	43	48	47	46	43	38	46	45	44 ± 4
PRA (ng/ml/hr)	1.31–3.95	17.15	10.29	47.13	6.32	50.00	31.07	38.35	29.04	30.35	29.14	28.9 ± 14.4
PAC (pg/ml)	70–350	252	206	140	147	134	266	304	320	288	237	229.4 ± 69.6
HCO3⁻ (mmol/L)	24	31.6	27.2	30.7	28.0	33.0	26.8	28.0	22.6	24.1	35.1	28.7 ± 3.9
Urine												
Creatinine (mmol/L)		10.6	9.4	7.9	5.7	7.3	2.1	7.9	6.2	4.7	5.2	8.6 ± 3.8
Sodium (mmol/L)		172	53	58	66	64	46	96	32	42	199	82.8 ± 57.1
Potassium (mmol/L)		45	21	27	48	43	26	17	56	37	49	36.9 ± 13.3
Chloride (mmol/L)		143	86	93	67	44	59	51	35	77	207	86.2 ± 52.4
Calcium (mmol/L)		0.58	0.55	0.25	1.28	0.23	0.05	0.10	0.63	0.38	0.53	0.46 ± 0.35
Magnesium (mmol/L)		3.09	2.55	2.34	3.58	3.17	0.86	0.62	2.26	1.52	4.61	2.46 ± 1.23
TTKG		7.15	7.28	7.10	10.80	12.51	12.61	7.13	41.13	22.67	6.23	13.46 ± 10.91

SBP, systolic blood pressure; DBP, diastolic blood pressure; PRA, plasma renin activity; PAC, plasma aldosterone concentration; TTKG, transtubular potassium gradient.

respectively. uEVs number was correlated strongly with urine creatinine (r^2 for 0.81, $P < 0.0001$) shown in **Figure 1C**. TEM also confirmed the quality of uEVs isolated by ultracentrifugation (**Figure 1D**). To further validate the uEVs purification protocol, we evaluated four commonly used uEVs makers including AQP2, TSG101, NSE, and CD9 in immunoblotting shown in **Figure 1E**. Expression pattern of selected renal transporters including NHE3, NKCC2, NCC, p-NCC, ENaCβ, pendrin, ROMK, and Maxi-K in healthy controls were shown in **Figure 1F**.

uEVs for Renal Tubular Na⁺ and K⁺ Associated Transporter Expression in GS

Compared with healthy controls, GS patients with different biallelic mutations exhibited a markedly attenuated expression of NCC and p-NCC protein isolated from their uEVs, indicative of an impaired NCC expression and function in GS (**Figures 2A,B**). The expression of NHE3, ENaCβ, and pendrin significantly increased although NKCC2 was not significantly increased. For uEVs associated renal tubular K⁺ associated transporter expression, GS patients had significantly increased ROMK and Maxi-K expression.

Renal Tubular Na⁺ and K⁺ Associated Transporter Expression From Kidney Tissues in GS

AQP2 used for a tubular maker of CD was clearly stained. Compared with control kidney tissue, the representative kidney

tissues from GS patients showed obviously diminished expression in both NCC and p-NCC. The expression of NHE3, ENaCβ and pendrin was significantly increased (**Figure 3**). The expression of ROMK was increased and the Maxi-K unexpressed in control kidney tissue without hypokalemia was also significantly enhanced in three GS patients. Overall, these finding from immunofluorescence of kidney tissues supported the findings of the isolated uEVs to examine Na⁺ and K⁺ associated renal transporter adaptation in GS patients.

Tubular Transporter Expression From uEVs and Kidney Tissue in Bulimic Patients

Three bulimic patients (male/female = 2/1, age 23.3 ± 4.0 years old) with normotension (systolic blood pressure 102 ± 17 mmHg, diastolic blood pressure 63 ± 5 mmHg) exhibited chronic hypokalemia (K⁺ 2.73 ± 0.55 mmol/L), metabolic alkalosis (HCO3⁻, 46.6 ± 11.9 mmol/L), with secondary hyperreninemia (PRA 4.3 ± 1.3 ng/mL/h) but normal to high PAC (127.6 ± 26.7 pg/mL). They all exhibited higher urinary K⁺ excretion, high Na⁺ (120.3 ± 80.4 mmol/L) but low Cl⁻ (18.7 ± 6.4 mmol/L), alkaline urine (bicarbonaturia), indicative of recent vomiting. As shown in **Figure 4A**, uEVs from them showed an increased abundance of NCC and p-NCC as well as NHE3, NKCC2, ENaCβ, pendrin, ROMK and Maxi-K. Immunofluorescence of the kidney tissue from a representative bulimic patient also had the similar finding to those in uEVs (**Figure 4B**).

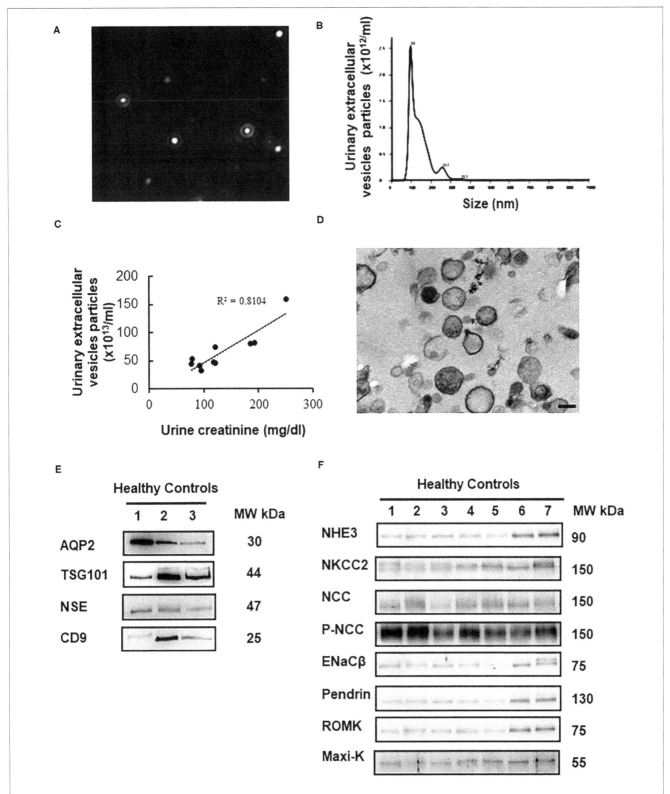

FIGURE 1 | Characterization of urinary extracellular vesicles (uEVs) from healthy controls. **(A)** Screen shot from 1:2,000 diluted urine sample reveals a range of particle sizes by nanoparticle tracking analysis (NTA). **(B)** Concentration and size distribution of uEVs (0–150 nm diameter) by NTA were shown. The concentration is expressed as number of particles per ml. **(C)** uEVs particles were correlated strongly with urine creatinine (r^2 for 0.81, $P < 0.0001$). **(D)** Transmission electron microscopy of uEVs was shown (scale bar 100 nm). **(E)** uEVs markers (AQP2, TSG101, NSE, and CD9) were assessed by immunoblotting. **(F)** Expression pattern of renal transporters including NHE3, NKCC2, NCC, p-NCC, ENaCβ, pendrin, ROMK, and Maxi-K from healthy controls was similar.

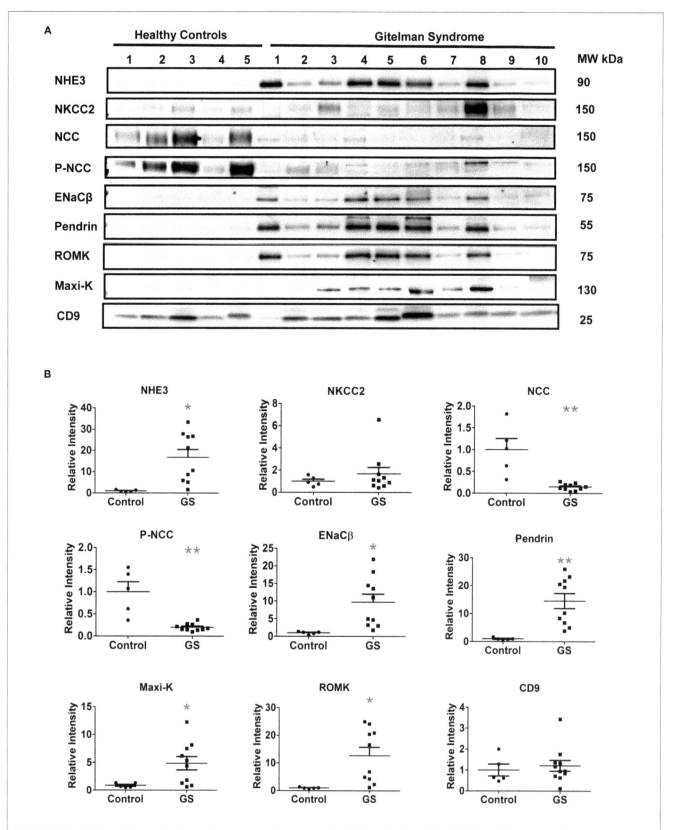

FIGURE 2 | Renal Na⁺ and K⁺ associated transporters expression from urinary extracellular vesicles in patients with GS ($n = 10$) compared with healthy controls. **(A)** Immunoblotting of renal transporters (NHE3, NKCC2, NCC, p-NCC, ENaCβ, pendrin, ROMK, Maxi-K, and CD9). **(B)** Quantification of immunoblotting of NHE3, NKCC2, NCC, p-NCC, ENaCβ, pendrin, ROMK, Maxi-K, and CD9. Error bars, standard deviation. $^*P < 0.05$, $^{**}P < 0.01$.

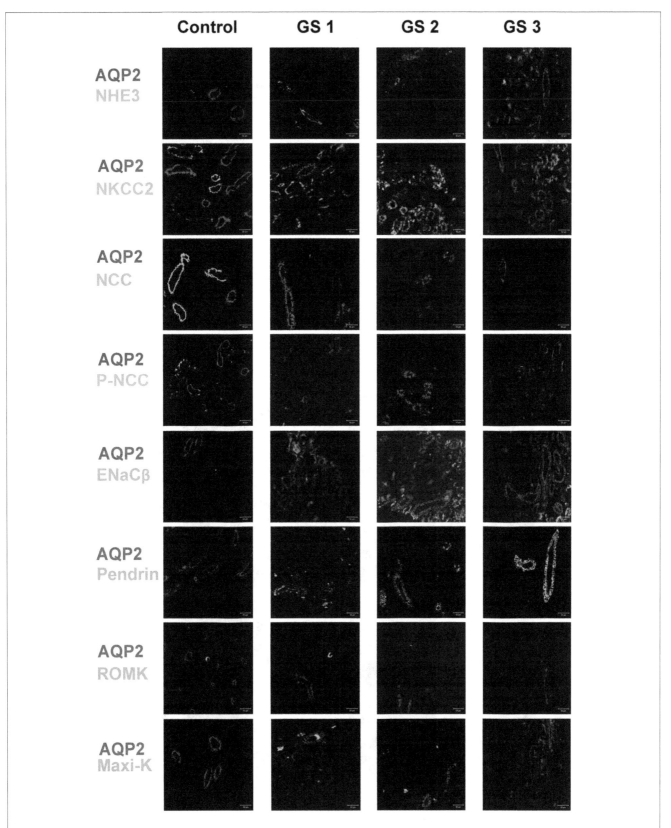

FIGURE 3 | Immunofluorescence of biopsied kidney tissues from another 3 representative GS patients (GS 1, GS 2, and GS 3) compared with the control kidney tissue. Renal transporters including NHE3, NKCC2, NCC, p-NCC, ENaCβ, pendrin, ROMK, Maxi-K were stained with green. AQP2 was stained with red for localization. Scale bar, 50 μm.

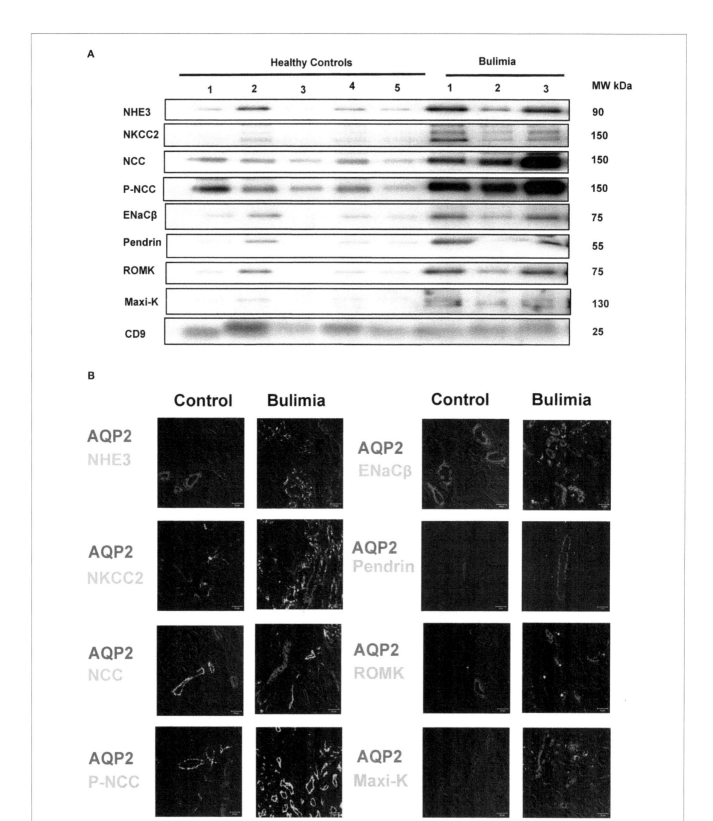

FIGURE 4 | Renal transporters expression from urinary extracellular vesicles (uEVs) and immunofluorescence of biopsied kidney tissues from bulimic patients. **(A)** Immunoblotting of renal transporters (NHE3, NKCC2, NCC, p-NCC, ENaCβ, pendrin, ROMK, Maxi-K, and CD9) from uEVs in bulimic patients ($n = 3$) compared with healthy control. **(B)** Immunofluorescence of NHE3, NKCC2, NCC, p-NCC (green, **right**) and ENaCβ, pendrin, ROMK, Maxi-K (green, **left**) from one representative bulimia patient compared with the control. AQP2 was stained with red for localization. Scale bar, 50 μm.

DISCUSSION

In this study, the isolated uEVs from GS patients with biallelic *SLC12A3* mutations showed the markedly attenuated expression of NCC and p-NCC whereas those from non-GS bulimic patients did a significantly enhanced abundance of NCC and p-NCC. In response to renal salt loss, the expression of upstream NHE3 and downstream ENaCβ, and pendrin were all accentuated. The abundance of ROMK and Maxi-K expression were also augmented for renal K^+ wasting in GS. Immunofluorescence of the representative kidney tissues from GS and bulimic patients also demonstrated similar findings to those from uEVs. This study might be the first to assess the abundance of renal tubular Na^+ and K^+ associated transporters from uEVs and kidney tissues in GS patients.

GS caused by inactivating *SLC12A3* mutations has an impaired NCC expression and/or activity as shown in both *vitro* and *vivo* studies. Although normal NCC expression with an impaired functional activity was shown in oocytes overexpressed T60M mutation at the critical NCC phosphorylation site, a markedly decreased total NCC and p-NCC protein abundance was evident in NccT58M/T58M GS knock-in mice and in the urine of human GS with homozygous T60M mutations (23). In addition, the reduced or abolished NCC abundance on the apical membrane of DCT from the human kidney tissues in GS patients with *SLC12A3* mutations were also demonstrated (24, 25). These findings supported the notion that the reduced expression of NCC was a biomarker for GS despite different mechanisms involved in the impaired NCC protein synthesis (24, 26), and sorting or trafficking defect of NCC (27). Accordingly, it is important to find a non-invasive method to faithfully represent NCC abundance in GS. Previous studies using uEVs to measure the mutated NCC by immunoblotting and enzyme-linked immunosorbent assays (ELISAs) in GS patients only showed the decreased NCC abundance (17, 18). In this study, the isolated uEVs from GS patients revealed that both NCC and p-NCC abundance were markedly diminished, also confirmed by the human kidney tissue of genetically-confirmed GS patients.

It is of great interest to understand and localize the tubular adaptation in the inherited renal tubular disorders. The traditional methods were the preparation of whole kidney sections for immunostaining and immunoblotting or biotinylating the rat or mice kidney tissues *in situ* under various chronic conditions in animal models. Tubular adaptation to renal Na^+ loss has been evaluated in the distal tubules in experimental models of GS but not human GS. Knepper et al. has used the LC-MS/MS to profile the proteome of human uEVs and suggested that uEVs analysis be a potential approach to discover adaptation in renal transporters (12). Using uEVs analysis in GS, we found that the abundance of upstream NHE3 in the proximal tubules (PT) necessary for bicarbonate reabsorption, salt and fluid homeostasis was significantly increased (28–30). Renal NHE3 abundance was markedly increased in K^+-depleted rats (31), indicating that NHE3 expression can be also regulated by the hypokalemia independent of volume depletion. Similarly, downstream ENaCβ in the principal cells of CD for tubular salt reabsorption was enhanced (32, 33). Of note, pendrin as a

Cl^-/HCO_3^- exchanger expressed in the apical region of distal tubules and involved in the tubular Cl^- absorption and HCO_3^- secretion was augmented (34). Activation of pendrin-mediated Cl^- absorption has also been reported in NCC KO mice (35). Although pendrin expression has been examined in many rodent treatment models such as NCC KO mice, an aldosterone infusion or the administration of $NaHCO_3$ to regulate acid-base and salt regulation, our study suggested the increased pendrin expression from uEVs and biopsied kidney tissues be responsive to renal salt wasting and also chronic metabolic alkalosis in GS patients.

K^+ excretion in distal nephron is driven by either voltage-dependent ROMK and/or flow dependent Maxi-K (36). ROMK is an inwardly rectifying K^+ channel (37) traditionally responsible for the main renal K^+ secretory channel, dependent on Na^+ delivery and driven by electrogenic ENaC-mediated Na^+ reabsorption (38–40). Maxi-K is flow-stimulated K^+ secretion and activated by an increase in intracellular calcium and membrane depolarization (41, 42). Defective NaCl absorption in DCT leads to the increased flow rate to downstream connecting tubules (CNT) and CD to naturally stimulate both ROMK and Maxi-K. In animal model of GS (Ser707X knockin mice), an enhanced expression of both ROMK and Maxi-K has been clearly shown (6). Our uEVs for the expression of both ROMK and Maxi-K abundance were significantly increased in GS patients, akin to the findings of their representative immunofluorescence of kidney tissues. Of note, the abundance of Maxi-K was extremely low in both uEVs and biopsied kidney in controls but higher in GS patients, indicating that Maxi-K expression was more augmented at the high urinary flow rate.

The above-mentioned findings with an increased protein expression related to Na^+ reabsorption, K^+ secretion and regulation of acid/base balance at distal nephron from the uEVs in our GS patients with diminished NCC expression consisted with current idea that distal tubules including CD are highly plastic. Tubular plasticity for adaptation is defined as structural remodeling of renal tubules via cell proliferation (hyperplasia) and cell growth (hypertrophy) (43, 44). In NCC-deficient mice, early DCT showed a remarkable atrophy but CNT exhibited a marked epithelial hypertrophy accompanied by an increased apical abundance of ENaC (45). In SPAK KO mice featuring GS-like phenotypes, a distal nephron remodeling process of the CNT/CD developed to produce an increase in the numbers of principle cells and β-intercalated cells (46). These two mice models with deficient NCC clearly demonstrated the markedly attenuated DCT along with the distinctly hypertrophic and/or hyperplastic CNT/CD. Our uEVs results in GS patients were similar to those from NCC deficient animal studies, also supporting the notion of nephron plasticity with compensatory increase in the CNT/CD size.

Bulimic patients, also called pseudo-GS syndrome (47, 48), exhibiting similar laboratory and clinical features to GS, were also evaluated for disease controls. In contrast to GS patients, uEVs from bulimic patients showed a markedly enhanced abundance of NCC and p-NCC. The increased NCC and p-NCC abundance may be secondary response to volume depletion and K^+ deficiency *per se*. In rat model of K^+ deficiency, enhanced abundance NCC and p-NCC has been clearly shown (49), closely linked to increased WNK body formation and activation of SPAK/OSR1 (50). Similarly, uEVs for upstream NHE3 and NKCC2 along with downstream ENaCβ and pendrin expression were also increased in response to salt-losing and metabolic alkalosis. Of interest, only the slightly increased ROMK and Maxi-K abundance from the isolated uEVs and biopsied kidney tissues may be associated with the interaction of bicarbonaturia to stimulate them as well as the enhanced NCC and chronic hypokalemia to suppress them.

Recently, uEVs has been emerged as a promising liquid biopsy biomarker in kidney disease research. Several novel biomarkers from uEVs including proteins, miRNA or noncoding RNA have been discovered in acute kidney injury (51, 52), chronic kidney disease (53, 54), diabetic nephropathy (55), focal segmental glomerulosclerosis (56), and lupus nephritis (57). In addition to GS and Bartter syndrome, uEVs is also utilized in some renal tubular disorders such as nephrogenic diabetes insipidus, and familial hyperkalemic hypertension due to *KLHL3* mutation (58). Accordingly, these evidence demonstrated the relevance of uEVs in understanding the pathophysiology of kidney diseases and the discovery of potential therapeutic targets. Our study provided a feasible way to analyze the differential expression proteins in renal tubular disorders and may be also applied to other non-tubular disorder such as cisplatin or drug induced tubulopathy.

There were some limitations of this study. First, the sample size of GS patients was still small due to the restricted loading wells of SDS/PAGE for immunoblotting. Second, other relevant transporters along the renal tubules such as TRPV5 and TRPM6 were not examined because of limited uEVs

proteins isolated from ultracentrifugation. Third, the localization of these transporters in renal tubules could not be identified using uEVs. Finally, the specificity and sensitivity of the antibodies used for this study might affect expression of renal transporters between immunoblotting and immunofluorescence (for example NKCC2). Using the detergent for immunoblotting is another approach to enhance intracellular epitope recognition in uEVs (22).

In conclusion, uEVs could be used as non-invasive diagnostic tool to evaluate the renal tubular Na$^+$ or K$^+$ associated transporters expression in GS patients. High-throughput proteomic studies from uEVs in GS patients will be anticipated in the further investigation.

AUTHOR CONTRIBUTIONS

C-CS, M-HC, and S-HL substantially contributed to study conception and design, acquisition of data, and analysis and interpretation of data. Y-ChaL, Y-ChuL, Y-JL, and S-SY substantially contributed to acquisition of data, and analysis and interpretation of data. All the authors revised the paper and approved the final version of the article to be published.

ACKNOWLEDGMENTS

The authors acknowledge technical services provided by Instrument Center of National Defense Medical Center.

REFERENCES

1. Blanchard A, Bockenhauer D, Bolignano D, Calò LA, Cosyns E, Devuyst O, et al. Gitelman syndrome: consensus and guidance from a Kidney Disease: Improving Global Outcomes (KDIGO) Controversies Conference. *Kidney Int.* (2017) 91:24–33. doi: 10.1016/j.kint.2016.09.046

2. Simon DB, Nelson-Williams C, Bia MJ, Ellison D, Karet FE, Molina AM, et al. Gitelman's variant of Bartter's syndrome, inherited hypokalaemic alkalosis, is caused by mutations in the thiazide-sensitive Na-Cl cotransporter. *Nat Genet.* (1996) 12:24–30. doi: 10.1038/ng0196-24

3. Lo Y-F, Nozu K, Iijima K, Morishita T, Huang C-C, Yang S-S, et al. Recurrent deep intronic mutations in the SLC12A3 gene responsible for Gitelman's syndrome. *Clin J Am Soc Nephrol.* (2011) 6:630–9. doi: 10.2215/CJN.06730810

4. Vargas-Poussou R, Dahan K, Kahila D, Venisse A, Riveira-Munoz E, Debaix H, et al. Spectrum of mutations in Gitelman syndrome. *J Am Soc Nephrol.* (2011) 22:693–703. doi: 10.1681/ASN.2010090907

5. Tseng MH, Yang SS, Hsu YJ, Fang YW, Wu CJ, Tsai JD, et al. Genotype, phenotype, and follow-up in Taiwanese patients with salt-losing tubulopathy associated with SLC12A3 mutation. *J Clin Endocrinol Metab.* (2012) 97:E1478–82. doi: 10.1210/jc.2012-1707

6. Yang SS, Lo YF, Yu IS, Lin SW, Chang TH, Hsu YJ, et al. Generation and analysis of the thiazide-sensitive Na+ -Cl- cotransporter (Ncc/Slc12a3) Ser707X knockin mouse as a model of Gitelman syndrome. *Hum Mutat.* (2010) 31:1304–15. doi: 10.1002/humu.21364

7. van Balkom BW, Pisitkun T, Verhaar MC, Knepper MA. Exosomes and the kidney: prospects for diagnosis and therapy of renal diseases. *Kidney Int.* (2011) 80:1138–45. doi: 10.1038/ki.2011.292

8. Pisitkun T, Shen RF, Knepper MA. Identification and proteomic profiling of exosomes in human urine. *Proc Natl Acad Sci USA.* (2004) 101:13368–73. doi: 10.1073/pnas.0403453101

9. Gonzales P, Pisitkun T, Knepper MA. Urinary exosomes: is there a future? *Nephrol Dial Transplant.* (2008) 23:1799–801. doi: 10.1093/ndt/gfn058

10. Knepper MA, Pisitkun T. Exosomes in urine: who would have thought? *Kidney Int.* (2007) 72:1043–5. doi: 10.1038/sj.ki.5002510

11. Bonifacino JS, Traub LM. Signals for sorting of transmembrane proteins to endosomes and lysosomes. *Annu Rev Biochem.* (2003) 72:395–447. doi: 10.1146/annurev.biochem.72.121801.161800

12. Gonzales PA, Pisitkun T, Hoffert JD, Tchapyjnikov D, Star RA, Kleta R, et al. Large-scale proteomics and phosphoproteomics of urinary exosomes. *J Am Soc Nephrol.* (2009) 20:363–79. doi: 10.1681/ASN.2008040406

13. van der Lubbe N, Jansen PM, Salih M, Fenton RA, van den Meiracker AH, Danser AH, et al. The phosphorylated sodium chloride cotransporter in urinary exosomes is superior to prostasin as a marker for aldosteronism. *Hypertension.* (2012) 60:741–8. doi: 10.1161/HYPERTENSIONAHA.112.198135

14. Salih M, Fenton RA, Zietse R, Hoorn EJ. Urinary extracellular vesicles as markers to assess kidney sodium transport. *Curr Opin Nephrol Hypertens.* (2016) 25:67–72. doi: 10.1097/MNH.0000000000000192

15. Salih M, Bovée DM, van der Lubbe N, Danser AHJ, Zietse R, Feelders RA, et al. Increased urinary extracellular vesicle sodium transporters in Cushing syndrome with hypertension. *J Clin Endocrinol Metab.* (2018) 103:2583–91. doi: 10.1210/jc.2018-00065

16. Wolley MJ, Wu A, Xu S, Gordon RD, Fenton RA, Stowasser M. In primary aldosteronism, mineralocorticoids influence exosomal sodium-chloride cotransporter abundance. *J Am Soc Nephrol.* (2017) 28:56–63. doi: 10.1681/ASN.2015111221

17. Corbetta S, Raimondo F, Tedeschi S, Syrèn ML, Rebora P, Savoia A, et al. Urinary exosomes in the diagnosis of Gitelman and Bartter syndromes. *Nephrol Dial Transplant.* (2015) 30:621–30. doi: 10.1093/ndt/gfu362

18. Isobe K, Mori T, Asano T, Kawaguchi H, Nonoyama S, Kumagai N, et al. Development of enzyme-linked immunosorbent assays for urinary thiazide-sensitive Na-Cl cotransporter measurement. *Am J Physiol Renal Physiol.* (2013) 305:F1374–81. doi: 10.1152/ajprenal.00208.2013

19. Vahia VN. Diagnostic and statistical manual of mental disorders 5: a quick glance. *Indian J Psychiatry.* (2013) 55:220–3. doi: 10.4103/0019-5545.117131

20. Sokolova V, Ludwig AK, Hornung S, Rotan O, Horn PA, Epple M, et al. Characterisation of exosomes derived from human cells by nanoparticle tracking analysis and scanning electron microscopy. *Colloids Surf B Biointerfaces.* (2011) 87:146–50. doi: 10.1016/j.colsurfb.2011.05.013

21. Abdeen A, Sonoda H, Oshikawa S, Hoshino Y, Kondo H, Ikeda M. Acetazolamide enhances the release of urinary exosomal aquaporin-1. *Nephrol Dial Transplant.* (2016) 31:1623–32. doi: 10.1093/ndt/gfw033

22. Blijdorp CJ, Tutakhel OAZ, Hartjes TA, van den Bosch TPP, van Heugten MH, Rigalli JP, et al. Comparing approaches to normalize, quantify, and characterize urinary extracellular vesicles. *J Am Soc Nephrol.* (2021) 32:1210–26. doi: 10.1681/ASN.2020081142

23. Yang SS, Fang YW, Tseng MH, Chu PY, Yu IS, Wu HC, et al. Phosphorylation regulates NCC stability and transporter activity in vivo. *J Am Soc Nephrol.* (2013) 24:1587–97. doi: 10.1681/ASN.2012070742

24. Joo KW, Lee JW, Jang HR, Heo NJ, Jeon US, Oh YK, et al. Reduced urinary excretion of thiazide-sensitive Na-Cl cotransporter in Gitelman syndrome: preliminary data. *Am J Kidney Dis.* (2007) 50:765–73. doi: 10.1053/j.ajkd.2007.07.022

25. Jang HR, Lee JW, Oh YK, Na KY, Joo KW, Jeon US, et al. From bench to bedside: diagnosis of Gitelman's syndrome – defect of sodium-chloride cotransporter in renal tissue. *Kidney Int.* (2006) 70:813–7. doi: 10.1038/sj.ki.5001694

26. Syrèn ML, Tedeschi S, Cesareo L, Bellantuono R, Colussi G, Procaccio M, et al. Identification of fifteen novel mutations in the SLC12A3 gene encoding the Na-Cl Co-transporter in Italian patients with Gitelman syndrome. *Hum Mutat.* (2002) 20:78. doi: 10.1002/humu.9045

27. De Jong JC, Van Der Vliet WA, Van Den Heuvel LP, Willems PH, Knoers NV, Bindels RJ. Functional expression of mutations in the human NaCl cotransporter: evidence for impaired routing mechanisms in Gitelman's syndrome. *J Am Soc Nephrol.* (2002) 13:1442–8. doi: 10.1097/01.ASN.0000017904.77985.03

28. Knepper MA, Brooks HL. Regulation of the sodium transporters NHE3, NKCC2 and NCC in the kidney. *Curr Opin Nephrol Hypertens.* (2001) 10:655–9. doi: 10.1097/00041552-200109000-00017

29. Bobulescu IA, Moe OW. Na^+/H^+ exchangers in renal regulation of acid-base balance. *Semin Nephrol.* (2006) 26:334–44. doi: 10.1016/j.semnephrol.2006.07.001

30. Fenton RA, Poulsen SB, de la Mora Chavez S, Soleimani M, Dominguez Rieg JA, Rieg T. Renal tubular NHE3 is required in the maintenance of water and sodium chloride homeostasis. *Kidney Int.* (2017) 92:397–414. doi: 10.1016/j.kint.2017.02.001

31. Elkjaer ML, Kwon TH, Wang W, Nielsen J, Knepper MA, Frøkiaer J, et al. Altered expression of renal NHE3, TSC, BSC-1, and ENaC subunits in potassium-depleted rats. *Am J Physiol Renal Physiol.* (2002) 283:F1376–88. doi: 10.1152/ajprenal.00186.2002

32. Khuri RN, Strieder WN, Giebisch G. Effects of flow rate and potassium intake on distal tubular potassium transfer. *Am J Physiol.* (1975) 228:1249–61. doi: 10.1152/ajplegacy.1975.228.4.1249

33. Malnic G, Berliner RW, Giebisch G. Flow dependence of K^+ secretion in cortical distal tubules of the rat. *Am J Physiol.* (1989) 256 (5 Pt 2):F932–41. doi: 10.1152/ajprenal.1989.256.5.F932

34. Wall SM, Verlander JW, Romero CA. The renal physiology of pendrin-positive intercalated cells. *Physiol Rev.* (2020) 100:1119–47. doi: 10.1152/physrev.00011.2019

35. Soleimani M, Barone S, Xu J, Shull GE, Siddiqui F, Zahedi K, et al. Double knockout of pendrin and Na-Cl cotransporter (NCC) causes severe salt wasting, volume depletion, and renal failure. *Proc Natl Acad Sci USA.* (2012) 109:13368–73. doi: 10.1073/pnas.1202671109

36. Subramanya AR, Ellison DH. Distal convoluted tubule. *Clin J Am Soc Nephrol.* (2014) 9:2147–63. doi: 10.2215/CJN.05920613

37. Hebert SC. An ATP-regulated, inwardly rectifying potassium channel from rat kidney (ROMK). *Kidney Int.* (1995) 48:1010–6. doi: 10.1038/ki.1995.383

38. Lee WS, Hebert SC. ROMK inwardly rectifying ATP-sensitive K+ channel. I. Expression in rat distal nephron segments. *Am J Physiol.* (1995) 268 (6 Pt 2):F1124–31. doi: 10.1152/ajprenal.1995.268.6.F1124

39. Giebisch G. Renal potassium transport: mechanisms and regulation. *Am J Physiol.* (1998) 274:F817–33. doi: 10.1152/ajprenal.1998.274.5.F817

40. Welling PA, Ho K. A comprehensive guide to the ROMK potassium channel: form and function in health and disease. *Am J Physiol Renal Physiol.* (2009) 297:F849–63. doi: 10.1152/ajprenal.00181.2009

41. Pluznick JL, Sansom SC. BK channels in the kidney: role in K(+) secretion and localization of molecular components. *Am J Physiol Renal Physiol.* (2006) 291:F517–29. doi: 10.1152/ajprenal.00118.2006

42. Rodan AR, Huang CL. Distal potassium handling based on flow modulation of maxi-K channel activity. *Curr Opin Nephrol Hypertens.* (2009) 18:350–5. doi: 10.1097/MNH.0b013e32832c75d8

43. Kaissling B, Bachmann S, Kriz W. Structural adaptation of the distal convoluted tubule to prolonged furosemide treatment. *Am J Physiol.* (1985) 248 (3 Pt 2):F374–81. doi: 10.1152/ajprenal.1985.248.3.F374

44. Kaissling B, Stanton BA. Adaptation of distal tubule and collecting duct to increased sodium delivery. I. Ultrastructure. *Am J Physiol.* (1988) 255 (6 Pt 2):F1256–68. doi: 10.1152/ajprenal.1988.255.6.F1256

45. Loffing J, Vallon V, Loffing-Cueni D, Aregger F, Richter K, Pietri L, et al. Altered renal distal tubule structure and renal Na^+ and Ca^{2+} handling in a mouse model for Gitelman's syndrome. *J Am Soc Nephrol.* (2004) 15:2276–88. doi: 10.1097/01.ASN.0000138234.18569.63

46. Grimm PR, Lazo-Fernandez Y, Delpire E, Wall SM, Dorsey SG, Weinman EJ, et al. Integrated compensatory network is activated in the absence of NCC phosphorylation. *J Clin Invest.* (2015) 125:2136–50. doi: 10.1172/JCI78558

47. Seyberth HW, Schlingmann KP. Bartter- and Gitelman-like syndromes: salt-losing tubulopathies with loop or DCT defects. *Pediatr Nephrol.* (2011) 26:1789–802. doi: 10.1007/s00467-011-1871-4

48. Matsunoshita N, Nozu K, Shono A, Nozu Y, Fu XJ, Morisada N, et al. Differential diagnosis of Bartter syndrome, Gitelman syndrome, and pseudo-Bartter/Gitelman syndrome based on clinical characteristics. *Genet Med.* (2016) 18:180–8. doi: 10.1038/gim.2015.56

49. Frindt G, Palmer LG. Effects of dietary K^+ on cell-surface expression of renal ion channels and transporters. *Am J Physiol Renal Physiol.* (2010) 299:F890–7. doi: 10.1152/ajprenal.00323.2010

50. Wade JB, Liu J, Coleman R, Grimm PR, Delpire E, Welling PA. SPAK-mediated NCC regulation in response to low-K+ diet. *Am J Physiol Renal Physiol.* (2015) 308:F923–31. doi: 10.1152/ajprenal.00388.2014

51. Sonoda H, Lee BR, Park K-H, Nihalani D, Yoon J-H, Ikeda M, et al. miRNA profiling of urinary exosomes to assess the progression of acute kidney injury. *Scientific Reports.* (2019) 9:4692. doi: 10.1038/s41598-019-40747-8

52. Awdishu L, Tsunoda S, Pearlman M, Kokoy-Mondragon C, Ghassemian M, Naviaux RK, et al. Identification of maltase glucoamylase as a biomarker of acute kidney injury in patients with cirrhosis. *Crit Care Res Pract.* (2019) 2019:5912804. doi: 10.1155/2019/5912804

53. Khurana R, Ranches G, Schafferer S, Lukasser M, Rudnicki M, Mayer G, et al. Identification of urinary exosomal noncoding RNAs as novel biomarkers in chronic kidney disease. *Rna.* (2017) 23:142–52. doi: 10.1261/rna.058834.116

54. Wang B, Zhang A, Wang H, Klein JD, Tan L, Wang ZM, et al. miR-26a limits muscle wasting and cardiac fibrosis through exosome-mediated microRNA transfer in chronic kidney disease. *Theranostics.* (2019) 9:1864–77. doi: 10.7150/thno.29579

55. Zang J, Maxwell AP, Simpson DA, McKay GJ. Differential expression of urinary exosomal microRNAs miR-21-5p and miR-30b-5p in individuals with diabetic kidney disease. *Sci Rep.* (2019) 9:10900. doi: 10.1038/s41598-019-47504-x

56. Gebeshuber CA, Kornauth C, Dong L, Sierig R, Seibler J, Reiss M, et al. Focal segmental glomerulosclerosis is induced by microRNA-193a and its downregulation of WT1. *Nat Med.* (2013) 19:481–7. doi: 10.1038/nm.3142

57. Garcia-Vives E, Solé C, Moliné T, Vidal M, Agraz I, Ordi-Ros J, et al. The urinary exosomal miRNA expression profile is predictive of clinical response in lupus nephritis. *Int J Mol Sci.* (2020) 21:1372. doi: 10.3390/ijms21041372

19

A Novel Prognostic Model Based on Ferroptosis-Related Gene Signature for Bladder Cancer

Libo Yang[1†], Chunyan Li[2†], Yang Qin[1], Guoying Zhang[1], Bin Zhao[1], Ziyuan Wang[3], Youguang Huang[3*] and Yong Yang[1*]

[1] Department of Urology, The Third Affiliated Hospital of Kunming Medical University, Kunming, China, [2] Second Department of Head and Neck Surgery, The Third Affiliated Hospital of Kunming Medical University, Kunming, China, [3] Department of Yunnan Tumor Research Institute, The Third Affiliated Hospital of Kunming Medical University, Kunming, China

*Correspondence:
Yong Yang
yongy1974@163.com
Youguang Huang
huangyouguang2008@126.com

[†]These authors have contributed equally to this work and share first authorship

Background: Bladder cancer (BC) is a molecular heterogeneous malignant tumor; the treatment strategies for advanced-stage patients were limited. Therefore, it is vital for improving the clinical outcome of BC patients to identify key biomarkers affecting prognosis. Ferroptosis is a newly discovered programmed cell death and plays a crucial role in the occurrence and progression of tumors. Ferroptosis-related genes (FRGs) can be promising candidate biomarkers in BC. The objective of our study was to construct a prognostic model to improve the prognosis prediction of BC.

Methods: The mRNA expression profiles and corresponding clinical data of bladder urothelial carcinoma (BLCA) patients were downloaded from The Cancer Genome Atlas (TCGA) and Gene Expression Omnibus (GEO) databases. FRGs were identified by downloading data from FerrDb. Differential analysis was performed to identify differentially expressed genes (DEGs) related to ferroptosis. Univariate and multivariate Cox regression analyses were conducted to establish a prognostic model in the TCGA cohort. BLCA patients from the GEO cohort were used for validation. Gene ontology (GO), Kyoto Encyclopedia of Genes and Genomes (KEGG), and single-sample gene set enrichment analysis (ssGSEA) were used to explore underlying mechanisms.

Results: Nine genes (ALB, BID, FADS2, FANCD2, IFNG, MIOX, PLIN4, SCD, and SLC2A3) were identified to construct a prognostic model. Patients were classified into high-risk and low-risk groups according to the signature-based risk score. Receiver operating characteristic (ROC) and Kaplan–Meier (K–M) survival analysis confirmed the superior predictive performance of the novel survival model based on the nine-FRG signature. Multivariate Cox regression analyses showed that risk score was an independent risk factor associated with overall survival (OS). GO and KEGG enrichment analysis indicated that apart from ferroptosis-related pathways, immune-related pathways were significantly enriched. ssGSEA analysis indicated that the immune status was different between the two risk groups.

Conclusion: The results of our study indicated that a novel prognostic model based on the nine-FRG signature can be used for prognostic prediction in BC patients. FRGs are potential prognostic biomarkers and therapeutic targets.

Keywords: ferroptosis, prognosis, biomarkers, bladder cancer, bladder urothelial carcinoma

INTRODUCTION

Bladder cancer is one of the leading causes of cancer-related death worldwide. As the second most frequent genitourinary malignancy, BC is the 10th most common cancer globally according to global cancer data, with 573,278 new cases diagnosed and 212,526 deaths in 2020 according to Globocan prediction (1). The incidence and mortality of BC have been continuing to increase. Urothelial carcinoma is the most common histologic type, accounting for approximately 90% of primary BC (2). Among the newly diagnosed BC, non-muscular invasive bladder cancer (NMIBC) accounts for approximately 70% and transurethral resection of bladder tumor (TURBT) is the main treatment (3, 4). About 63.24% and 11.76% of the NMIBC patients after TURBT have tumor recurrence and progression (5). Likewise, nearly 50% of muscular invasive bladder cancer (MIBC) patients undergoing radical cystectomy still have local recurrence or distant metastasis, with a 5-year survival rate of only 66% (6). Furthermore, for 30 years, clinicians were stuck with the same, limited range of therapeutics to offer patients with BC, and 5-year survival rates were flat (7). Onset of BC is a complex process, which a multi-factor, multi-step, and multi-gene participation in (8). Therefore, a better understanding of the molecular characterization involved in tumorigenesis and the identification of novel prognostic biomarkers are essential for improving the clinical outcome of patients. The complex etiologic factors, along with the high-level heterogeneity of BC (9), make the prognosis significantly different and prognostic prediction challenging. This calls for the development of novel prognostic models.

Ferroptosis is a newly discovered iron-dependent form of regulated cell death (RCD) that is driven by the lethal accumulation of lipid peroxidation (10, 11). In 2012, it was firstly described that ferroptosis differs from apoptosis, necrosis, and autophagy in terms of morphology, biochemistry, and genetics. Ferroptosis is characterized by the rupture and blistering of cell membranes, mitochondrial shrinkage, increased membrane density, decreased or disappearance of mitochondrial ridges, rupture of outer mitochondrial membranes, and normal-sized nuclei without condensed chromatin (10). Studies have demonstrated strong association of ferroptosis with mammalian neurodegenerative diseases, cancer, and stroke (12). Since the first demonstration in 2012, ferroptosis has received widespread attention as a potential therapeutic pathway for cancer treatment. In recent years, the induction of ferroptosis has emerged as a promising therapeutic alternative to trigger cancer cell death, especially for malignancies that are resistant to traditional treatments (13, 14). Various studies have determined the key role of ferroptosis

in killing tumor cells and inhibiting tumor growth (15, 16). A large number of studies demonstrated the potential clinical value of utilizing these deregulated proteins as prognostic biomarkers of malignancy (17–19). Some previous studies have also confirmed the important significance of ferroptosis for the treatment of bladder cancer (20, 21), However, whether these ferroptosis-related genes (FRGs) are correlated with BC patient prognosis remains unclear.

The objective of this study was to determine the prognostic value of FRGs in BC. mRNA expression profiles and corresponding clinical data of bladder urothelial carcinoma (BLCA) were extracted from the public databases. Ferroptosis-related differentially expressed genes (DEGs) closely associated with the prognosis were identified to construct predictive models for the prognosis of BLCA in the TCGA cohort. Then, we validated it in the GEO cohort. Besides this, functional enrichment analysis was performed to explore the underlying mechanisms.

MATERIALS AND METHODS

Data Acquisition TCGA Cohort and GEO Cohort

All datasets used in this study were available to the public. Therefore, ethical approval for this study was not required. This study followed the policies and guidelines for data access and publication specified by the TCGA and GEO databases. Data cutoff was January 20, 2020.

Patients who met the following selection criteria were included: (a) histologically diagnosed with transitional cell carcinoma; (b) available gene expression data; and (c) available survival information. Patients with no complete clinical information were excluded. The RNA sequencing (RNA-seq) dataset and corresponding clinical information of 430 BCLA patients were downloaded from GDC (https://cancergenome.nih.gov/) as training cohort. The gene expression profile was standardized using the variance stabilizing transformation method provided by the "DEseq2" R package. Gene expression annotation information was obtained from the Ensembl website (https://asia.ensembl.org/index.html/). Similarly, the other RNA sequencing (RNA-seq) dataset and corresponding clinical information of 165 BCLA patients were downloaded from the Gene Expression Omnibus database portal website (https://www.ncbi.nlm.nih.gov/geo/) as a validation cohort. Internal standardization was performed *via* the "limma" package. Gene sequencing data annotation was performed with the R package "illuminaHumanv2 GPL6102 platform" from Bioconductor. Then, difference analysis was performed *via* the "Deseq2" R package.

FRGs and Immune-Related Data

The list of FRGs was download from the FerrDb web portal (http://www.zhounan.org/ferrdb), which contains six datasets. A total of 259 FRGs were identified with the following criteria: driver, suppressor, and marker of ferroptosis. We provided the list in **Supplementary Table S1**. The immune-related data were obtained from the ImmPort web portal (https://immport.org/shared/home).

Establishment and Validation of a Prognostic Model of FRGs Signature

DEGs related to ferroptosis in tumor tissues and adjacent normal tissues in the TCGA cohort were selected using the "Deseq2" R package, with an absolute log2-fold change (FC) ≥ 1 and an adjusted p-value < 0.05. The Venn diagram and heatmap were drawn using the Venn diagrams analysis online website (http://bioinformatics.psb.ugent.be/webtools/Venn/) and the "heatmap" R package. An interaction network for the candidate prognostic DEGs was generated by the online STRING database (version 3.7.1). Plots in the present study were drawn by ggplot2.

FRGs associated with overall survival (OS) were identified with univariate Cox regression analysis. P values were adjusted by Benjamini and Hochberg (BH) method. Multivariate Cox regression model analysis was performed to identify covariates with independent prognostic values for patient survival. Based on a multivariate Cox regression for these genes, a prognostic gene signature using ferroptosis-related DEGs was established.

To reflect the comprehensive effects of the ferroptosis, a risk score of each patient was calculated according to the normalized expression level of each gene and its corresponding regression coefficients. The formula was established as follows: risk score = Σ (Coefi * Expi). The optimal cutoff values for gene expression were determined using the "surv-cutpoint" function of the "Surviminer" package in R. Patients in TCGA training and GEO validation cohorts were divided into high-risk and low-risk groups based on the median risk score as the cutoff value. Kaplan–Meier survival analysis and log-rank test were used to compare difference in the OS between the stratified groups. Then, receiver operating characteristic (ROC) curve analysis and the area under the ROC curve (AUC) was applied to test the predictive power of the prognostic risk score model. The difference in gene expression between tumor tissues and normal tissues and its correlation with prognosis was further validated by the GEPIA online database (http://gepia.cancer-pku.cn/).

Construction and Evaluation of a Predictive Nomogram

During the quantification of the risk on individuals in a clinical setting with the integration of multiple risk factors, the nomogram was an excellent tool in the assessment. The independent predictive factors identified by multivariate Cox regression were integrated to construct a predictive nomogram and corresponding calibration curves using the "rms" R package. The closer the calibration curve is to the 45° line, which represents the best prediction, the better is the prognostic prediction performance of the nomogram.

Function Enrichment Analysis

We applied the "limma" R package to analyze the correlations of DEGs between the high-risk and low-risk groups in TCGA and GEO cohorts, respectively. Gene ontology (GO) and Kyoto Encyclopedia of Genes and Genomes (KEGG) enrichment analysis for DEGs were conducted using the "clusterProfiler" package in R. For differential infiltrating score analysis between the high- and low-risk groups, infiltrating scores of 16 immune cells and 13 immune-related pathways were calculated by single-sample gene set enrichment analysis (ssGSEA) using the "gsva" package in R. The genes related to immune cell infiltration are provided in **Supplementary Table S2**.

Statistical Analysis

Statistical analyses were carried out with the R software (Version 3.5.3). The Student's t-test was used to compare the gene expression between tumor tissues and adjacent normal tissues. Patients in TCGA training and GEO validation cohorts were divided into high-risk and low-risk groups based on the median risk score. Chi-square test was adopted to compare differences in age, gender, T stage, N (lymph node metastasis) status, M (tumor metastasis) status, diagnosis subtype, and histologic grade between the high- and low-risk groups. Mann–Whitney test with p-values adjusted by the BH method was used to compare the ssGSEA scores of immune cells or pathways between the high- and low-risk groups. Kaplan–Meier survival analysis and log-rank test were used to compare difference in the OS between the stratified groups. Univariate and multivariate Cox regression analyses were used to determine independent prognostic factors. $p < 0.05$ was considered statistically significant.

RESULTS

To systematically describe our study, the flow chart of the study is shown in **Figure 1**. From the TCGA RNA-seq dataset, we obtained expression data of 430 BLCA patients from the TCGA cohort and 165 patients from GEO (GSE13507). A total of 372 BLCA patients with complete clinical information were finally enrolled in the TCGA cohort. Baseline demographic and clinical characteristics of the included patents are shown in **Table 1**.

Identification of Prognostic DEGs Related to FRGs of BLCA in the TCGA Cohort

The RNA expression data of 411 BLCA tumor samples and 19 adjacent normal samples were obtained from TCGA. Differential expression analysis was conducted with the DEseq2 package. A total of 4610 DEGs were screened out and a total of 67 FRGs (25.9%) were differentially expressed between tumor tissues and adjacent normal tissues (**Figures 2A, B**). Twelve candidate FRGs associated with OS were identified with univariate Cox regression analysis (**Figures 2C, D**). The protein–protein interaction network provided interactive information among these DEGs (**Figure 2E**). *BID*, *FADS2*, and *SCD* were identified as hub genes with "igraph" R package. The correlation network of these genes is presented in **Figure 2F**.

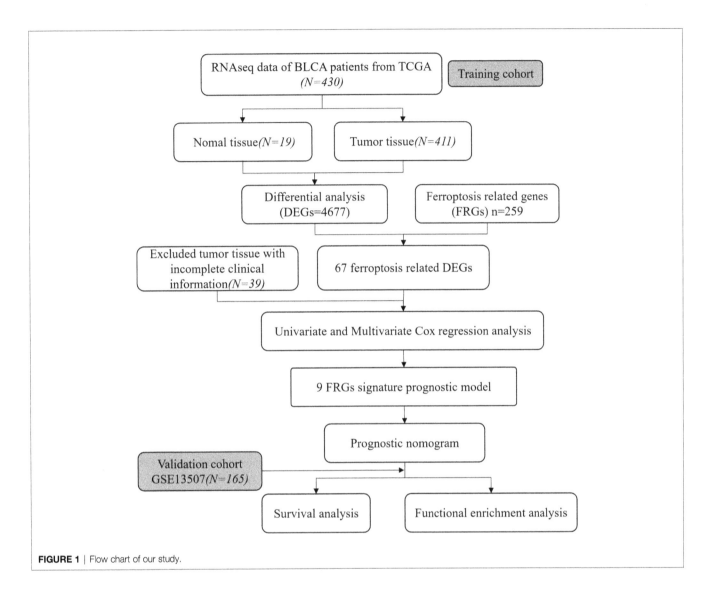

FIGURE 1 | Flow chart of our study.

Establishment of a Prognostic Model of FRGs in TCGA Cohort

The expression profiles of the 12 candidate genes mentioned above were incorporated into a prognostic model using multivariate Cox regression analysis. A nine-gene signature, namely, *ALB, BID, FADS2, FANCD2, IFNG, MIOX, PLIN4, SCD,* and *SLC2A3*, was constructed (**Figure 3A**). Patients in the TCGA training cohort were classified as high risk (*n* = 186) or low risk (*n* = 186) based on the median cutoff value of risk score (**Figure 3B**). The risk score was calculated as follows: risk score= (−0.065* expression level of *ALB*) + (−0.165* expression level of *BID*) + (0.0898* expression level of *FADS2*) + (−0.3198* expression level of *FANCD2*) + (−0.14* expression level of *IFNG*) + (−0.085* expression level of *MIOX*) + (−0.087* expression level of PLIN4) + (0.1324* expression level of *SCD*) + (0.17* expression level of *SLC2A3*). The heatmap result showed high-risk group patients with higher expression levels of *FADS2, SCD,* and *SLC2A3* (**Figure 3C**). Patients in the high-risk group had a shorter survival time than those in the low-risk

group (**Figure 3D**). Likewise, Kaplan–Meier survival curves show that OS of high-risk patients was significantly worse than OS of low-risk patients (**Figure 3E**). The predictive performance of the prognostic risk score model was evaluated by time-dependent ROC curves and the area under the curve (AUC). As shown in **Figure 3F**, the AUC reached 0.694 at 1 year, 0.723 at 3 years, and 0.757 at 5 years, suggesting a favorable predictive value of the risk score model in short- and long-term follow-up.

Validation of the Prognostic Model based on Nine-FRG Signature in the GEO Cohort

The reliability of the model constructed from the TCGA cohort was validated in the GEO cohort. A total of 165 patients from the GEO cohort were divided into high-risk (*n* = 83) and low-risk (*n* = 82) groups by the median value calculated using the same risk formula and cutoff point obtained from the TCGA cohort (**Figure 4B**). The results are consistent with results obtained from the TCGA cohort. Patients in the high-risk group had a shorter survival time than those in the low-risk group

TABLE 1 | Clinical characteristics of BLCA patients in the TCGA cohort and GEO GSE13507.

Characteristics		TCGA Total (n = 372)	GEO Total (n = 165)
Age (years)	<60	79 (21.2%)	42 (25.5%)
	≥60	293 (78.7%)	123 (74.5%)
Gender	Male	276 (74.2%)	135 (81.8%)
	Female	96 (25.8%)	30 (18.2%)
T stage 1	T0	1 (0.3%)	0
	T1	4 (1.1%)	80 (48.5%)
	T2	116 (31.2%)	31 (18.8%)
	T3	193 (51.9%)	19 (11.5%)
	T4	57 (15.3%)	11 (6.7%)
	Tx	1 (0.3%)	24 (14.5%)
T stage 2	T0–2	121 (32.5%)	111 (67.3%)
	T3–4	251 (67.5%)	30 (18.2%)
	Tx	1 (0.3%)	24 (14.5%)
Lymph node metastasis	Yes	124 (33.3%)	15 (9.1%)
	No	221 (59.4%)	149 (90.3%)
	Unknown	27 (7.0%)	1 (0.61%)
Metastasis	Yes	8 (2.2%)	7 (4.2%)
	No	183 (49.2%)	158 (95.8%)
	Unknown	181 (48.7%)	0
Diagnosis subtype	Papillary	117 (31.5%)	NA
	Non-papillary	250 (67.2%)	NA
	Unknown	5 (1.3%)	NA
Histologic grade	High	351 (94.4)	60 (36.4%)
	Low	19 (5.1%)	105 (63.6%)
	Unknown	2 (0.5%)	0
Vital status	Dead	166 (44.6%)	69 (41.8%)
	Alive	206 (55.4%)	96 (58.2%)

NA, Not Applicable.

(**Figure 4A**). Likewise, Kaplan–Meier survival curves show that OS of high-risk patients was significantly worse than OS of low-risk patients (**Figure 4D**). ROC curves also suggest a good predictive value of the risk score model (**Figure 4E**).

Prognostic Analysis of the BLCA Patients Based on the Expression of the Nine-FRG Signature

To further determine the accuracy of the prognostic model of FRGs, the Gene Expression Profiling Interactive Analysis (GEPIA) database was used to analyze the OS of BLCA patients based on the expression of FRGs. Cutoff for high value and low value is set to 50%. $p < 0.05$ was considered statistically significant. In the signature genes, four genes, namely, *FADS2, SCD, IFNG*, and *PLIN4*, were significantly correlated with the OS of BLCA (**Figures 5C, E, G, H**). *FADS2* and *SCD* were unfavorable factors for OS of BLCA patients, whereas *IFNG* and *PLIN4* were favorable factors for OS of BLCA patients. This was consistent with results of multivariate Cox regression.

Independent Prognostic Analysis of the Prognostic Model

Univariate and multivariate Cox regression analyses were conducted to evaluate whether the signature-based risk score was an independent predictor of OS (**Figure 6**). Hazard ratios (HRs) and 95% confidence intervals (CIs) for each variable were calculated. $p < 0.05$ was considered statistically significant. In both TCGA and GEO data, results show that the risk scores were

independent prognostic predictors for OS in the univariate and multivariate Cox regression analyses.

Construction and Validation of the Nomogram in the TCGA Cohort

Nomogram was generated based on several independent predictive factors to predict the probability of 1-year, 2-year, and 3-year OS rates with the TCGA Training dataset. Different factors were scored based on the proportion of contribution to survival risk as shown in **Figure 7A**. The calibration curve for the 1-year, 3-year, and 5-year OS probability results showed that the predicted survival rate is closely related to the actual survival rate (**Figure 7B**). These results indicated that the signature of the nine FRGs was a reliable prognostic indicator in BLCA patients.

GO and KEGG Enrichment Analysis of the TCGA Cohort

To investigate the potential biological characteristics of the DEGs in high-risk and low-risk patients in the TGCA cohort, GO enrichment and KEGG pathway analyses were performed using the ClusterProfile R package. GO analysis indicated that DEGs were obviously enriched in some ferroptosis-related, immune-related biological processes and molecular functions (adjusted $p < 0.05$; **Figures 8A, C**). KEGG functional enrichment analysis suggested that DEGs were mostly enriched in the ferroptosis-related pathway, immune-related pathways, and bladder cancer (**Figures 8B, D**).

To further explore the relationship between the risk score and immune status, we quantified the infiltrating scores of immune-

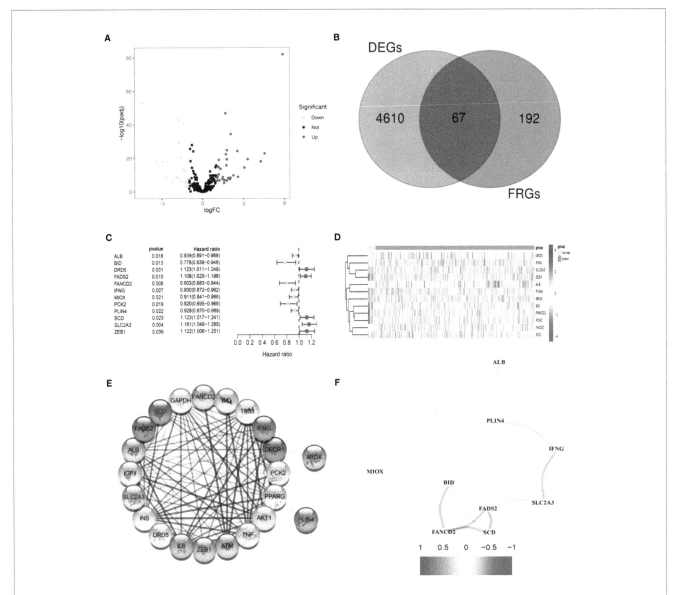

FIGURE 2 | Identification of prognostic DEGs related to FRGs in the TCGA cohort. **(A)** The 67 overlapping genes were shown in the volcano map. Forty genes were upregulated and 27 genes were downregulated in tumor tissues. **(B)** Venn diagram to identify DEGs related to FRGs. **(C)** Univariate Cox proportional regression analysis showed that the 12 genes were significantly associated with OS. **(D)** A heatmap showing the expressions of the 12 prognostic genes in the tumors and normal tissues. **(E)** PPI network provided interactive information among the candidate prognostic genes. **(F)** The correlation network of candidate genes. Different colors represented the correlation coefficients.

cell and immunity-related pathways with ssGSEA. The correlations between ssGSEA scores and different risk groups showed that the scores of aDCs, mast cells, NK cells, APC co-inhibition, cytolytic activity, MHC class I, and type I IFN response were significantly different between the low-risk and high-risk groups in the TCGA cohort (**Figures 9A, B**). Interestingly, the scores of aDCs, DCs, macrophages, Tfh, Tfh1 cells, TIL, Treg, APC co-stimulation, CCR, checkpoint, cytolytic activity, inflammation promoting, MHC class I, parainflammation, T-cell co-inhibition, and T-cell co-stimulation were significantly different between the low-risk and high-risk groups in GEO cohorts (**Figures 9C, D**).

Moreover, although the expression of immune checkpoint molecules including programmed cell death protein 1 (PD1), PD1 ligand 1 (PDL1), and cytotoxic T lymphocyte antigen 4 (CTLA4) was no statistical difference in TCGA cohort (**Figure 10A**), it significantly higher in the high-risk group in GEO cohort (**Figure 10B**).

DISCUSSION

Bladder cancer is a molecular heterogeneous malignant tumor; the treatment strategies for advanced-stage patients are limited.

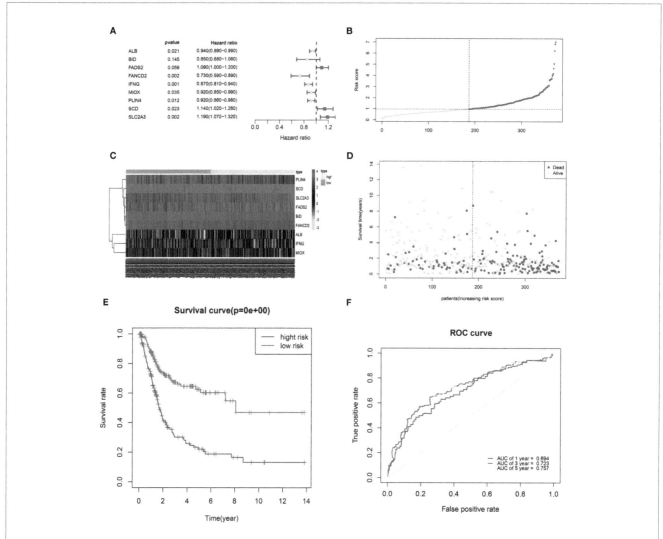

FIGURE 3 | Establishment of a prognostic model of FRGs in the TCGA cohort. **(A)** A nine-gene signature was generated by Multivariate Cox regression analysis. **(B)** Distribution of signature-based risk scores. **(C)** The differences in the expression of the prognostic signature in different risk groups. **(D)** Survival status of high-risk and low-risk patients. **(E)** Kaplan–Meier curves indicated that the OS in the high-risk group was markedly poorer than that in the low-risk group (*p* < 0.0001). **(F)** Time-dependent ROC curve analysis for measuring the prognostic performance of the signature-based risk score on OS.

The molecular characteristics are closely related to prognosis of bladder cancer. Therefore, it is vital for improving the clinical outcome of BC patients to identify key biomarkers and targets affecting prognosis. The development of high-throughput array technology provides an opportunity to explore novel genes involved in the occurrence and development of BC. Increasing evidence has shown that ferroptosis plays a crucial role in tumorigenesis and cancer therapeutics (22). In this study, the differential expression of FRGs between BLCA tumor tissues and adjacent normal tissues were systematically investigated. FRGs associated with the prognosis of BLCA were determined by Cox proportional hazards regression analysis. Results significantly indicated the feasibility of building a prognostic model with these FRGs.

A novel prognostic model integrating nine ferroptosis-related DEGs was, for the first time, constructed and externally validated. These genes that make up the prognostic model were *ALB*, *BID*, *FADS2*, *FANCD2*, *IFNG*, *MIOX*, *PLIN4*, *SCD*, and *SLC2A3*. It was reported that *ALB* (albumin) may act synergistically with transferrin to limit iron supply, which may lead to the promotion of ferroptosis (23). The expression level of *ALB* was upregulated in BLCA tumor tissue compared with normal tissues (**Figure 5A**). The OS of the high-expression group was better than that of the low-expression group, which was consistent with the expression in the different risk groups based on the prognostic signature (**Figure 3C**). Ferroptosis is defined as an oxidative and iron-dependent pathway of regulated cell death, which is different from caspase-dependent apoptosis. Mitochondrial transactivation of *BID* links ferroptosis to mitochondrial damage as the last execution step of oxidative cell death (24). Overexpression of *BID* may promote the suppression of ferroptosis, indicating a worse prognosis

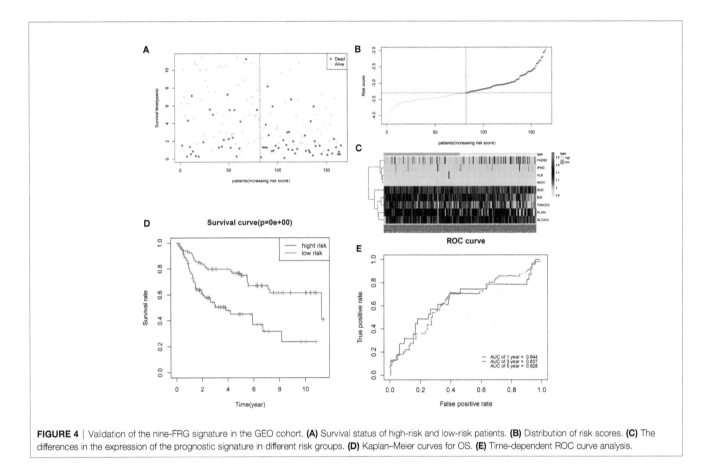

FIGURE 4 | Validation of the nine-FRG signature in the GEO cohort. **(A)** Survival status of high-risk and low-risk patients. **(B)** Distribution of risk scores. **(C)** The differences in the expression of the prognostic signature in different risk groups. **(D)** Kaplan–Meier curves for OS. **(E)** Time-dependent ROC curve analysis.

(**Figure 5B**). *FADS2* is abnormally expressed in many malignant tumors, and its expression is significantly correlated with tumor proliferation, cell migration invasion, and ferroptosis (25). Activation of *FADS2* involved in the Warburg effect inhibits ferroptosis (26). Upregulation of *FADS2* was associated with poor prognosis in BLCA (**Figure 5C**). *SCD*, like *FADS2*, was involved in Warburg effect (26). A study (27) confirmed that *SCD* was an enzyme that catalyzes the rate-limiting step in monounsaturated fatty acid synthesis in ovarian cancer cells; inhibition of *SCD1* could induce both ferroptosis and apoptosis. *SCD* was highly expressed in ovarian cancer tissue. The expression levels of *SCD* in BLCA was also high (**Figure 5H**). *FANCD2*, a protein that mediates DNA repair, suppresses ferroptosis by transcription and transcription-independent mechanisms (28). *FANCD2* is closely correlated to tumorigenesis and progression (29). A study indicated that *FANCD2* expression correlated with the activation of apoptotic, cell cycle, and EMT pathways in clear cell renal cell carcinoma (30). The high expression level of *FANCD2* was related to better prognosis in BLCA (**Figure 4C, 5D**), which suggests that the role of *FANCD2* in BLCA may be consistent with other studies. *IFNG* (interferon gamma, *INFγ*)released from CD8+ T cells downregulates the expression of *SLC3A2* and *SLC7A11*, two subunits of the glutamate-cystine antiporter system xc-, inhibits the uptake of cystine by tumor cells, and consequently promotes tumor cell lipid peroxidation and

ferroptosis (31). Expression of *IFNG* was negatively associated, in BCLA patients, with patient outcome (**Figure 5E**). Overexpression of myo-inositol oxygenase (*MIOX*) exacerbates cellular redox injury in cisplatin-induced acute kidney injury (AKI) by accelerating ferroptosis (32). It is reasonable to assume that *MIOX* may play an anti-cancer role by promoting ferroptosis in BLCA. This could explain why *MIOX* is highly expressed in the low-risk group (**Figure 3C**). *PLIN4* (Perilipins4) is one of the families of lipid droplet-associated proteins that participate in lipid metabolism regulation. It can be used as diagnostic markers of liposarcoma and to differentiate liposarcoma subtypes (33). Compared with the corresponding normal tissues, the expression of *PLIN4* in BLCA tumor tissues was downregulated (**Figure 5G**), and higher expression of *PLIN4* was associated with better prognosis (**Figure 5G**). *PLIN4* could also be used as prognostic markers. Upregulation of the *SLC2A* gene that encodes the glucose transporter (GLUT) protein is associated with poor prognosis in many cancers. It was observed that upregulation of the *SLC2A3* genes is associated with decreased OS and DFS in colorectal cancer patients (34). Likewise, we found that *SLC2A3* expression was high in the high-risk group (**Figure 4C**). The nine FRGs were either positively or negatively correlated with ferroptosis. They were differentially expressed in different risk groups, which was consistent with their gene functions in cancers. However, not all nine genes had expression levels consistent with their

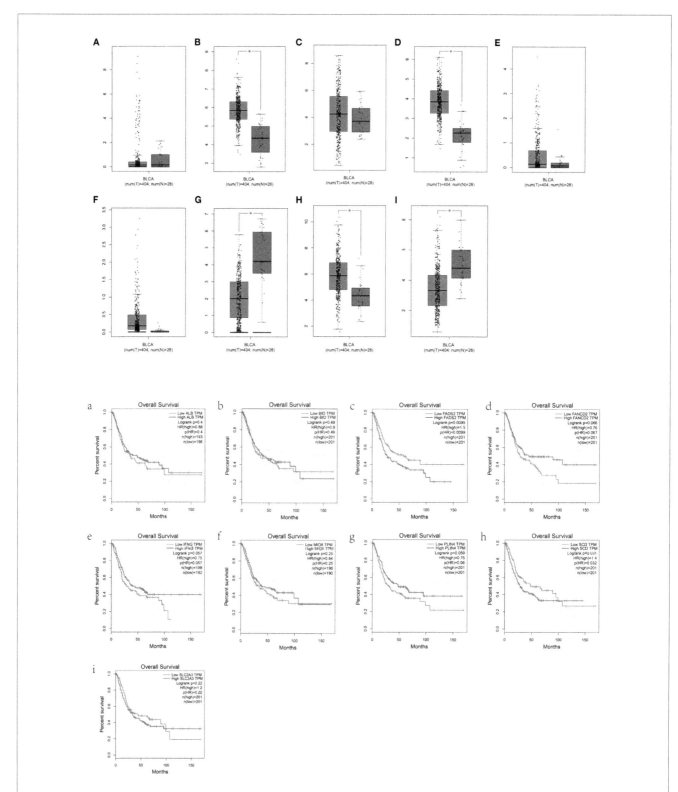

FIGURE 5 | Prognostic analysis of the BLCA patients based on the expression of FRGs. **(A–I)** Box plots show the differences in the expression of nine different ferroptosis-related genes in the tumor and normal tissues from the GEPIA dataset. **(a–i)** The overall survival of BLCA patients based on the expression of the nine FRGs is shown.

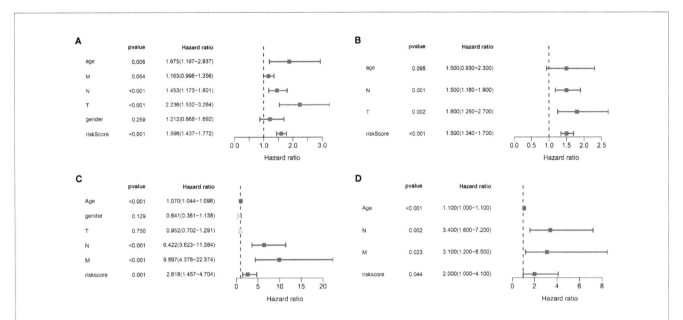

FIGURE 6 | Univariate and multivariate Cox regression analyses. Results showing the signature-based risk score was an independent predictor of OS. **(A)** The univariate Cox regression analysis in the TCGA cohort. **(B)** The multivariate Cox regression analysis in the TCGA cohort. **(C)** The univariate Cox regression analysis in the GEO cohort. **(D)** The multivariate Cox regression analysis in the GEO cohort.

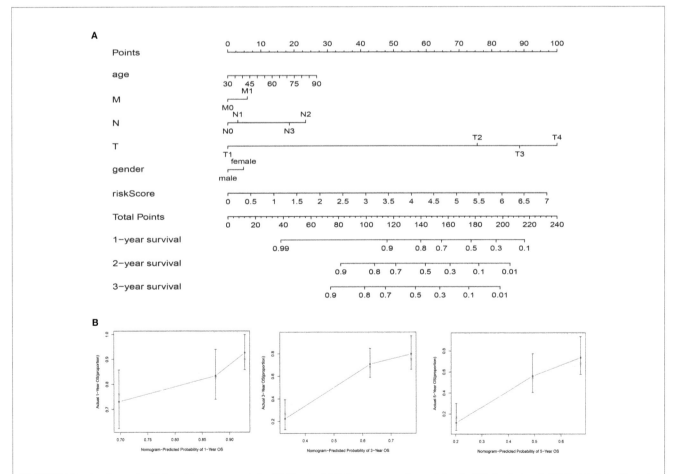

FIGURE 7 | Construction and validation of the nomogram in the TCGA cohort. **(A)** The nomogram for predicting the OS of patients with BLCA at 1, 2, and 3 years in the TCGA dataset. **(B)** Calibration curves of the nomogram for OS prediction at 1, 3, and 5 years in the TCGA dataset.

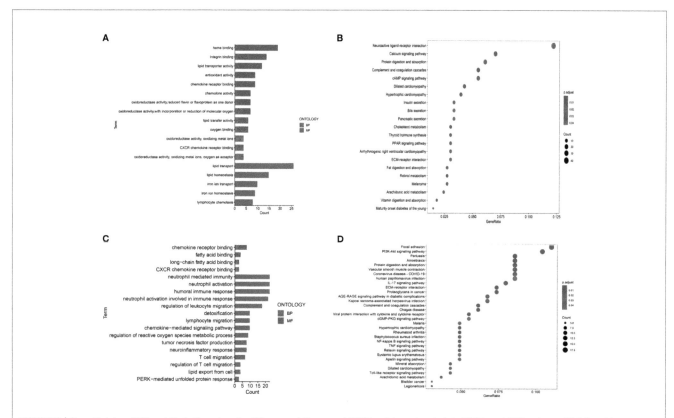

FIGURE 8 | Gene Ontology (GO) and Kyoto Encyclopedia of Genes and Genomes (KEGG) enrichment analysis in TCGA and GEO cohorts. **(A)** GO enrichment analysis in the TCGA cohort. **(B)** KEGG enrichment analysis in the TCGA cohort. **(C)** GO enrichment analysis in the GEO cohort. **(D)** KEGG enrichment analysis in the GEO cohort.

functions in BLCA (**Figure 5**). Therefore, the specific role of these genes in BLCA has to be further investigated.

We further demonstrated that the risk score of the nine-gene signature was an independent prognostic indicator of OS for patients with BLCA. The high-risk group was found to have a significantly higher percentage of BLCA patients with worse clinicopathological features, such as an advanced T stage, lymph node metastasis, and histologic grade (**Table 2**). In addition, micropapillary carcinoma of the bladder (MPBC) is a variant type of infiltrating urothelial carcinoma, which portends a poor biological behavior in terms of disease stage at first diagnosis and clinical outcome (35). We tried to assess the risk of MPBC patients by our risk score, but unfortunately, the correlation between risk score and diagnosis subtype was not statistically significant. Thereafter, an individualized prognostic prediction model was constructed with nomograms, where the risks of individuals in the clinical context were quantified by integrating multiple risk factors including risk score. Calibration curves suggested high consistency between the actual and predicted OS rates. According to the aforementioned results, it was suggestive that the prognostic risk score model based on the nine-gene signature was a powerful prognostic indicator in BLCA patients.

To determine the role of ferroptosis-related classical signaling pathways in different risk groups, GO and KEGG enrichment analysis of DEGs in the high-risk and low-risk groups. Expectedly, the results indicated that DEGs were significantly enriched in biological oxidation, fatty acid metabolism, and iron metabolism (**Figure 5C**). These biological processes are all critical for the execution of ferroptosis (13, 17). Interestingly, many immunity-related functions and pathways were significantly enriched, such as chemokine receptor binding, humoral immune response, IL-17 signaling pathway, protein interaction with cytokine–cytokine receptor, and toil-like receptor signaling pathway (**Figures 8C, D**). ssGSEA revealed that the infiltrating scores of immune-cell and immunity-related pathways were significantly different in different risk groups. At present, many researchers have proven that ferroptosis is related to immunity. We found that NK cells, CD8+ T cells, and MHC class I molecules were significantly higher in the low-risk group (**Figures 9A, B**). A study indicated that ferritin heavy chain in tumor cells may modulate the expression of MHC class I molecules and influence NK cells (36). MHC class I molecules enable CD8+ T cells to recognize and kill tumor cells (37). CD8+ T cells release interferon (IFN)γ, and (IFN)γ can regulate the lipid peroxidation and ferroptosis pathways in tumors (31). In addition, studies have demonstrated that increased tumor-associated macrophages (38, 39) or Treg cells (39, 40) are related to poor prognosis in HCC patients due to their role in

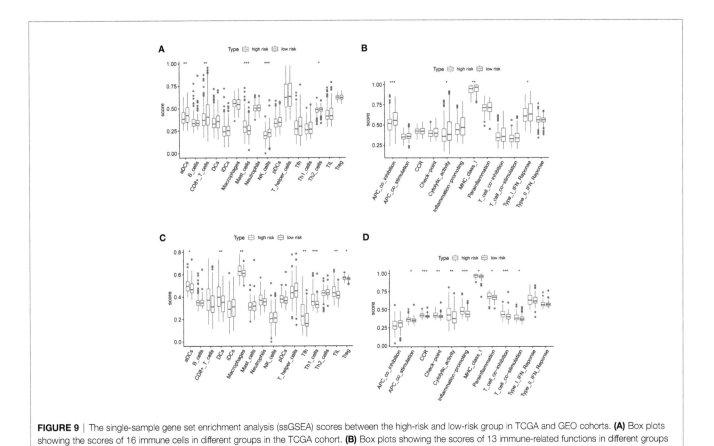

FIGURE 9 | The single-sample gene set enrichment analysis (ssGSEA) scores between the high-risk and low-risk group in TCGA and GEO cohorts. **(A)** Box plots showing the scores of 16 immune cells in different groups in the TCGA cohort. **(B)** Box plots showing the scores of 13 immune-related functions in different groups in the TCGA cohort. **(C)** Box plots showing the scores of 16 immune cells in different groups in the GEO cohort. **(D)** Box plots showing the scores of 13 immune-related functions in different groups in the GEO cohort. Adjusted p-values are shown as follows: *p < 0.05; **p < 0.01; ***p < 0.001.

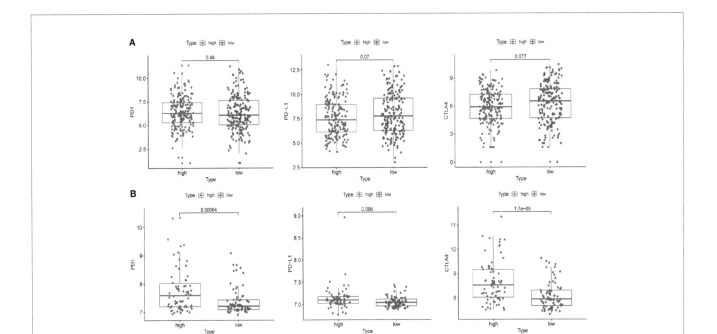

FIGURE 10 | The expression of immune checkpoint molecules including PD1, PDL1, and CTLA4 between the high-risk and the low-risk group in TCGA and GEO cohorts. **(A)** Box plots show the differences in the expression of PD1, PDL1, and CTLA4 between the high-risk and low-risk group in the TCGA cohort. **(B)** Box plots show the differences in the expression of PD1, PDL1, and CTLA4 between the high-risk and the low-risk group in the GEO cohort.

TABLE 2 | Baseline characteristics of the patients in different risk groups in the TCGA cohort and the GEO cohort.

Characteristics		TCGA cohort (N = 372)			GEO cohort (N = 165)		
		High risk	Low risk	p-value	High risk	Low risk	p-value
Age (years)				0.205			0.033
	<60	34	45		15	27	
	≥60	152	141		68	55	
Gender				0.075			0.84
	Male	130	146		67	68	
	Female	56	40		16	14	
T stage				<0.001			0.002
	T0–2	42	79		53	58	
	T3–4	143	107		23	7	
	Tx	1	0		7	17	
Lymph node metastasis				<0.001			0.243
	Yes	76	48		10	5	
	No	104	117		72	77	
	Unknown	8	21		1	0	
Metastasis				0.775			0.443
	Yes	5	3		5	2	
	No	91	92		78	80	
	Unknown	90	91		0	0	
Diagnosis subtype				0.075			
	Papillary	49	68		NA	NA	
	Non-papillary	135	115		NA	NA	
	Unknown	2	3		NA	NA	
Histologic grade				0.108			0.015
	High	180	171		38	22	
	Low	5	14		45	60	
	Unknown	1	1				

NA, Not Applicable.

immune invasion. The fractions of macrophages and Treg cells were higher in high-risk group BLCA patients in the GEO cohort (**Figure 9C**), which were consistent with the abovementioned research results.

In recent years, immune checkpoint inhibitor treatment has become a new and promising therapy for BC. The recent IMvigor010 study (41) was designed to evaluate the role of a checkpoint inhibitor in muscle-invasive urothelial carcinoma (MIUC). Although the trial did not meet its primary endpoint of improved disease-free survival (DFS) in the atezolizumab group over observation because of higher frequencies of adverse events, we also could find that adjuvant checkpoint inhibitor therapy may have some advantages in muscle-invasive urothelial carcinoma. The stirring CheckMate274 study presented by Dean Bajorin at the 2021 ASCO Genitourinary Cancers Symposium indicated that the adjuvant nivolumab, a PD-1 immune checkpoint inhibitor, significantly improved DFS in patients with high-risk MIUC after radical surgery, especially in PD-L1≥1% patients. There was significant difference in checkpoint between the high-risk and low-risk patients in our study (**Figure 9D**). The expression of immune checkpoint molecules including PD1, PDL1, and CTLA4 was significantly higher in the high-risk group in GEO cohorts (**Figure 10B**). This indicates that patients in the high-risk group may benefit more from immune checkpoint inhibitor therapy than patients in the low-risk group and provides new insight for BC immunotherapy. Considered together, these

findings suggest that poor prognosis of patients with high risk might be correlated with immunosuppression, and ferroptosis could play a role in the immunotherapy of BC.

Despite the confirmation of our prognostic model in various datasets, this study was limited because it was a retrospective study. A further well-designed prospective study is necessary to validate the clinical value of the developed model. Besides, it was inevitable that by merely considering a single hallmark to build a prognostic model, many prominent prognostic genes in BC might have been excluded.

In conclusion, a novel prognostic model based on the nine-FRG signature in BLCA was the first established and validated. The prognostic models exhibited superior predictive performance and could independently predict the prognosis of BC patients. Understanding the roles of the signature and the relationship between ferroptosis and tumor immunity can provide insights into prognostic and therapeutic implications for BC patients.

AUTHOR CONTRIBUTIONS

YY and YH conceived and designed the study. LY and CL provided equal contributions to research design, data analysis and article writing. YQ, GZ, BZ, and ZW revised the manuscript. All authors contributed to the article and approved the submitted version.

REFERENCES

1. Sung H, Ferlay J, Siegel RL, Laversanne M, Soerjomataram I, Jemal A, et al. Global Cancer Statistics 2020: GLOBOCAN Estimates of Incidence and Mortality Worldwide for 36 Cancers in 185 Countries. *CA Cancer J Clin* (2021) 71(3):209–49. doi: 10.3322/caac.21660

2. Fleshner NE, Herr HW, Stewart AK, Murphy GP, Mettlin C, Menck HR. The National Cancer Data Base Report on Bladder Carcinoma. The American College of Surgeons Commission on Cancer and the American Cancer Society. *Cancer* (1996) 78(7):1505–13. doi: 10.1002/(sici)1097-0142 (19961001)78:7<1505::aid-cncr19>3.0.co;2-3

3. Ro JY, Staerkel GA, Ayala AG. Cytologic and Histologic Features of Superficial Bladder Cancer. *Urol Clin North Am* (1992) 19(3):435–53. doi: 10.1016/S0094-0143(21)00412-2

4. Babjuk M, Bohle A, Burger M, Capoun O, Cohen D, Comperat EM, et al. EAU Guidelines on Non-Muscle-Invasive Urothelial Carcinoma of the Bladder: Update 2016. *Eur Urol* (2017) 71(3):447–61. doi: 10.1016/ j.eururo.2016.05.041

5. Divrik RT, Yildirim U, Zorlu F, Ozen H. The Effect of Repeat Transurethral Resection on Recurrence and Progression Rates in Patients With T1 Tumors of the Bladder Who Received Intravesical Mitomycin: A Prospective, Randomized Clinical Trial. *J Urol* (2006) 175(5):1641–4. doi: 10.1016/ S0022-5347(05)01002-5

6. Alfred Witjes J, Lebret T, Comperat EM, Cowan NC, De Santis M, Bruins HM, et al. Updated 2016 EAU Guidelines on Muscle-Invasive and Metastatic Bladder Cancer. *Eur Urol* (2017) 71(3):462–75. doi: 10.1016/ j.eururo.2016.06.020

7. Grayson M. Bladder Cancer. *Nature* (2017) 551(7679):S33. doi: 10.1038/ 551S33a

8. Zhao M, He XL, Teng XD. Understanding the Molecular Pathogenesis and Prognostics of Bladder Cancer: An Overview. *Chin J Cancer Res* (2016) 28 (1):92–8. doi: 10.3978/j.issn.1000-9604.2016.02.05

9. Gerlinger M, Catto JW, Orntoft TF, Real FX, Zwarthoff EC, Swanton C. Intratumour Heterogeneity in Urologic Cancers: From Molecular Evidence to Clinical Implications. *Eur Urol* (2015) 67(4):729–37. doi: 10.1016/ j.eururo.2014.04.014

10. Dixon SJ, Lemberg KM, Lamprecht MR, Skouta R, Zaitsev EM, Gleason CE, et al. Ferroptosis: An Iron-Dependent Form of Nonapoptotic Cell Death. *Cell* (2012) 149(5):1060–72. doi: 10.1016/j.cell.2012.03.042

11. Stockwell BR, Friedmann Angeli JP, Bayir H, Bush AI, Conrad M, Dixon SJ, et al. Ferroptosis: A Regulated Cell Death Nexus Linking Metabolism, Redox Biology, and Disease. *Cell* (2017) 171(2):273–85. doi: 10.1016/ j.cell.2017.09.021

12. Yang WS, Stockwell BR. Ferroptosis: Death by Lipid Peroxidation. *Trends Cell Biol* (2016) 26(3):165–76. doi: 10.1016/j.tcb.2015.10.014

13. Hassannia B, Vandenabeele P, Vanden Berghe T. Targeting Ferroptosis to Iron Out Cancer. *Cancer Cell* (2019) 35(6):830–49. doi: 10.1016/ j.ccell.2019.04.002

14. Liang C, Zhang X, Yang M, Dong X. Recent Progress in Ferroptosis Inducers for Cancer Therapy. *Adv Mater* (2019) 31(51):e1904197. doi: 10.1002/ adma.201904197

15. Ooko E, Saeed ME, Kadioglu O, Sarvi S, Colak M, Elmasaoudi K, et al. Artemisinin Derivatives Induce Iron-Dependent Cell Death (Ferroptosis) in Tumor Cells. *Phytomedicine* (2015) 22(11):1045–54. doi: 10.1016/ j.phymed.2015.08.002

16. Yamaguchi H, Hsu JL, Chen CT, Wang YN, Hsu MC, Chang SS, et al. Caspase-Independent Cell Death is Involved in the Negative Effect of EGF Receptor Inhibitors on Cisplatin in Non-Small Cell Lung Cancer Cells. *Clin Cancer Res* (2013) 19(4):845–54. doi: 10.1158/1078-0432.CCR-12-2621

17. Lelievre P, Sancey L, Coll JL, Deniaud A, Busser B. Iron Dysregulation in Human Cancer: Altered Metabolism, Biomarkers for Diagnosis, Prognosis, Monitoring and Rationale for Therapy. *Cancers (Basel)* (2020) 12(12):3524. doi: 10.3390/cancers12123524

18. Zhang S, Chang W, Wu H, Wang YH, Gong YW, Zhao YL, et al. Pan-Cancer Analysis of Iron Metabolic Landscape Across the Cancer Genome Atlas. *J Cell Physiol* (2020) 235(2):1013 24. doi: 10.1002/jcp.29017

19. Zhao B, Li R, Cheng G, Li Z, Zhang Z, Li J, et al. Role of Hepcidin and Iron Metabolism in the Onset of Prostate Cancer. *Oncol Lett* (2018) 15(6):9953–8. doi: 10.3892/ol.2018.8544

20. Jasim KA, Gesquiere AJ. Ultrastable and Biofunctionalizable Conjugated Polymer Nanoparticles With Encapsulated Iron for Ferroptosis Assisted Chemodynamic Therapy. *Mol Pharm* (2019) 16(12):4852–66. doi: 10.1021/ acs.molpharmaceut.9b00737

21. Martin-Sanchez D, Fontecha-Barriuso M, Sanchez-Nino MD, Ramos AM, Cabello R, Gonzalez-Enguita C, et al. Cell Death-Based Approaches in Treatment of the Urinary Tract-Associated Diseases: A Fight for Survival in the Killing Fields. *Cell Death Dis* (2018) 9(2):118. doi: 10.1038/s41419-017-0043-2

22. Liu HJ, Hu HM, Li GZ, Zhang Y, Wu F, Liu X, et al. Ferroptosis-Related Gene Signature Predicts Glioma Cell Death and Glioma Patient Progression. *Front Cell Dev Biol* (2020) 8:538. doi: 10.3389/fcell.2020.00538

23. Konopka K, Neilands JB. Effect of Serum Albumin on Siderophore-Mediated Utilization of Transferrin Iron. *Biochemistry* (1984) 23(10):2122–7. doi: 10.1021/bi00305a003

24. Neitemeier S, Jelinek A, Laino V, Hoffmann L, Eisenbach I, Eying R, et al. BID Links Ferroptosis to Mitochondrial Cell Death Pathways. *Redox Biol* (2017) 12:558–70. doi: 10.1016/j.redox.2017.03.007

25. Li YL, Tian H, Jiang J, Zhang Y, Qi XW. Multifaceted Regulation and Functions of Fatty Acid Desaturase 2 in Human Cancers. *Am J Cancer Res* (2020) 10(12):4098–111.

26. Jiang Y, Mao C, Yang R, Yan B, Shi Y, Liu X, et al. EGLN1/c-Myc Induced Lymphoid-Specific Helicase Inhibits Ferroptosis Through Lipid Metabolic Gene Expression Changes. *Theranostics* (2017) 7(13):3293–305. doi: 10.7150/ thno.19988

27. Tesfay L, Paul BT, Konstorum A, Deng Z, Cox AO, Lee J, et al. Stearoyl-CoA Desaturase 1 Protects Ovarian Cancer Cells From Ferroptotic Cell Death. *Cancer Res* (2019) 79(20):5355–66. doi: 10.1158/0008-5472.CAN-19-0369

28. Song X, Xie Y, Kang R, Hou W, Sun X, Epperly MW, et al. FANCD2 Protects Against Bone Marrow Injury From Ferroptosis. *Biochem Biophys Res Commun* (2016) 480(3):443–9. doi: 10.1016/j.bbrc.2016.10.068

29. Han B, Shen Y, Zhang P, Jayabal P, Che R, Zhang J, et al. Overlooked FANCD2 Variant Encodes a Promising, Portent Tumor Suppressor, and Alternative Polyadenylation Contributes to its Expression. *Oncotarget* (2017) 8(14):22490–500. doi: 10.18632/oncotarget.14989

30. Wu G, Wang Q, Xu Y, Li Q, Cheng L. A New Survival Model Based on Ferroptosis-Related Genes for Prognostic Prediction in Clear Cell Renal Cell Carcinoma. *Aging (Albany NY)* (2020) 12(14):14933–48. doi: 10.18632/ aging.103553

31. Wang W, Green M, Choi JE, Gijon M, Kennedy PD, Johnson JK, et al. CD8(+) T Cells Regulate Tumour Ferroptosis During Cancer Immunotherapy. *Nature* (2019) 569(7755):270–4. doi: 10.1038/s41586-019-1170-y

32. Deng F, Sharma I, Dai Y, Yang M, Kanwar YS. Myo-Inositol Oxygenase Expression Profile Modulates Pathogenic Ferroptosis in the Renal Proximal Tubule. *J Clin Invest* (2019) 129(11):5033–49. doi: 10.1172/JCI129903

33. Zhang Q, Zhang P, Li B, Dang H, Jiang J, Meng L, et al. The Expression of Perilipin Family Proteins Can Be Used as Diagnostic Markers of Liposarcoma and to Differentiate Subtypes. *J Cancer* (2020) 11(14):4081–90. doi: 10.7150/ jca.41736

34. Kim E, Jung S, Park WS, Lee JH, Shin R, Heo SC, et al. Upregulation of SLC2A3 Gene and Prognosis in Colorectal Carcinoma: Analysis of TCGA Data. *BMC Cancer* (2019) 19(1):302. doi: 10.1186/s12885-019-5475-x

35. Sanguedolce F, Russo D, Mancini V, Selvaggio O, Calo B, Carrieri G, et al. Prognostic and Therapeutic Role of HER2 Expression in Micropapillary Carcinoma of the Bladder. *Mol Clin Oncol* (2019) 10(2):205–13. doi: 10.3892/mco.2018.1786

36. Sottile R, Federico G, Garofalo C, Tallerico R, Faniello MC, Quaresima B, et al. Iron and Ferritin Modulate MHC Class I Expression and NK Cell Recognition. *Front Immunol* (2019) 10:224. doi: 10.3389/fimmu.2019.00224

37. Joffre OP, Segura E, Savina A, Amigorena S. Cross-Presentation by Dendritic Cells. *Nat Rev Immunol* (2012) 12(8):557–69. doi: 10.1038/nri3254

38. Zhang Q, He Y, Luo N, Patel SJ, Han Y, Gao R, et al. Landscape and Dynamics of Single Immune Cells in Hepatocellular Carcinoma. *Cell* (2019) 179(4):829–45 e20. doi: 10.1016/j.cell.2019.10.003

39. Zhou SL, Zhou ZJ, Hu ZQ, Huang XW, Wang Z, Chen EB, et al. Tumor-Associated Neutrophils Recruit Macrophages and T-Regulatory Cells to Promote Progression of Hepatocellular Carcinoma and Resistance to Sorafenib. *Gastroenterology* (2016) 150(7):1646–58 e17. doi: 10.1053/j.gastro.2016.02.040

40. Fu J, Xu D, Liu Z, Shi M, Zhao P, Fu B, et al. Increased Regulatory T Cells Correlate With CD8 T-Cell Impairment and Poor Survival in Hepatocellular Carcinoma Patients. *Gastroenterology* (2007) 132(7):2328–39. doi: 10.1053/j.gastro.2007.03.102

41. Bellmunt J, Hussain M, Gschwend JE, Albers P, Oudard S, Castellano D, et al. Adjuvant Atezolizumab Versus Observation in Muscle-Invasive Urothelial Carcinoma (IMvigor010): A Multicentre, Open-Label, Randomised, Phase 3 Trial. *Lancet Oncol* (2021) 22(4):525–37. doi: 10.1016/S1470-2045(21)00004-8

20

Comprehensive Analysis of the Immune Infiltrates of Pyroptosis in Kidney Renal Clear Cell Carcinoma

Zhuolun Sun[1], Changying Jing[2], Xudong Guo[3], Mingxiao Zhang[4], Feng Kong[3], Zhenqing Wang[4], Shaobo Jiang[3]* and Hanbo Wang[3]*

[1] Department of Urology, Third Affiliated Hospital, Sun Yat-sen University, Guangzhou, China, [2] School of Medicine, Technical University of Munich, Munich, Germany, [3] Department of Urology, Shandong Provincial Hospital Affiliated to Shandong First Medical University, Jinan, China, [4] Department of Urology, The First Affiliated Hospital of Sun Yat-sen University, Guangzhou, China

*Correspondence:
Shaobo Jiang
jiangshaobo@sdu.edu.cn
Hanbo Wang
wanghanbo0709@163.com

Kidney renal clear cell carcinoma (KIRC) has long been identified as a highly immune-infiltrated tumor. However, the underlying role of pyroptosis in the tumor microenvironment (TME) of KIRC remains poorly described. Herein, we systematically analyzed the prognostic value, role in the TME, response to ICIs, and drug sensitivity of pyroptosis-related genes (PRGs) in KIRC patients based on The Cancer Genome Atlas (TCGA) database. Cluster 2, by consensus clustering for 24 PRGs, presented a poor prognosis, likely because malignancy-related hallmarks were remarkably enriched. Additionally, we constructed a prognostic prediction model that discriminated well between high- and low-risk patients and was further confirmed in external E-MTAB-1980 cohort and HSP cohort. By further analyzing the TME based on the risk model, higher immune cell infiltration and lower tumor purity were found in the high-risk group, which presented a poor prognosis. Patients with high risk scores also exhibited higher ICI expression, indicating that these patients may be more prone to profit from ICIs. The sensitivity to anticancer drugs that correlated with model-related genes was also identified. Collectively, the pyroptosis-related prognosis risk model may improve prognostic information and provide directions for current research investigations on immunotherapeutic strategies for KIRC patients.

Keywords: pyroptosis, kidney renal clear cell carcinoma, tumor microenvironment, survival analysis, prognostic model

INTRODUCTION

Renal cell carcinoma (RCC) is one of the most prevalent urologic malignancies worldwide, with an estimated annual incidence of 14,000 cancer-related deaths in the United States (1). Approximately 30% of patients harbor distant metastases at the time of diagnosis (2). Patients with metastatic RCC (mRCC) present a poor prognosis and have a 10% 5-year survival rate, in contrast to that of non-RCC with an estimated rate of over 55% (3). Kidney renal clear cell carcinoma (KIRC) is the most frequent histological type and is responsible for approximately 70% of all cases of RCC in adults (4). Surgical resection remains the primary treatment modality in most patients with KIRC; however,

30%–40% of patients with localized disease develop metastatic recurrence during follow-up following surgical resection (2). The role of immune infiltrations in cancer development has become the focus of much research. Numerous studies have demonstrated that the different immune cell infiltrates present in the tumor are closely related to the clinical outcomes in some human malignancies (5). KIRC has long been identified and proven to be a highly infiltrated tumor in genomic studies and clinical settings (6). It has been estimated that up to 1% of spontaneous KIRC regression is accompanied by signs of immune mediation (7). Historically, KIRC is one of the first malignant tumors to respond to immunotherapy and remains one of the most sensitive (8). The recent development of cancer immunotherapies such as immune checkpoint inhibitors (ICIs) has revolutionized traditional cancer therapy because of its safety and efficacy (9). However, the response of KIRC to immunotherapy has been unsatisfactory, as expected, and effective disease control and therapeutic strategies are required for further improvements (10). The tumor microenvironment (TME) represents the primary site of continuous interaction between neoplastic and immune system cells, and its various components are associated with tumor progression and therapeutic outcomes (11, 12). Additionally, multiple cytokines and various immunosuppressive cells are involved in tumor immune escape in the KIRC microenvironment (13). Thus, understanding the regulatory mechanism of the TME is critical to identify efficient prognostic biomarkers and optimize individualized immunotherapy regimens against cancer.

The inflammasome is a large cytosolic multiprotein complex that forms a key component of the innate immune system (14). Pyroptosis, recognized as a highly specific inflammatory programmed cell death, is triggered by caspase-1 and -11 (also known as caspase-4 or -5 in humans) in the canonical and noncanonical pathways, respectively (15). Pyroptosis results in cell and organelle swelling, membrane lysis, DNA cleavage, and the release of intracellular proinflammatory contents such as interleukin-1β (IL-1β), which induces local or systemic inflammatory effects (16). Recently, pyroptosis was proven to be closely related to various human diseases, particularly malignant tumors. Pyroptosis plays a dual role during tumor progression (17). During pyroptosis, the various inflammatory mediators derived from the activation of signaling pathways affect tumorigenesis. For example, as an essential part of pyroptosis, NLRP1 mediates caspase-1-dependent secretion of IL-1β and IL-18 cytokines, which promote skin cancer (18). Miguchi et al. confirmed that TGFBR2 mutation upregulates the expression of GSDMC, facilitating colorectal tumor cell proliferation and tumorigenesis (19). Additionally, as a type of death, pyroptosis suppresses tumor development and progression. Wang et al. reported that the downregulation of GSDMD accelerated the S/G$_2$ cell transition to accelerate gastric cancer cell proliferation by regulating cell cycle-related proteins (20).

Currently, most studies have focused primarily on the intrinsic oncogenic pathways of malignant tumors, and the function and underlying mechanism of pyroptosis in the TME

remain unelucidated. Erkes et al. demonstrated that an intact immune system, particularly CD4+ and CD8+ T cells, is required for the efficacy of BRAF inhibitors and MEK inhibitors (BRAFi + MEKi) in melanoma (21). BRAFi + MEKi trigger the activation of caspase-3, causing the cleavage of GSDME, which is a hallmark of pyroptosis of tumor cells and is essential for T-cell activation and tumor regression. The secondary pyroptosis mediated by the caspase 3-dependent cleavage of GSDME could be an indispensable intermediary of immune-driven treatment responsiveness, revealing a potential therapeutic target in enhancing immunotherapy efficacy. Accordingly, pyroptosis-related genes (PRGs) involved in regulating the tumor immune response might be recognized as potential targets in potentiating the clinical activity of immunotherapies. Nevertheless, a complete understanding of pyroptosis in KIRC, including the interactions between pyroptosis and the TME, remains limited.

In the current work, the constructed clustering subtypes and pyroptosis-related risk model were essential for improving clinical risk stratification to make management decisions and predict prognosis for patients with KIRC. Additionally, we thoroughly analyzed the prognostic value, role in the TME, response to ICIs, and drug sensitivity of PRGs in KIRC patients based on the pyroptosis-related prognosis model to further study the effects of pyroptosis on the TME. We performed the present study to provide a novel perspective and a more detailed understanding of the immune infiltrates of pyroptosis and identify reliable prognostic predictors for KIRC patients.

MATERIALS AND METHODS

Data Source
RNA sequencing transcriptome data harmonized to the fragments per kilobase million (FPKM) of 539 KIRC samples and 72 normal kidney tissues were downloaded from the TCGA database (https://tcga-data.nci.nih.gov/tcga/). The corresponding clinical characteristics, including age, gender, grade, AJCC stage, TNM stage, and survival status, were also extracted from TCGA. Patients with simultaneously available mRNA expression profiles and survival times (OS and DFS) > 0 days were enrolled in the study. In total, 525 patients were randomly split into a training cohort (60%; n = 317) and a testing cohort (40%; n = 208) via a 10-fold cross-validation method using the R package "caret". The training cohort was used to construct the prognostic risk model, and the testing cohort and entire cohort were used to verify the predictive reliability and accuracy of the model. Additionally, the E-MTAB-1980 cohort downloaded from the ArrayExpress database (https://www.ebi.ac.uk/arrayexpress/) and Shandong Provincial Hospital (HSP) cohort were used as the external validation cohorts. The clinical characteristics of these patients are shown in **Table 1**.

Next, 24 PRGs were retrieved from the previously published literature (22–24). The "limma" package was used to analyze

TABLE 1 | Characteristics of all patients included in this study.

Variable	Training cohort (n = 317)	Testing cohort (n = 208)	Entire cohort (n = 525)
	Number (%)	Number (%)	Number (%)
Age			
≤60	158(49.84)	106(50.96)	264(50.29)
>60	159(50.16)	102(49.04)	261(49.71)
Gender			
Female	109(34.38)	73(35.1)	182(34.67)
Male	208(65.62)	135(64.9)	343(65.33)
Grade			
G1	8(2.52)	5(2.40)	13(2.48)
G2	131(41.32)	95(46.67)	226(43.05)
G3	127(40.06)	77(37.02)	204(38.86)
G4	47(14.83)	27(12.98)	74(14.10)
unknow	4(1.26)	4(1.92)	8(1.52)
AJCC stage			
I	147(46.37)	114(71.28)	26149.71)
II	42(13.25)	14(6.73)	56(10.67)
III	75(23.66)	48(23.08)	123(23.43)
IV	52(16.40)	30(14.42)	82(15.62)
unknow	1(0.32)	2(0.96)	3(0.57)
T stage			
T1	150(47.32)	117(56.25)	267(50.86)
T2	49(15.46)	19(9.13)	68(12.95)
T3	111(35.02)	68(23.69)	179(34.1)
T4	7(2.21)	4(1.92)	11(2.10)
N stage			
N0	138(43.53)	99(47.6)	237(45.14)
N1-3	11(3.47)	5(2.4)	16(3.05)
unknow	168(53)	104(50)	272(51.81)
M stage			
M0	252(79.5)	165(79.33)	417(79.43)
M1	49(15.46)	29(13.94)	78(14.86)
unknow	16(5.05)	14(3.76)	30(5.71)

Variable	E-MTAB-1980 cohort (n = 101)	HSP cohort (n = 186)
	Number (%)	Number (%)
Age		
≤60	44(41.90)	132(70.96)
>60	57(58.10)	54(29.04)
Gender		
Female	24(23.76)	121(65.05)
Male	77(76.24)	55(34.95)
Grade		
G1	13(12.87)	44(23.66)
G2	59(58.41)	102(54.84)
G3	22(21.78)	28(15.05)
G4	5(4.96)	12(6.45)
unknow	0(0.00)	0(0.00)
AJCC stage		
I	66(64.35)	102(54.54)
II	10(9.90)	36(19.36)
III	13(12.87)	24(12.90)
IV	12(11.88)	24(12.90)
unknow	0(0.00)	0(0.00)
T stage		
T1	68(67.33)	110(59.14)
T2	11(10.89)	42(22.58)
T3	21(20.79)	25(13.44)
T4	1(0.99)	9(4.84)

(Continued)

TABLE 1 | Continued

Variable	E-MTAB-1980 cohort (n = 101)	HSP cohort (n = 186)
	Number (%)	Number (%)
N stage		
N0	11(90.10)	176(94.62)
N1-3	10(9.90)	10(5.38)
unknow	0(0.00)	0(0.00)
M stage		
M0	94(93.07)	171(91.94)
M1	7(6.93)	15(8.06)
unknow	0(0.00)	0(0.00)

differentially expressed PRGs between tumor tissues and adjacent normal pairs from TCGA.

Consensus Clustering Analysis of PRGs

To investigate the biological characteristics of PRGs in KIRC patients, we classified the patients into different subtypes using the "ConsensusClusterPlus" package with a resampling rate of 80% and 50 iterations. PCA was performed to detect differences in gene expression patterns in distinct KIRC subtypes. The differentially expressed genes in different subtypes were subjected to biological process term GO functional annotation. To illustrate the functions associated with different subtypes of KIRC, GSEA was performed using the Hallmark gene set "h.all.v7.2.symbols.gmt" from the MSigDB database (http://www.broadinstitute.org/gsea) as previously described (25). GSEA significance was determined as a false discovery rate (FDR) ≤ 0.25 and nominal $p ≤ 0.05$.

Construction and Evaluation of the Pyroptosis-Related Prognostic Risk Model

Univariate Cox proportional hazards regression analysis was used to assess the prognostic implication of every differentially expressed PRG, and then the features with a p value < 0.05 in the training cohort were defined as prognosis-related factors. Next, LASSO Cox regression analysis was performed to screen out the optimal gene combination to construct the risk model. The optimal values of the penalty parameter λ were finally determined by 10-fold cross-validation to construct an optimal LASSO regression model. The coefficient calculated by LASSO regression and gene expression level were applied to obtain the risk score formula as follows: Risk score = $(expr_{gene1} × Coef_{gene1}) + (expr_{gene2} × Coef_{gene2}) + ... + (expr_{genen} × Coef_{genen})$. Every KIRC patient in the training and validation cohorts (including the testing cohort, entire cohort, E-MTAB-1980 cohort, and HSP cohort) received an individual risk score according to this equation. The subjects were subsequently assigned into high- and low-risk groups using the median cutoff risk score as a threshold. Subsequently, Kaplan-Meier curves and ROC curves were applied to assess the prognostic role of the model. To verify the clinical application value of the constructed model, we analyzed the association between the model-based risk score and clinicopathological features based on the TCGA database. Additionally, survival analysis was performed using different subgroups of patients.

Protein Network Construction

GeneMANIA (http://genemania.org/), a multifunctional and user-friendly web interface, was utilized for predicting interactions and functions of genes and gene sets (26). In this study, we used this web tool to develop a 6-PRG-involved network and to screen other potential binding partners in the regulatory network.

Evaluation of the Immune Status, Immune Cell Infiltration Fractions, and ICIs Between the Low- and High-Risk Groups

To investigate the immune status of the different groups, we first quantified the enrichment levels of the 29 immune markers in each sample by ssGSEA. The estimated score, stromal score, immune score, and corresponding tumor purity for each patient were subsequently calculated using the ESTIMATE algorithm (27). The expression of HLA-genes was also analyzed. Next, we estimated the relative abundance of LM22 for each contained sample based on gene expression data through CIBERSORT (6). Patients with a P value < 0.05 were included, and significance was assessed based on 1,000 permutations. The proportion of immune cells was depicted in the violin map to compare the distributions of LM22 between the subtypes grouped by clustering analysis. To understand the association between the model and tumor immune microenvironment, the expression levels of 17 ICIs were analyzed between the low- and high-risk groups (28).

Somatic Mutation Analysis

Somatic mutation information of KIRC was downloaded from the TCGA database. The data which included somatic variants were extract from Mutation Annotation Format (MAF) form, and then analyzed by using "maftools" package (29). The waterfall was used to present the mutation landscapes in patients with high- and low-risk groups in the KIRC patients. In this study, the TMB score of each sample was calculated as the number of mutations/length of exons (30Mb). All KIRC samples with somatic mutations were divided into the high- and the low-TMB groups according the median data. Kaplan-Meier analysis was performed to compare the survival difference between low- and high-TMB groups. Moreover, we further assessed the associations of TMB levels with risk score *via* Wilcoxon test.

TIMER Database and GDSC Database

TIMER (https://cistrome.shinyapps.io/timer/) is a reliable database to analyze the abundance of tumor-infiltrating immune cells (30). The "SCNA" module of the TIMER database was employed to explore the SCNA of risk model-related genes and effect on the infiltration levels of six immune cells.

GDSC (https://www.cancerrxgene.org/) is a public online database for information on drug sensitivity in cancer cells and molecular markers of drug response, providing a unique resource to facilitate the discovery of novel targets for cancer therapies (31). We used GDSC to explore the sensitivity to anticancer drugs associated with the selected risk signature genes.

Patients and Specimens

From January 2012 and May 2019, 186 KIRC tissue samples were collected from patients at SPH. No patients received chemotherapy or radiotherapy before surgery. The pathological diagnosis was confirmed by two independent pathologists after surgery. All patients were informed of the importance of follow-up and were regularly followed every three months after surgery. All samples were subjected to quantitative real-time polymerase chain reaction (qRT-PCR) analysis. The study was approved by the Ethics Committee of SPH, and all patients signed the informed consents for using their pathological tissues and related information.

RNA Extraction and qRT-PCR

Total RNA from 186 fresh-frozen KIRC tissue samples was extracted using the RNAiso plus kit (TAKARA) according to the manufacturer's instructions, and the expression of the model-related genes was further examined by qRT-PCR. The complementary DNA (cDNA) was synthesized with PrimeScript RT Reagent kit (TAKARA) according to the manufacturer's instructions. The qRT-PCR was performed on LightCycler 480 II System (Roche) using an SYBR Green Master Kit (Roche). Human β-actin was introduced as an internal reference gene to normalize mRNA levels. Expression levels of each mRNA were calculated using the $-\triangle$Ct method. All trials were conducted in triplicate. The primers are presented in **Supplementary Table 1**.

Statistical Analysis

The Mann-Whitney U test was used to compare gene expression between tumor tissues and adjacent nontumorous tissues. The Wilcoxon test was used to compare two groups, and the Kruskal-Wallis test was used to compare more than two groups. Chi-squared tests were performed to compare the categorical variables. Qualitative variables were compared using Pearson's test, where appropriate. Kaplan-Meier analysis was used to evaluate OS, and the log-rank test was used to compare the OS between groups. Univariate and multivariate Cox regression analyses were implemented to identify independent predictors of OS. All statistical analyses were conducted using R version 4.01 and SPSS 24.0 (IBM, NY, USA). If not specified above, $P < 0.05$ was considered statistically significant.

RESULTS

The Expression Level of PRGs Is Upregulated in KIRC

To explore the biological functions of PRGs and their significance in KIRC, we initially measured the expression patterns of 24 PRGs in 72 pairs of KIRC samples and adjacent non-tumor samples based on The Cancer Genome Atlas (TCGA) database. Differential analysis revealed that the expression levels of PRGs between KIRC and normal samples were distinct (**Figures 1A, B**). Twenty-one genes were identified as differentially expressed PRGs, including 20 downregulated genes (NLRP6, GSDMD, GSDMB, GSDMC, NLRP7, GSDMA, NLRP1, MEFV, NLRP12,

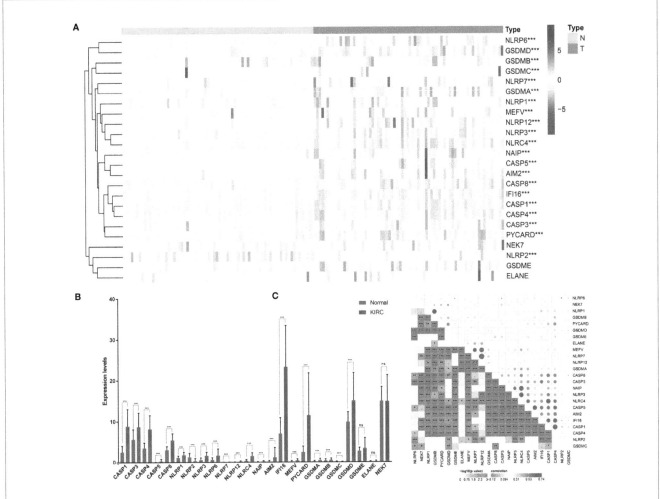

FIGURE 1 | Expression of PRGs in KIRC tissues compared with normal kidney tissues and their interactions. **(A)** Heatmap of the expression of the 24 PRGs in the tumors and normal tissues of the TCGA dataset. **(B)** The expression of PRGs was significantly increased in 72 KIRC compared with that in normal kidney pairs. **(C)** Interaction analysis among the 24 PRGs. *$P < 0.05$, **$P < 0.01$, ***$P < 0.001$. ns, no significance.

NLRP3, NLRC4, NAIP, CASP5, AIM2, CASP8, IFI16, CASP1, CASP4, CASP3, and PYCARD) and 1 downregulated gene (NLRP2) in KIRC compared with normal adjacent tissues ($P < 0.001$). Additionally, no significant difference was found in the expression of NEK7, GSDME, and ELANE between KIRC and normal tissues ($P > 0.05$). Collectively, these findings suggest that pyroptosis plays an important biological role during tumorigenesis and disease progression.

To further explore the nature of the interactions among PRGs, we examined the correlation among 24 PRGs. Most of the interactions exhibited a significantly positive correlation between two quantities (**Figure 1C**). Additionally, NLRP7 was most correlated with NLRP12 among all the interactions of 24 PRGs.

Two Subgroups Are Different in Clinicopathological Features and Survival in KIRC by Consensus Clustering of PRGs

We found that the K-means clustering algorithm with 2 clusters achieved the clearest population clusters and was considered the

optimal value. According to the expression levels of the PRGs from the TCGA database, the KIRC samples were clustered into 2 subtypes (cluster 1, n = 383 and cluster 2, n = 142) (**Figures 2A–C**). We then employed principal component analysis (PCA) to study the gene expression pattern between the two subtypes and observed that the distribution pattern of gene expression profiles within the two groups differed (**Figure 2D**). Next, the relationships between the clustering and clinicopathological features were evaluated (**Figure 2E**). Cluster 2 was preferentially associated with a higher M stage ($P < 0.01$), T stage ($P < 0.01$), AJCC stage ($P < 0.001$), and grade ($P < 0.001$), while no significant difference was observed for other parameters, such as age and gender. Additionally, we noticed that cluster 2 showed a shorter overall survival (OS; $P = 7.979e$-10) and disease-free survival (DFS; $P = 2.29e$-07) than cluster 1 (**Figures 2F, G**).

The genes that were significantly altered between the two groups were subjected to gene ontology (GO) analysis. The results were closely related to immune-related biological processes, including leukocyte migration, neutrophil activation, and neutrophil-

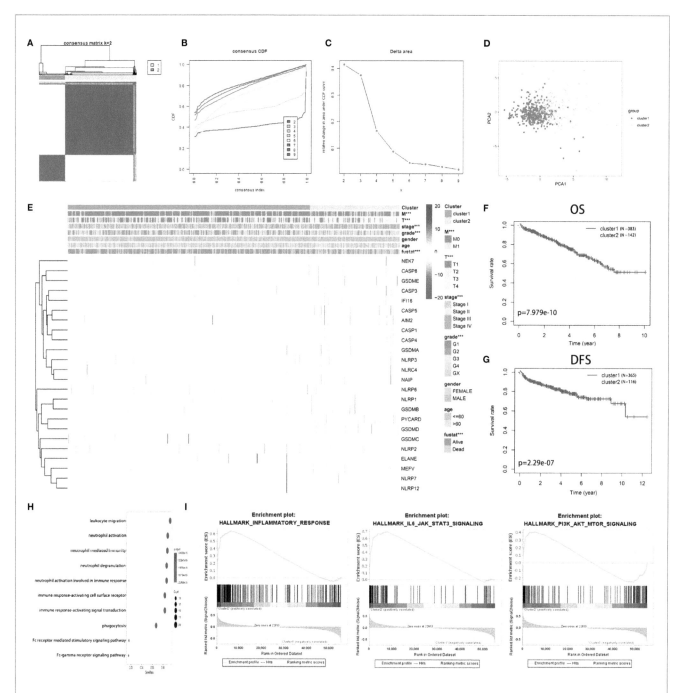

FIGURE 2 | Diverse clinical characteristics and survival of KIRC between cluster 1 and cluster 2 subtypes in the TCGA cohort. **(A)** The TCGA KIRC cohort was divided into two distinct clusters when k = 2. **(B)** Consensus clustering cumulative distribution function (CDF) for k = 2 to 9. **(C)** Relative change in the area under the CDF curve for k = 2 to 9. **(D)** PCA of the TCGA dataset based on the expression profiles of the 24 PRGs. **(E)** Heatmap and distribution of clinicopathological variables between the two clusters. **(F, G)** Kaplan-Meier curves of OS **(F)** and DFS **(G)** for patients with KIRC between the two clusters. **(H)** Biological processes of the genes with different expression between the two clusters. **(I)** GSEA showed that the inflammatory response, IL6-JAK-STAT3 signaling, and PI3K-AKT-mTOR signaling were significantly enriched in cluster 2. ***P < 0.001.

mediated immunity (**Figure 2H**). Subsequently, gene set enrichment analysis (GSEA) was conducted, indicating that immune- and cancer-related hallmarks, including the inflammatory response, IL6-JAK-STAT3 signaling, and epithelial-mesenchymal transitions signaling, had significant correlations with cluster 2 (**Figure 2I**). The above results demonstrated that the two subgroups determined based on the expression of the PRGs were strongly linked to the malignancy of KIRC.

Construction of the Prognostic Risk Model Based on the TCGA Training Cohort

Because we identified distinct expression patterns in KIRC patients, we next considered that constructing a pyroptosis-related risk signature might be useful for predicting prognosis. We first conducted a univariate Cox regression analysis and identified 8 PRGs (CASP4, CASP5, NLRP1, NLRP6, AIM2, IFI16, PYCARD, GSDMB) that were correlated with OS in the training cohort ($P < 0.05$) (**Figure 3A**). All eight PRGs, except NLRP6, were considered risk genes with HRs > 1. Based on the above results, to further clarify the prognostic potential, we

subsequently conducted LASSO analysis on the expression values of 8 prognostic PRGs (**Figures 3B, C**). Ultimately, 6 genes, CASP4, NLRP6, AIM2, IFI16, PYCARD, and GSDMB, were identified to construct the prediction model. The prognostic risk model was established based on the following formula: risk score = (0.0137 × expression value of CASP4) – (0.0624 × expression value of NLRP6) + (0.0227 × expression value of AIM2) + (0.0149 × expression value of IFI16) + (0.0059 × expression value of PYCARD) + (0.2049 × expression value of GSDMB). The risk score for each patient in the TCGA training cohort was calculated, and the patients were stratified into

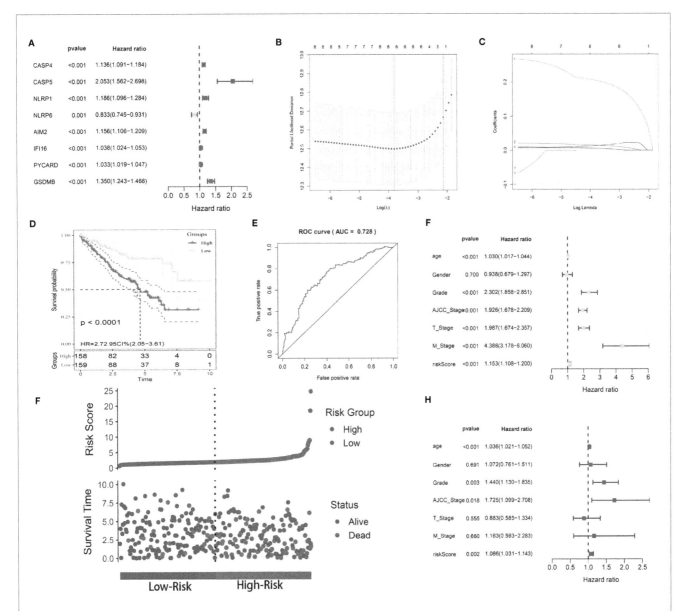

FIGURE 3 | Construction of the prognostic risk model based on the TCGA training cohort. **(A)** Forest map of 8 PRGs significantly correlated with OS and identified by Cox univariate analysis. **(B)** Screening of optimal parameters (lambda) in the LASSO regression model based on the TCGA training cohort. **(C)** LASSO coefficient profiles of the 8 PRGs determined by the optimal lambda. **(D)** Kaplan-Meier curve for the OS of KIRC patients in the high- and low-risk groups in the TCGA training cohort. **(E)** ROC analysis of the prognostic model regarding the OS and survival status in the TCGA training cohort. **(F)** Scatterplots in the top and bottom panels illustrate the distribution of the risk score and survival status in the TCGA training patients, respectively. **(G, H)** Univariate **(G)** and multivariate **(H)** Cox regression analyses of the risk score and clinicopathological parameters in the TCGA training cohort.

a high-risk group and a low-risk group according to the median risk score. Kaplan-Meier analysis showed that the prognosis of the KIRC patients in the high-risk group was poorer than that in the low-risk group (P < 0.0001; **Figure 3D**). The prognostic model showed a satisfactory prediction efficiency, with an area under the ROC curve (AUC) value of 0.728 (**Figure 3E**). Additionally, the risk score distributions and patient survival status are shown in **Figure 3F**.

Univariable and multivariable Cox regression analyses were utilized to identify whether the model-based risk score could be an independent predictor of OS. The results showed that age, grade, AJCC stage, T stage, M stage, and risk score were closely related to OS (P < 0.001) in univariate analysis (**Figure 3G**). Likewise, age (P < 0.001), grade (P = 0.003), AJCC stage (P = 0.018), and risk score (P = 0.002) maintained their prognostic values in multivariate Cox analysis (**Figure 3H**). Therefore, these data demonstrated that the risk score was an independent prognostic indicator for patients with KIRC.

Internal and External Validation of the Prognostic Risk Model in KIRC Patients

To explore whether the prognostic model was generalizable and harbored similar prognostic value in different populations, we applied it to the internal (TCGA testing and entire) and independent external (E-MTAB-1980 and HSP) validation cohorts. Regarding the predictions in the TCGA testing cohort,

Kaplan-Meier analysis showed that patients with high risk scores had worse OS (P < 0.001) (**Figure 4A**). The AUC value for predicting OS in the TCGA testing cohort was 0.717 (**Figure 4E**). For the TCGA entire cohort, the model could still separate analytic samples into various subgroups of clinical importance. The Kaplan-Meier survival curve indicated that patients in the high-risk group exhibited a significantly lower OS than those in the low-risk group (P < 0.001) (**Figure 4B**). The AUC value of the entire TCGA cohort was 0.772, which was comparable to the model results described above (**Figure 4F**). Next, External validation using the E-MTAB-1980 and HSP cohorts was performed to validate the robustness and validity of the constructed model. Consistent with TCGA analysis, Kaplan-Meier analysis suggested that the patients in the high-risk group had a significantly shorter OS within both the E-MTAB-1980 cohort and HSP cohort (**Figures 4C, D**). The AUC values of the E-MTAB-1980 cohort and HSP cohort were found to be 0.711 and 0.705, respectively (**Figures 4G, H**). The risk score distributions and patient survival status in four cohorts were shown in **Supplementary Figure 1**. Overall, the risk score showed favorable discrimination ability in all four cohorts.

Clinical Evaluation of the Prognostic Risk Model Based on the TCGA Entire Cohort

To validate the clinical value of the prognostic model, we evaluated the relationship between the risk score and clinical features.

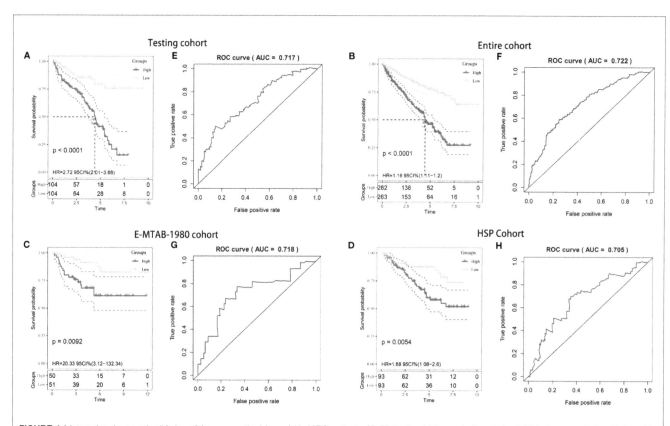

FIGURE 4 | Internal and external validation of the prognostic risk model in KIRC patients. **(A–D)** Kaplan–Meier survival analysis of OS between patients with low-risk scores and high-risk scores in the TCGA testing cohort **(A)**, TCGA entire cohort **(B)**, E-MTAB-1980 cohort **(C)**, and HSP cohort **(D)**. **(E–H)** ROC analysis of the prognostic model in the TCGA testing cohort **(E)**, TCGA entire cohort **(F)**, E-MTAB-1980 cohort **(G)**, and HSP cohort **(H)**.

A heatmap was used to visualize differences in the expression levels of the six genes between the low- and high-risk groups. The analysis demonstrated that risk genes (CASP4, AIM2, IFI16, PYCARD, GSDMB) were upregulated in the high-risk group, while the expression of protective genes (NLRP6) was downregulated (**Figure 5A**). Additionally, a significant difference was found among the diverse groups in terms of the M stage ($P < 0.001$), T stage ($P < 0.001$), AJCC stage ($P < 0.001$), and grade ($P < 0.001$). We also noticed that the risk score increased with the progression or severity of the tumor (**Figure 5B**).

Subsequently, stratified survival analyses were performed to examine the good applicability of our prognostic model. As expected, the patients with Grade 1 disease showed the best prognosis, followed by those with Grade 2, Grade 3, and Grade 4 disease. Furthermore, similar trends were presented in the AJCC stage, T stage, and M stage (**Figure 5C**). We next conducted stratified survival analyses according to the different clinical features. Excitingly, we observed that the patients with high-risk scores were associated with a shorter OS across all the subgroups (**Supplementary Figure 2**). Thus, the dysregulation of pyroptosis is critically involved in the development and progression of KIRC.

Analysis of Network and Gene Set Enrichment Analysis (GSEA)

A gene interaction network was visualized using GeneMANIA to gain further insight into the possible relationships between the

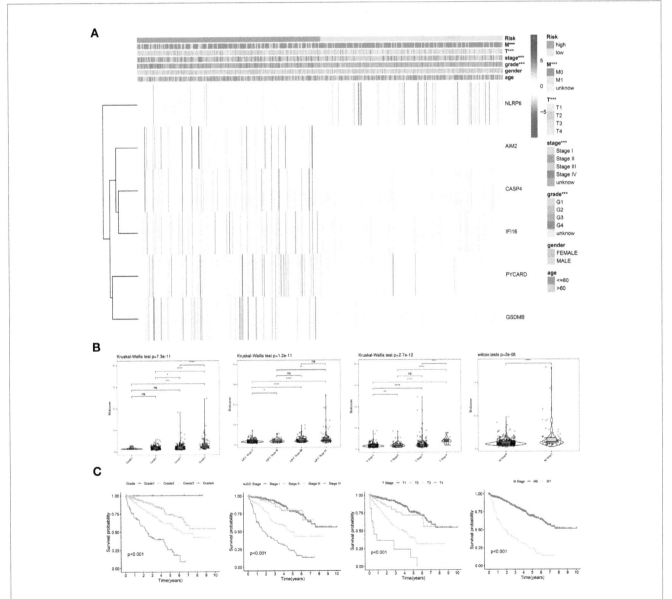

FIGURE 5 | Clinical evaluation of the prognosis risk model based on the TCGA entire cohort. **(A)** Heatmap of the expression of 6 PRGs and distribution of clinical features between the low- and high-risk groups. **(B, C)** Expression of the model-based risk score **(B)** and Kaplan-Meier survival analysis **(C)** in KIRC patients stratified by different clinicopathological characteristics (grade, AJCC stage, T stage, and M stage). *$P < 0.05$, **$P < 0.01$, ***$P < 0.001$, ****$P < 0.0001$. ns, no significance.

six PFRs and their potential binding partners. The regulatory network carried twenty-six genes, including six target PFRs and additional twenty genes that were recognized automatically through GeneMANIA (**Figure 6A**). We then analyzed the correlation of the six genes in KIRC and found that the interaction between CASP4 and IFI16 (r = 0.61) was most significant and displayed a positive correlation (**Figure 6B**).

GSEA was performed to investigate the relevant biological processes and signaling pathways using the pyroptosis model based risk score for classification. The results suggested that cancer- and immune-related 'Hallmark' gene sets, such as epithelial-mesenchymal transition, inflammatory response, PI3K/AKT/mTOR signaling pathway, and Wnt/β-catenin signaling pathway that were highly enriched in the high–risk phenotype (**Figure 6C**). Moreover, several classical pathways from KEGG, Reactome, BioCarta, PID gene sets, including the cell cycle, caspase pathway, Myc pathway were also related to the high–risk group (**Figures 6D–G**).

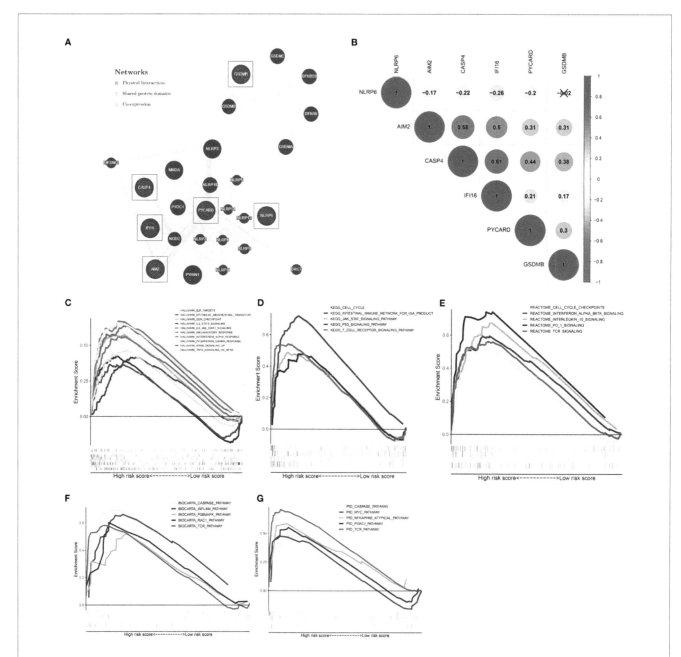

FIGURE 6 | Analysis of the regulatory network and gene sets associated with high-risk groups. **(A)** The regulatory network involving six model-related genes and twenty potential binding proteins was constructed through GeneMANIA. **(B)** Correlation analysis of the six genes. **(C–G)** GSEA showed the significantly enriched Hallmark **(C)**, KEGG **(D)**, Reactome **(E)**, BioCarta **(F)**, and PID **(G)** gene sets in high-risk score based on the TCGA database.

Prognostic Risk Scores Related to Different Immune Statuses, Immune Cell Infiltration and ICIs

According to the results shown above, to further assess the relationship between immune status between the groups, the relative quantities of 29 immune markers were systematically evaluated using single-sample GSEA (ssGSEA). A heatmap was constructed to depict a more comprehensive immune infiltration landscape for the TCGA KIRC cohort (**Figure 7A**). We used the ESTIMATE algorithm to successfully generate the tumor purity score, estimate score, immune score, and stromal score. Notably,

patients with a low-risk score presented a higher level of tumor purity ($P < 0.001$) and a lower estimate score ($p < 0.001$), immune score ($P < 0.001$), and stromal score ($P < 0.001$) than those with a high-risk score ($P < 0.001$) (**Figures 7B–E**), consistent with previous study findings that a lower estimate score represents higher tumor purity. Considering that human leukocyte antigen (HLA)-related genes play an essential role in regulating the immune response, we then compared the expression of HLA-related genes between different groups and found that most of the HLA-related genes were upregulated in the high-risk group (**Figure 7F**).

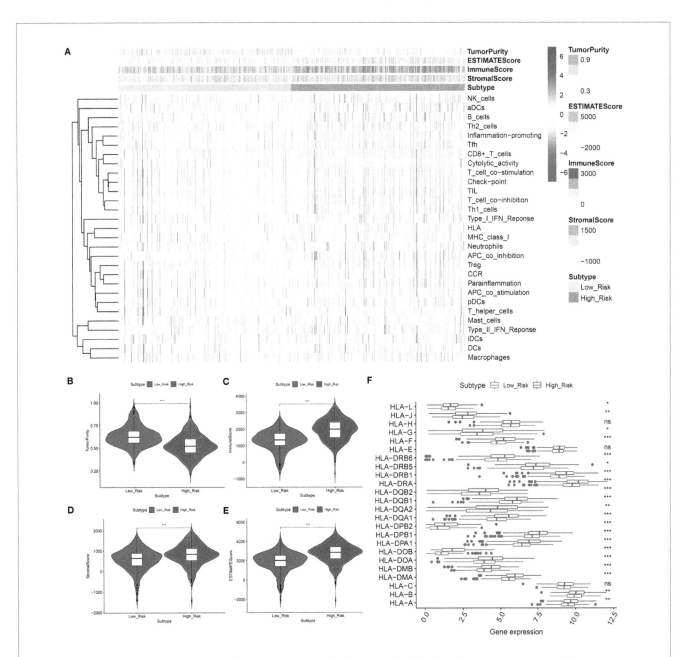

FIGURE 7 | The low- and high-risk groups display different immune statuses. **(A)** Heatmap of the distribution of 29 immune-related genes between the low-and high-risk groups using ssGSEA. **(B–F)** Expression level of the tumor purity **(B)**, ESTIMATE score **(C)**, immune score **(D)**, stromal score **(E)**, and HLA-related genes between the low- and high-risk groups. *$P < 0.05$, **$P < 0.01$, ***$P < 0.001$. ns, no significance.

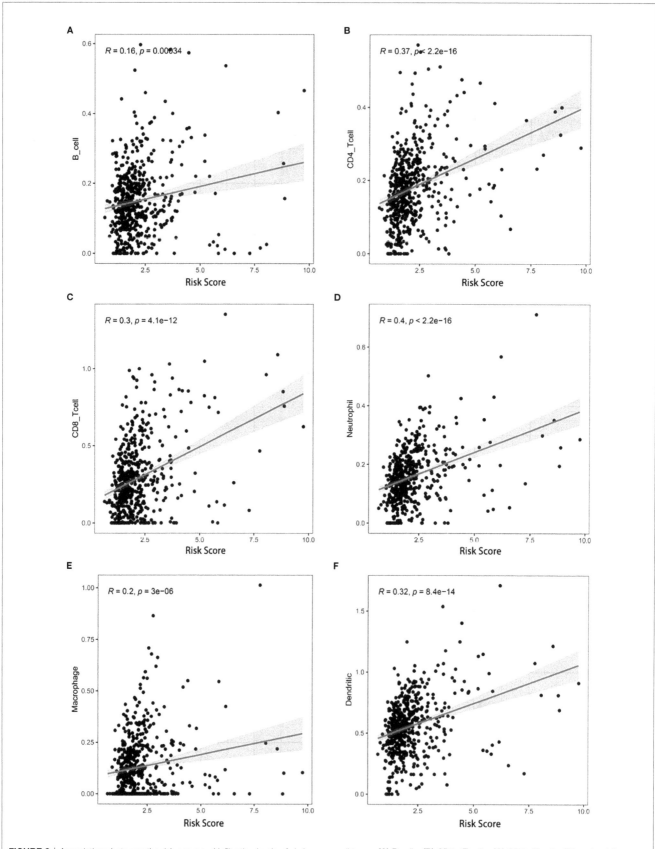

FIGURE 8 | Associations between the risk score and infiltration levels of six immune cell types. **(A)** B cells, **(B)** CD4+ T cells, **(C)** CD8+ T cells, **(D)** neutrophils, **(E)** macrophages, and **(F)** dendritic cells.

Additionally, we analyzed the relationship between the risk score and infiltration levels of six immune cell types (B cells, CD4+ T cells, CD8+ T cells, neutrophils, macrophages, and dendrites). Interestingly, a significantly positive correlation was found between the risk score and content of the six immune cell types (**Figure 8**). The pyroptosis-related risk model effectively reflected the status of the immune microenvironment for KIRC patients.

Subsequently, we estimated the fraction of 22 tumor-infiltrating immune cells (LM22) in the low- and high-risk groups using CIBERSORT. The bar plot illustrates the specific fractions of LM22 in each KIRC sample (**Supplementary Figure 3A**). Additionally, we depicted the distributions of LM22 between the two groups in the heatmap (**Supplementary Figure 3B**). We observed a dependency among the various immunocyte subpopulation fractions (**Supplementary Figure 3C**). Finally, we compared the differential infiltration of 22 immune cells between the groups. The low-risk group had higher infiltration levels of resting CD4 memory T cells, gamma delta T cells, monocytes, M2 macrophages, resting dendritic cells, activated dendritic cells, resting mast cells, and eosinophils, whereas infiltration was more correlated with plasma cells, CD8 T cells, activated CD4 memory

T cells, follicular helper T cells, and regulatory T cells (Tregs) (**Supplementary Figure 3D**).

Recent breakthroughs in tumor immunology have generated substantial interest in the potential of ICIs to treat other solid tumors. To further understand the relationship between the model and ICIs, 17 ICIs (B7-H3, B7-H4, CTLA4, CD27, ICOS, TIGIT, PD-1, LAG3, CD58, CD86, PD-L1, PD-L2, TIM-3, CD270, CD70, CD40, and IDO1) were analyzed as reported previously. We discovered that high risk scores were positively correlated with high expression of ICIs, in addition to B7-H4, PD-L1, and CD40 (**Supplementary Figure 4**).

Tumor Somatic Mutational Landscape and Effect of Genetic Mutants of Model-Related PRGs on Immune Cell Infiltration

Giving that gene mutations are an important cause of tumorigenesis, we explored the differences in the distribution of somatic mutations between high- and low-risk groups. The top 30 most frequently mutated genes of these two groups were displayed in **Figures 9A, B**, respectively. The Kaplan-Meier curves for OS indicated that the patients with high-TMB group had significantly worse OS than those with low-TMB group (**Figure 9C**). In addition,

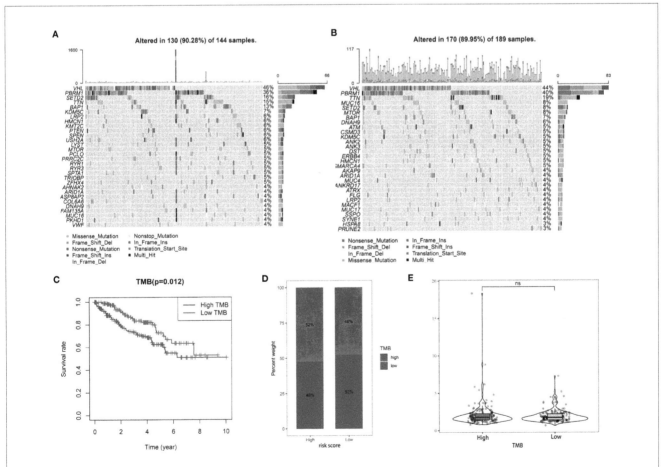

FIGURE 9 | Tumor somatic mutational analyses between high- and low-risk scores. **(A, B)** Waterfall plot shows the mutation distribution of the top 30 most frequently mutated genes in the high-risk group **(A)** and low-risk group **(B)**. **(C)** Survival analysis of OS in KIRC patients between high- and low-TMB groups. **(D)** Difference in TMB between the high- and low-risk groups. **(E)** Difference in risk scores between the high- and low- TMB groups. ns, no significance.

the high-risk group presented more extensive TMB than the low-risk group (**Figure 9D**). Interestingly, however, there was no statistical difference in the expression level of risk score between the low- and high-TMB groups (**Figure 9E**).

We further investigated the underlying relationships between the somatic cell copy number alternations (CNAs) of these model-related genes and different immune cell infiltrations using the Tumor Immune Estimation Resource (TIMER) database. The mutants of these six genes were strongly associated with the immune infiltration microenvironment in KIRC. Compared with the immune infiltration levels in samples with wild-type genes, diverse forms of mutations carried by these six genes displayed lower levels of immune infiltrates. Among the CNAs of the six identified model-related genes, arm-level deletion and arm-level gain exhibited a statistically significant effect on the immune cell infiltration levels in KIRC (**Figure 10**). In addition, to further understand the relationship between six model-related genes and immune infiltration in KIRC microenvironment, we explored the correlation ship in TIMER. The results illuminated that the expression of these genes were positively correlated with the infiltrating levels of immune cells (**Figure 11**).

Drug Sensitivity Analysis of Model-Related PRGs

We next used the Genomics of Drugs Sensitivity in Cancer (GDSC) database to identify an association between sensitivity to anticancer drugs and the expression levels of the six genes. The results indicated that the six genes were frequently associated with the resistance or sensitivity of kidney cancer cells to multiple targeted drugs (**Figure 12**). Among these six genes, NLRP6, IFI16, and GSDM8 were relatively important because their expression levels were closely associated with sunitinib. Moreover, the expression of NLRP6 and GSDM8 was negatively correlated with sunitinib resistance. However, the expression of IFI16 was positively correlated with sunitinib resistance.

DISCUSSION

Pyroptosis is a highly inflammatory form of programmed cell death that is characterized by inflammasome activation and the secretion of IL-1β and IL-18 (32, 33). Dysregulation of pyroptosis may cause dysfunction in the stimulation of adaptive immune defenses and contribute to the initiation and progression of multiple tumors

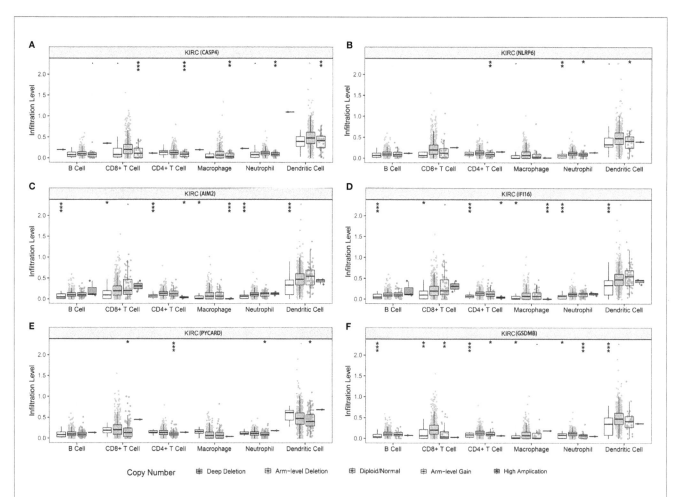

FIGURE 10 | Relationship between the mutants of six model-related PRGs and immune cell infiltration. **(A)** CASP4, **(B)** NLRP6, **(C)** AIM2, **(D)** IFI16, **(E)** PYCARD, and **(F)** GSDMB. *P < 0.05, **P < 0.01, ***P < 0.001.

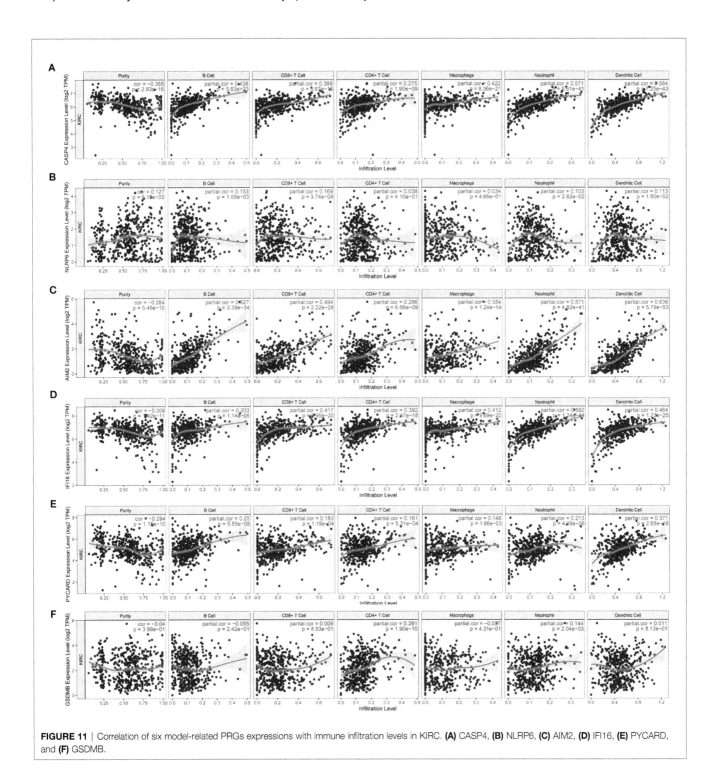

FIGURE 11 | Correlation of six model-related PRGs expressions with immune infiltration levels in KIRC. **(A)** CASP4, **(B)** NLRP6, **(C)** AIM2, **(D)** IFI16, **(E)** PYCARD, and **(F)** GSDMB.

(17, 34). However, controversies exist concerning the role of PRGs as tumor suppressors or tumor promoters. For example, Wang et al. (20) reported that GSDMD was downregulated in gastric cancer and exerted a tumor suppressor role by inhibiting the PI3K/AKT signaling pathway. Conversely, Gao et al. (35) found that GSDMD protein was significantly upregulated and promoted cell proliferation and a poor prognosis by potentiating the EGFR/AKT signaling pathway in lung cancer. The distinct effect of PRGs in different tumor cells reflects the overwhelmingly complex molecular regulation mechanism of pyroptosis. Because most of the studies primarily concentrated on the intrinsic oncogenic pathways of malignant tumors, it is indispensable to elucidate the potential regulatory mechanisms of pyroptosis that may significantly affect the characteristics of the cancer treatment response, particularly precision immunotherapy. Furthermore, the detailed effects of pyroptosis on the TME of KIRC remain to be fully investigated.

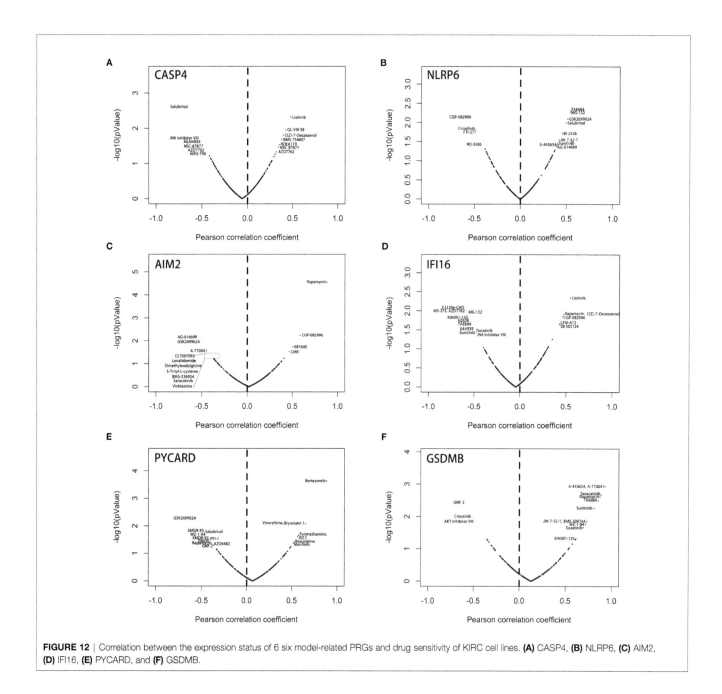

FIGURE 12 | Correlation between the expression status of 6 six model-related PRGs and drug sensitivity of KIRC cell lines. **(A)** CASP4, **(B)** NLRP6, **(C)** AIM2, **(D)** IFI16, **(E)** PYCARD, and **(F)** GSDMB.

In this study, we sought to explore the expression patterns of pyroptosis in KIRC and its prognostic value and effect on the TME. The expression of NLRP2 was significantly decreased in KIRC tissues compared with that in normal tissues, whereas NEK7, GSDME, and ELANE were not significantly different. The expression levels of other PRGs were higher in KIRC tissues than in noncancerous tissues. Next, we then determined two subtypes of KIRC—namely, cluster 1 and cluster 2—by consensus clustering based on the expression profiles of PRGs from the TCGA database. The diverse subtypes affected the prognosis and showed significant differences in clinicopathological features and tumor immune infiltrations. The patients in cluster 2 were found to be closely related to a more advanced tumor stage and grade.

As predicted, cluster 1 presented better OS and DFS than cluster 2. GO enrichment analysis and GSEA were conducted to further explore the functions associated with different subgroups. Several biological processes correlated with immunity were identified, including leukocyte migration, neutrophil activation, and neutrophil-mediated immunity. A previous study suggested that leukocyte migration might contribute to the pathogenesis of many human diseases, including tumors (36). Additionally, increasing evidence has revealed that the immune system is involved in carcinogenesis and tumor progression by promoting cancer cell proliferation, migration, immune escape and chemotherapy resistance (37). GSEA revealed that the characteristic features of malignant tumors, including IL6-JAK-STAT3 signaling and PI3K/

AKT/mTOR signaling, were obviously related to cluster 2. Wang et al. found that the downregulation of GSDMD markedly promoted the proliferation of gastric cancer through inactivating the STAT3 and PI3K/AKT pathways (20). Similarly, Chen et al. found that downregulated AIM2 expression may be involved in the PI3K/AKT signaling pathway in colorectal cancer (38). Here, we suggest that pyroptosis is related to many biological processes and signaling pathways, revealing their significant roles in the initiation and development of KIRC.

We then constructed a prognostic prediction model in the training cohort. The risk scoring system based on six genes predicted the prognosis of KIRC patients, and the patients were effectively stratified into high- and low-risk groups. Patients in the high-risk group had a significantly shorter OS than those in the low-risk group. The performance of the prognostic pyroptosis-relevant model was confirmed in two internal cohorts. The independent external E-MTAB-1980 and HSP cohorts also yielded consistent results. Additionally, the risk score increased with the progression or severity of the tumor. Univariate and multivariate Cox analyses indicated that the six-gene prognosis model is an independent factor. Among these six model-related PRGs, the expression of NLRP6 was significantly decreased in high-risk KIRC patients. Surprisingly, NLRP6 was upregulated in normal tissue samples compared with that in KIRC tissue, likely because of the different effects of NLRP6 at different stages in KIRC tumorigenesis and development. Chen et al. suggested that NLRP6 plays a fundamental role in maintaining intestinal homeostasis, thus preventing intestinal tissue from aberrant inflammation and tumors (39). AIM2 has been identified as a tumor-suppressive gene in human colorectal cancer (38), but Zhang et al. (40) showed that AIM2 promotes non-small cell lung cancer progression through an inflammasome-dependent pathway. One previous study found that caspase-4 is highly expressed in the lamina propria of colorectal cancer compared with that in normal tissues, indicating that caspase-4 may represent a biomarker of colon carcinoma (41). IFI16 and PYCAED serve as oncogenes in cervical cancer and gastric cancer, respectively (42, 43). Accumulated evidence indicates that GSDMB is overexpressed in several cancer types and may be involved in cancer progression and metastasis (44). These studies revealed that the dysregulation of pyroptosis might play divergent roles in different types of cancer.

The tumor microenvironment plays a critical regulatory role in carcinogenesis and tumor progression (45). According to our scoring system, the difference in the TME between the low-risk and high-risk groups was notable. The immune score and expression levels of HLA-related genes in the high-risk group were significantly higher than those in the low-risk group, while the tumor purity exhibited the opposite trend, likely explaining why the low-risk group patients had a higher survival. Our observation agreed with that reported by Zeng et al. (46), suggesting that the OS of patients with low immune scores is better than that of patients with high immune scores. By contrast, low tumor purity was responsible for glioma's aggressive phenotype and poor prognosis (47). KIRC is considered an immunogenic tumor; however, to a large extent, it mediates immune dysfunction by inducing immunosuppressive cells to infiltrate the tumor microenvironment (48). Currently, the investigation of PRGs in the TME in KIRC is insufficient. In the present study, the model-based risk score was positively associated with the infiltration of six immune cell types. This finding is consistent with a previous study finding that high-risk glioma patients with higher immune cell infiltration levels show a poorer prognosis (49). These findings indicated that pyroptosis was, in part, involved in the regulation of the TME. Additionally, our research suggested that the CNAs of PRGs might affect the immune cell infiltration levels in KIRC, providing new insights for future TME studies. Taken together, the results show that the prognostic model may serve as an indicator for outcome and immune cell infiltration, holding promising prospects in modern clinical practice.

Presently, numerous clinical trials are underway that evaluate the effect of ICIs in KIRC patients. By exploring the correlation between the risk score and expression of critical ICIs, we further noticed that most ICIs (14/17) presented higher expression in the high-risk group. Based on these observations, we strongly suggest the critical role of the immunosuppressive microenvironment in these patients with a poor prognosis. Hence, patients with high risk scores might benefit most from ICIs compared with patients with low risk scores. We also found that these six model-related genes were associated with targeted therapies. NLRP6, IFI16, and GSDMB were associated with sensitivity to sunitinib. Moreover, some were associated with other targeted therapies, thereby determining a superior agent or treatment strategy for individual patients and expanding insights into future therapeutics for treating KIRC.

Our research had limitations. First, the prospective, larger multicenter trials are required to provide high-level evidence for clinical application. Moreover, the underlying mechanisms of the selected genes in our model should be explored to better study the molecular mechanisms involved in tumorigenesis and the development of KIRC.

In summary, we systematically analyzed the prognostic value, roles in the TME, response to ICIs, and drug sensitivity of PGRs in KIRC. Two KIRC subtypes (clusters 1/2) with diverse outcomes were identified by consensus clustering based on the expression profile of PRGs. The pyroptosis-related prognostic risk model developed from six PRGs can stratify KIRC patients into low- and high-risk subgroups with diverse prognoses and immune cell infiltration. The signature also suggests that the patients with high-risk scores might benefit most from ICIs. Pyroptosis may be involved in targeted therapies for patients with KIRC. Our findings may provide new insight into the role of pyroptosis in the TME in KIRC patients. In conclusion, our prognostic model showed potential clinical usefulness that may improve survival and even develop new therapeutic strategies for KIRC patients.

AUTHOR CONTRIBUTIONS

ZS designed the study and drafted the manuscript. CJ collected and analyzed the data. MZ and ZW prepared tables and figures. XG and FK revised the manuscript. SJ and HW supervised the study. All authors contributed to the article and approved the submitted version.

ACKNOWLEDGMENTS

The authors would like to thank the TCGA, ArrayExpress, TIMER, and GDSC databases for the availability of the data.

REFERENCES

1. Vuong L, Kotecha RR, Voss MH, Hakimi AA. Tumor Microenvironment Dynamics in Clear-Cell Renal Cell Carcinoma. *Cancer Discov* (2019) 9 (10):1349–57. doi: 10.1158/2159-8290.cd-19-0499

2. Choueiri TK, Motzer RJ. Systemic Therapy for Metastatic Renal-Cell Carcinoma. *N Engl J Med* (2017) 376(4):354–66. doi: 10.1056/NEJMra1601333

3. Leibovich BC, Lohse CM, Crispen PL, Boorjian SA, Thompson RH, Blute ML, et al. Histological Subtype Is an Independent Predictor of Outcome for Patients With Renal Cell Carcinoma. *J Urol* (2010) 183(4):1309–15. doi: 10.1016/j.juro.2009.12.035

4. Shuch B, Amin A, Armstrong AJ, Eble JN, Ficarra V, Lopez-Beltran A, et al. Understanding Pathologic Variants of Renal Cell Carcinoma: Distilling Therapeutic Opportunities From Biologic Complexity. *Eur Urol* (2015) 67 (1):85–97. doi: 10.1016/j.eururo.2014.04.029

5. Shao N, Tang H, Mi Y, Zhu Y, Wan F, Ye D. A Novel Gene Signature to Predict Immune Infiltration and Outcome in Patients With Prostate Cancer. *Oncoimmunology* (2020) 9(1):1762473. doi: 10.1080/2162402x.2020.1762473

6. Newman AM, Liu CL, Green MR, Gentles AJ, Feng W, Xu Y, et al. Robust Enumeration of Cell Subsets From Tissue Expression Profiles. *Nat Methods* (2015) 12(5):453–7. doi: 10.1038/nmeth.3337

7. Janiszewska J, Poletajew S, Wasiutyński A. Spontaneous Regression of Renal Cell Carcinoma. *Contemp Oncol (Poznan Poland)* (2013) 17(2):123–7. doi: 10.5114/wo.2013.34613

8. Inman BA, Harrison MR, George DJ. Novel Immunotherapeutic Strategies in Development for Renal Cell Carcinoma. *Eur Urol* (2013) 63(5):881–9. doi: 10.1016/j.eururo.2012.10.006

9. Desbois M, Udyavar AR, Ryner L, Kozlowski C, Guan Y, Dürrbaum M, et al. Integrated Digital Pathology and Transcriptome Analysis Identifies Molecular Mediators of T-Cell Exclusion in Ovarian Cancer. *Nat Commun* (2020) 11 (1):5583. doi: 10.1038/s41467-020-19408-2

10. Motzer RJ, Rini BI, McDermott DF, Redman BG, Kuzel TM, Harrison MR, et al. Nivolumab for Metastatic Renal Cell Carcinoma: Results of a Randomized Phase II Trial. *J Clin Oncol: Off J Am Soc Clin Oncol* (2015) 33 (13):1430–7. doi: 10.1200/jco.2014.59.0703

11. Zou W, Wolchok JD, Chen L. PD-L1 (B7-H1) and PD-1 Pathway Blockade for Cancer Therapy: Mechanisms, Response Biomarkers, and Combinations. *Sci Trans Med* (2016) 8(328):328rv4. doi: 10.1126/scitranslmed.aad7118

12. Binnewies M, Roberts EW, Kersten K, Chan V, Fearon DF, Merad M, et al. Understanding the Tumor Immune Microenvironment (TIME) for Effective Therapy. *Nat Med* (2018) 24(5):541–50. doi: 10.1038/s41591-018-0014-x

13. Zhang C, Duan Y, Xia M, Dong Y, Chen Y, Zheng L, et al. TFEB Mediates Immune Evasion and Resistance to mTOR Inhibition of Renal Cell Carcinoma *via* Induction of PD-L1. *Clin Cancer Res: An Off J Am Assoc Cancer Res* (2019) 25(22):6827–38. doi: 10.1158/1078-0432.ccr-19-0733

14. Rathinam VA, Fitzgerald KA. Inflammasome Complexes: Emerging Mechanisms and Effector Functions. *Cell* (2016) 165(4):792–800. doi: 10.1016/j.cell.2016.03.046

15. He WT, Wan H, Hu L, Chen P, Wang X, Huang Z, et al. Gasdermin D Is an Executor of Pyroptosis and Required for Interleukin-1β Secretion. *Cell Res* (2015) 25(12):1285–98. doi: 10.1038/cr.2015.139

16. Bergsbaken T, Fink SL, Cookson BT. Pyroptosis: Host Cell Death and Inflammation. *Nat Rev Microbiol* (2009) 7(2):99–109. doi: 10.1038/nrmicro2070

17. Xia X, Wang X, Cheng Z, Qin W, Lei L, Jiang J, et al. The Role of Pyroptosis in Cancer: Pro-Cancer or Pro-"Host"? *Cell Death Dis* (2019) 10(9):650. doi: 10.1038/s41419-019-1883-8

18. Awad F, Assrawi E, Louvrier C, Jumeau C, Giurgea I, Amselem S, et al.

19. Miguchi M, Hinoi T, Shimomura M, Adachi T, Saito Y, Niitsu H, et al. Gasdermin C Is Upregulated by Inactivation of Transforming Growth Factor β Receptor Type II in the Presence of Mutated Apc, Promoting Colorectal Cancer Proliferation. *PloS One* (2016) 11(11):e0166422. doi: 10.1371/journal.pone.0166422

20. Wang WJ, Chen D, Jiang MZ, Xu B, Li XW, Chu Y, et al. Downregulation of Gasdermin D Promotes Gastric Cancer Proliferation by Regulating Cell Cycle-Related Proteins. *J Dig Dig* (2018) 19(2):74–83. doi: 10.1111/1751-2980.12576

21. Erkes DA, Cai W, Sanchez IM, Purwin TJ, Rogers C, Field CO, et al. Mutant BRAF and MEK Inhibitors Regulate the Tumor Immune Microenvironment *via* Pyroptosis. *Cancer Discov* (2020) 10(2):254–69. doi: 10.1158/2159-8290.cd-19-0672

22. Wang Y, Gao W, Shi X, Ding J, Liu W, He H, et al. Chemotherapy Drugs Induce Pyroptosis Through Caspase-3 Cleavage of a Gasdermin. *Nature* (2017) 547(7661):99–103. doi: 10.1038/nature22393

23. Khanova E, Wu R, Wang W, Yan R, Chen Y, French SW, et al. Pyroptosis by Caspase11/4-Gasdermin-D Pathway in Alcoholic Hepatitis in Mice and Patients. *Hepatol (Baltimore Md)* (2018) 67(5):1737–53. doi: 10.1002/hep.29645

24. Kovacs SB, Miao EA. Gasdermins: Effectors of Pyroptosis. *Trends Cell Biol* (2017) 27(9):673–84. doi: 10.1016/j.tcb.2017.05.005

25. Estrella MA, Du J, Chen L, Rath S, Prangley E, Chitrakar A, et al. The Metabolites NADP(+) and NADPH Are the Targets of the Circadian Protein Nocturnin (Curled). *Nat Commun* (2019) 10(1):2367. doi: 10.1038/s41467-019-10125-z

26. Warde-Farley D, Donaldson SL, Comes O, Zuberi K, Badrawi R, Chao P, et al. The GeneMANIA Prediction Server: Biological Network Integration for Gene Prioritization and Predicting Gene Function. *Nucleic Acids Res* (2010) 38(Web Server issue):W214–20. doi: 10.1093/nar/gkq537

27. Yoshihara K, Shahmoradgoli M, Martínez E, Vegesna R, Kim H, Torres-Garcia W, et al. Inferring Tumour Purity and Stromal and Immune Cell Admixture From Expression Data. *Nat Commun* (2013) 4:2612. doi: 10.1038/ncomms3612

28. Liu J, Nie S, Wu Z, Jiang Y, Wan Y, Li S, et al. Exploration of a Novel Prognostic Risk Signatures and Immune Checkpoint Molecules in Endometrial Carcinoma Microenvironment. *Genomics* (2020) 112(5):3117–34. doi: 10.1016/j.ygeno.2020.05.022

29. Mayakonda A, Lin DC, Assenov Y, Plass C, Koeffler HP. Maftools: Efficient and Comprehensive Analysis of Somatic Variants in Cancer. *Genome Res* (2018) 28(11):1747–56. doi: 10.1101/gr.239244.118

30. Li T, Fan J, Wang B, Traugh N, Chen Q, Liu JS, et al. TIMER: A Web Server for Comprehensive Analysis of Tumor-Infiltrating Immune Cells. *Cancer Res* (2017) 77(21):e108–10. doi: 10.1158/0008-5472.can-17-0307

31. Yang W, Soares J, Greninger P, Edelman EJ, Lightfoot H, Forbes S, et al. Genomics of Drug Sensitivity in Cancer (GDSC): A Resource for Therapeutic Biomarker Discovery in Cancer Cells. *Nucleic Acids Res* (2013) 41(Database issue):D955–61. doi: 10.1093/nar/gks1111

32. Xiao J, Wang C, Yao JC, Alippe Y, Xu C, Kress D, et al. Gasdermin D Mediates the Pathogenesis of Neonatal-Onset Multisystem Inflammatory Disease in Mice. *PloS Biol* (2018) 16(11):e3000047. doi: 10.1371/journal.pbio.3000047

33. Mai W, Xu Y, Xu J, Zhao D, Ye L, Yu G, et al. Berberine Inhibits Nod-Like Receptor Family Pyrin Domain Containing 3 Inflammasome Activation and Pyroptosis in Nonalcoholic Steatohepatitis *via* the ROS/TXNIP Axis. *Front Pharmacol* (2020) 11:185. doi: 10.3389/fphar.2020.00185

Photoaging and Skin Cancer: Is the Inflammasome the Missing Link? *Mech Ageing Dev* (2018) 172:131–7. doi: 10.1016/j.mad.2018.03.003

34. Fang Y, Tian S, Pan Y, Li W, Wang Q, Tang Y, et al. Pyroptosis: A New Frontier in Cancer. *Biomed Pharmacother = Biomed Pharmacother* (2020) 121:109595. doi: 10.1016/j.biopha.2019.109595

35. Gao J, Qiu X, Xi G, Liu H, Zhang F, Lv T, et al. Downregulation of GSDMD Attenuates Tumor Proliferation *via* the Intrinsic Mitochondrial Apoptotic Pathway and Inhibition of EGFR/Akt Signaling and Predicts a Good Prognosis in Non–Small Cell Lung Cancer. *Oncol Rep* (2018) 40(4):1971–84. doi: 10.3892/or.2018.6634

36. Susek KH, Karvouni M, Alici E, Lundqvist A. The Role of CXC Chemokine Receptors 1-4 on Immune Cells in the Tumor Microenvironment. *Front Immunol* (2018) 9:2159. doi: 10.3389/fimmu.2018.02159

37. Li D, Yuan X, Liu J, Li C, Li W. Prognostic Value of Prognostic Nutritional Index in Lung Cancer: A Meta-Analysis. *J Thorac Dis* (2018) 10(9):5298–307. doi: 10.21037/jtd.2018.08.51

38. Chen J, Wang Z, Yu S. AIM2 Regulates Viability and Apoptosis in Human Colorectal Cancer Cells *via* the PI3K/Akt Pathway. *OncoTargets Ther* (2017) 10:811–7. doi: 10.2147/ott.s125039

39. Chen GY, Liu M, Wang F, Bertin J, Núñez G. A Functional Role for Nlrp6 in Intestinal Inflammation and Tumorigenesis. *J Immunol (Baltimore Md: 1950)* (2011) 186(12):7187–94. doi: 10.4049/jimmunol.1100412

40. Zhang M, Jin C, Yang Y, Wang K, Zhou Y, Zhou Y, et al. AIM2 Promotes Non-Small-Cell Lung Cancer Cell Growth Through Inflammasome-Dependent Pathway. *J Cell Physiol* (2019) 234(11):20161–73. doi: 10.1002/jcp.28617

41. Flood B, Oficjalska K, Laukens D, Fay J, O'Grady A, Caiazza F, et al. Altered Expression of Caspases-4 and -5 During Inflammatory Bowel Disease and Colorectal Cancer: Diagnostic and Therapeutic Potential. *Clin Exp Immunol* (2015) 181(1):39–50. doi: 10.1111/cei.12617

42. Cai H, Yan L, Liu N, Xu M, Cai H. IFI16 Promotes Cervical Cancer Progression by Upregulating PD-L1 in Immunomicroenvironment Through STING-TBK1-NF-kB Pathway. *Biomed Pharmacother = Biomed Pharmacother* (2020) 123:109790. doi: 10.1016/j.biopha.2019.109790

43. Deswaerte V, Nguyen P, West A, Browning AF, Yu L, Ruwanpura SM, et al. Inflammasome Adaptor ASC Suppresses Apoptosis of Gastric Cancer Cells by an IL18-Mediated Inflammation-Independent Mechanism. *Cancer Res* (2018) 78(5):1293–307. doi: 10.1158/0008-5472.can-17-1887

44. Li L, Li Y, Bai Y. Role of GSDMB in Pyroptosis and Cancer. *Cancer Manag Res* (2020) 12:3033–43. doi: 10.2147/cmar.s246948

45. Itoh H, Kadomatsu T, Tanoue H, Yugami M, Miyata K, Endo M, et al. TET2-Dependent IL-6 Induction Mediated by the Tumor Microenvironment Promotes Tumor Metastasis in Osteosarcoma. *Oncogene* (2018) 37 (22):2903–20. doi: 10.1038/s41388-018-0160-0

46. Zeng D, Zhou R, Yu Y, Luo Y, Zhang J, Sun H, et al. Gene Expression Profiles for a Prognostic Immunoscore in Gastric Cancer. *Br J Surg* (2018) 105 (10):1338–48. doi: 10.1002/bjs.10871

47. Zhang C, Cheng W, Ren X, Wang Z, Liu X, Li G, et al. Tumor Purity as an Underlying Key Factor in Glioma. *Clin Cancer Res: An Off J Am Assoc Cancer Res* (2017) 23(20):6279–91. doi: 10.1158/1078-0432.ccr-16-2598

48. Díaz-Montero CM, Rini BI, Finke JH. The Immunology of Renal Cell Carcinoma. *Nat Rev Nephrol* (2020) 16(12):721–35. doi: 10.1038/s41581-020-0316-3

49. Yin W, Jiang X, Tan J, Xin Z, Zhou Q, Zhan C, et al. Development and Validation of a Tumor Mutation Burden-Related Immune Prognostic Model for Lower-Grade Glioma. *Front Oncol* (2020) 10:1409. doi: 10.3389/fonc.2020.01409

21

Urinary Exosomes Diagnosis of Urological Tumors

Yipeng Xu[1†], Jianmin Lou[2†], Mingke Yu[2], Yingjun Jiang[3], Han Xu[4], Yueyu Huang[2], Yun Gao[5,6], Hua Wang[1], Guorong Li[7,8], Zongping Wang[1*] and An Zhao[5,6*]

[1] Department of Urology, Cancer Hospital of University of Chinese Academy of Sciences, Zhejiang Cancer Hospital, Hangzhou, China, [2] Zhejiang Chinese Medical University, Hangzhou, China, [3] Hangzhou Traditional Chinese Medicine Hospital, Zhejiang Chinese Medical University, Hangzhou, China, [4] Central Research Laboratory, Children's Hospital of Nanchang University, Nanchang, China, [5] Experimental Research Center, Cancer Hospital of University of Chinese Academy of Sciences, Zhejiang Cancer Hospital, Hangzhou, China, [6] Institute of Cancer and Basic Medicine (ICBM), Chinese Academy of Sciences, Hangzhou, China, [7] Department of Urology, North Hospital, CHU of Saint-Etienne, University of Jean-Monnet, Saint-Etienne, France, [8] Inserm U1059, Faculty of Medicine, University of Jean-Monnet, Saint-Etienne, France

*Correspondence:
An Zhao
zhaoan@zjcc.org.cn
Zongping Wang
wangzp@zjcc.org.cn

[†]These authors have contributed equally to this work and share first authorship

Purpose: Exosomes could be released directly into the urine by the urological tumoral cells, so testing urinary exosomes has great potential for non-invasive diagnosis and monitor of urological tumors. The objective of this study is to systematically review and meta-analysis of urinary exosome for urological tumors diagnosis.

Materials and Methods: A systematic review of the recent English-language literature was conducted according to the PRISMA statement recommendations (CRD42021250613) using PubMed, Embase, Cochrane Library, Web of Science, and Scopus databases up to April 30, 2021. Risk-of-bias assessment was performed according to the QUADAS 2 tool. The true diagnostic value of urinary exosomes by calculating the number of true positive, false positive, true negative, and false negative, diagnoses by extracting specificity and sensitivity data from the selected literature.

Results: Sixteen eligible studies enrolling 3224 patients were identified. The pooled sensitivity and specificity of urinary exosomes as a diagnostic tool in urological tumors were 83% and 88%, respectively. The area under the summary receiver operating characteristic curve was 0.92 (95% CI: 0.89–0.94). Further subgroup analyses showed that our results were stable irrespective of the urinary exosome content type and tumor type.

Conclusion: Urinary exosomes may serve as novel non-invasive biomarkers for urological cancer detection. Future clinical trial designs must validate and explore their utility in treatment decision-making.

Systematic Review Registration: [https://www.crd.york.ac.uk/prospero/], identifier [CRD42021250613].

Keywords: urological tumor, exosomes, urine, diagnosis, liquid biopsy

INTRODUCTION

Tissue biopsy is the current standard method for pathological diagnosis of urological cancer. However, based on one single needle biopsy is limited in reflecting the complete genomic landscape of cancer accurately and is inappropriate for early tumor screening (1). To detect cell-free biomarkers (such as circulating nucleic acids, circulating tumor cells and circulating exosomes) in the body fluid, also called "Liquid biopsy", has recently show its value in clinical application (2). Collecting the circulating tumor related gene has the potential to provide molecular characterization of primary or metastatic tumor, and these cell-free biomarkers may be used to manage the post-treatment process of tumor (3).

One of the main types of liquid biopsies, circulating exosome, is extracellular vesicles enclosed by a lipid bilayer membrane range from 40 to 150 nm. Exosomes contain a complex cargo of contents derived from the original cell, including nucleic acids, lipids, and proteins (4). The exosome released by tumor cells has been shown to play an important role in microenvironment, immune regulation, and other malignant processes (5). Compared with other tumors, urological tumors can direct release exosomes into the urine, so urinary exosomes may be more sensitive and specific to reflect the status of urological tumors (6). Since then, several studies assessing the diagnostic value of urinary exosome in urological tumor have been published (5, 7). But the diagnostic performance of this novel biomarker has not been evaluated systematically. Therefore, the purpose of this study was to assess the diagnostic performance of urinary exosome for the detection of urological cancer including renal cancer (RCa), bladder cancer (BCa), and prostate cancer (PCa).

MATERIALS AND METHODS

The protocol has been registered in the International Prospective Register of Systematic Reviews database (registration number: CRD42021250613).

Search Strategy

This systematic review and meta-analysis were performed according to the Preferred Reporting Items for Systematic Reviews and Meta-analyses (PRISMA) statement (8). A comprehensive literature search was followed the PRISMA 2009 checklist, and the PubMed, Embase, Cochrane Library, Web of Science, and Scopus databases were searched systematically in April 30, 2021.

The search strategy included the following terms: ("exosomes" or "extracellular vesicle") AND "urine" AND ("diagnosis" OR "biomarker") AND ("urological cancer" OR "urologic neoplasms" OR "urogenital neoplasms") AND ("kidney neoplasms" OR "kidney cancer" OR "renal cancer") AND ("prostate neoplasms" OR "prostate cancer") AND ("bladder cancer" OR "bladder neoplasms"). Two researchers (Yipeng Xu and Jianmin Lou) independently assessed the eligibility of each potentially relevant study by screening the titles and abstracts. Disagreements between the two researchers were resolved by discussion with two additional researchers (An Zhao and Zongping Wang). Other publications were identified by searching the list of references of the selected papers.

Inclusion and Exclusion Criteria

Inclusion criteria for primary studies were as follows: (1) The research article was a diagnostic study using urinary exosomes; (2) Subjects included cancer patients and healthy controls; (3) The data was sufficient to generate a two-by-two table consisting of true negative (TN), and false negative (FN), true positive (TP), and false positive (FP).

The exclusion criteria were as follows: (1) repeated or overlapped publications which included the same study population and genes; (2) experiments based exclusively on cell lines or tumor tissue rather than clinical samples; and (3) studies with a poor sample size (≤10).

Data Extraction and Quality Assessment

We extracted the following data from the selected studies: the first author's last name, year of publication, country of study, cancer type, sample sizes, exosome extraction method, type of exosome content/detection method, target molecular detection, diagnostic results (numbers of FP, FN, TP, and TN), and diagnostic performance (sensitivity and specificity).

Deek's funnel plot and Quality Assessment of Diagnostic Accuracy Studies (QUADAS) 2 tool were adopted to analyze qualitative publication bias, and a P-value of <0.05 was considered statistically significant. Risk-of-bias assessment was performed independently by two authors (YJ, YX) according to the QUADAS 2 tool. Disagreement was solved by a third party (AZ). This tool provides a measure of the risk of bias and applicability over four domains (index test, reference standard, flow, and timing) of interest (9).

Data Synthesis and Analysis

All statistical analyses were performed using STATA software (version 12.0, STATA Corp, MIDAS module). Quality assessment was managed with Review Manager 5.3 (Cochrane Collaboration, Copenhagen, Denmark). The number of diagnoses (TP, TN, FP, and FN) from each study was extracted to calculate diagnostic sensitivity, specificity, positive likelihood ratio (PLR), negative likelihood ratio (NLR), and diagnostic odds ratio (DOR) with 95% confidence interval (CIs). PLR is calculated as sensitivity/(1-specifcity), and NLR is calculated as (1-sensitivity)/specificity. The DOR value is used as a measure of the effectiveness of a diagnostic test and is calculated as PLR/NLR. Summary ROC curves (SROC) and AUCs of the SROC were measured. All P values were two sided, and a P value < 0.05 was considered as statistically significant.

RESULTS

Literature Search

Four hundred and thirty studies were confirmed through systematic search and manual review for initial screening, and 354 studies were remained after duplicates removed. After titles and abstracts were checked, 104 articles of the non-duplicate records were subjected to further full-text review, of which 88 were excluded according to the exclusion criteria. Finally, 22 studies from 16 articles were included in the present meta-analysis (10–25). No additional studies were identified *via* screening the bibliographies of these 16 articles. The process of literature inclusion and selection is presented in **Figure 1**.

Characteristics of Included Studies

Among them, 5 eligible studies featured a total of 408 patients with bladder cancer, 9 eligible studies featured a total of 1277 patients with prostate cancer, and 2 eligible studies featured a total of 179 patients with renal cell carcinoma. The main extraction methods of urinary exosome are ultracentrifugation or commercial exosome extraction kit. The technique for molecular examination depends on the type of exosome contents, nucleic acid exosome cargo was detected using methods such as qRT-PCR or sequencing, and non-nucleic acid exosomal cargo (proteins or lipids) was detected using methods such as enzyme-linked immunosorbent assay (ELISA) or mass spectrometry (MS). In total, all main characteristics of the eligible studies were summarized (**Table 1**).

Risk of Bias Within Studies

The quality of the selected studies was evaluated in accordance with the QUADAS-2 criteria; the results of these evaluations are shown in **Figure 2**. Five studies were considered to be low-risk with regards to bias and applicability, and the other 11 studies were estimated as suboptimal for unclear risk in several areas, including patient selection, reference standards, and index testing. Deek's funnel plot was also used to evaluate the publication bias of included studied, and no publication bias was found (P = 0.81) (**Supplementary Figure 1**).

In addition, meta-regression analyses were performed to analyze the heterogeneity with the potential variables, and the type of exosome content (nucleic acid/non-nucleic acid), the type of urological cancer (BCa/PCa/RCa), and proportion of patients with urological cancer (>50%/≤50%) were not significant factors affecting the heterogeneity (P > 0.05, **Supplementary Table 1**).

Meta Analysis of Diagnostic Value

All 22 eligible studies were used to evaluate the diagnostic accuracy between urinary exosome expression and urological tumors. As shown in **Figure 3**, the overall diagnostic sensitivity and specificity were 0.83 (95% CI, 0.78–0.88) and 0.88 (95% CI, 0.81–0.92), respectively. Urinary exosome was significantly correlated with sensitivity (P < 0.01, $I^2 = 87.89\%$) and specificity (P < 0.01, $I^2 = 92.10\%$) (**Figure 3**). The area under the SROC curve was 0.92 (95% CI: 0.89–0.94) (**Figure 4**). The pooled PLR was 6.94 (95% CI: 4.29–11.22), and the pooled NLR was 0.19 (95% CI: 0.14–0.26) through random effect model (**Supplementary Figure 2**).

Subgroup Analysis

When the studies were separately assessed according to the type of exosome content, nucleic acid analysis group of 12 studies yielded pooled sensitivity of 0.84 (95% CI 0.78–0.89) with specificity of 0.89 (95% CI 0.82–0.93), whereas non-nucleic acid analysis group of four studies yielded pooled sensitivity of 0.83 (95% CI 0.71–0.91) with specificity of 0.85 (95% CI 0.63–0.95) (**Figure 5A**).

Regarding the type of urological tumor, the pooled sensitivity of 0.82 (95% CI 0.71–0.90) with specificity of 0.86 (95% CI 0.80–0.90) in five studies of BCa, the pooled sensitivity of 0.86 (95% CI 0.79–0.91) with specificity of 0.88 (95% CI 0.78–0.94) in nine studies of PCa yielded (**Figure 5B**). The pooled

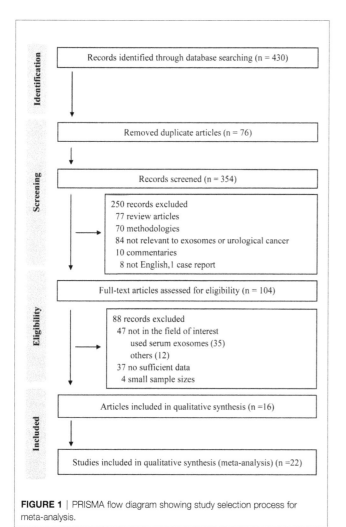

FIGURE 1 | PRISMA flow diagram showing study selection process for meta-analysis.

TABLE 1 | Characteristics of studies evaluating the urinary exosomes of patients with urological tumor.

Study ID (Ref/Region)	Sample size (case/control)	Exosome extraction method	Type of exosome content/detection method	Target molecular detection	TP	FP	TN	FN	Sensitivity	Specificity
Bladder cancer										
10/China	104/104 (Training set)	Urine Exosome RNA Isolation Kit (Norgen Biotek, Thorold, Canada)	Nucleic acid/ qRT-PCR	Panel of lncRNAs (MALAT1+PCAT-1+SPRY4-IT1)	75	19	89	29	72.1%	85.6%
	80/80 (Validation set)				50	12	68	30	62.5%	85.0%
11/Iran	59/24	Urine Exosome RNA Isolation Kit (Norgen Biotek, Thorold, Canada)	Nucleic acid/ qRT-PCR	Panel of lncRNAs (UCA1-201+UCA1-203+ MALAT1+LINC00355)	54	2	22	5	91.5%	91.7%
12/Turkey	59/34	Urine Exosome RNA Isolation Kit (Norgen Biotek, Thorold, Canada)	Nucleic acid/ qRT-PCR	Panel of miRNAs (miR-19b1-5p+miR-136-3p+ miR139-5p)	52	7	27	7	80.0%	88.1%
13/Egypt	70/12	Centrifugation, Filtration	Non-Nucleic acid/ Elisa	CD9 protein	65	2	10	5	92.6%	83.3%
14/Japan	36/24	Ultracentrifugation	Nucleic acid/ qRT-PCR/	miR-21-5p	27	1	23	9	75.0%	95.8%
Renal cell carcinoma										
15/China	70/30	Ultracentrifugation	Nucleic acid/ qRT-PCR	miR-30c-5p	48	0	30	22	68.6%	100.0%
16/Canada	28/18 (Discovery set)	Urine Exosome RNA Isolation Kit (Norgen Biotek, Thorold, Canada)	Nucleic acid/ qRT-PCR	Panel of miRNAs (miR-126-3p+miR-449a, the best combination)	23	5	13	5	82.8%	70.0%
	81/33 (Validation set)				68	12	21	13	83.8%	62.5%
Prostate cancer										
17/USA	568/268 (Training set)	Exosome RNA Isolation Kits (Norgen Biotek, Ontario, Canada)	Nucleic acid/ QuantStudio OpenArray	Panel of sncRNAs (Selected miRNAs+ selected snoRNAs)	533	11	257	35	93.8%	95.9%
	300/300 (Validation set)				281	25	275	19	93.7%	91.7%
18/Norway	20/9	Sequential centrifugation	Nucleic acid/ NGS	miR-196a	20	1	8	0	100.0%	88.9%
19/Russia	14/20 (TEV set)	Ultracentrifugation	Nucleic acid/ qRT-PCR	miR-19b	13	0	20	1	92.9%	100.0%
	14/20 (ERV set)				11	1	19	3	78.6%	95.0%
20/USA	89/106	Urine exosome clinical sample concentrator kit (Exosome Diagnostics, Cambridge, MA, USA)	Nucleic acid/ qRT-PCR	Panel of mRNAs (PCA3 and ERG)	67	49	57	22	75.3%	53.8%
21/Canada	28/28	Sucrose cushion ultracentrifugation	Nucleic acid/ qRT-PCR	Panel of mRNAs and miRNAs (ANXA3, CD24, TMPRSS2-ERG, SLC45A3, FOLH1, HPN, ITSN1, miR-375-3p, miR-574-3p)	22	3	25	6	78.6%	89.3%
22/	48/26	Ultracentrifugation	Nucleic acid/ qRT-PCR	Panel of miRNA isoforms (isomiRs of miR-21, miR-204 and miR-375)	35	3	23	13	72.9%	88.5%
Netherlands										
23/Belgium	85/122 (Overall population set)	N-butanol (Sigma-Aldrich, St. Louis, Missouri, USA), Ultracentrifugation	Non-Nucleic acid/ ECLIA	Urinary vesicle-associated PSA extraction ratio	60	55	67	25	70.6%	54.9%
	61/56 (sPSA between 4 ug/L and 10 ug/L set)				39	22	34	22	63.9%	60.7%

(Continued)

TABLE 1 | Continued

Study ID (Ref/Region)	Sample size (case/control)	Exosome extraction method	Type of exosome content/detection method	Target molecular detection	TP	FP	TN	FN	Sensitivity	Specificity
24/Norway	15/15	Sequential centrifugation	Non-Nucleic acid/MS	Panel of lipids (LacCer; d18:1/16:0, PS; 18:1/18:1 and 18:0/18:2)	14	0	15	1	93.3%	100%
25/Norway	16/16	Sequential centrifugation	Non-Nucleic acid/WB, ELISA	Flotillin 2 protein	14	1	15	2	87.5%	93.8%
	19/15			Panel of proteins (Flotillin 2 and PARK7)	13	1	14	6	68.4%	93.3%

TP, true positive; FP, false positive; TN, true negative; FN, false negative; qRT-PCR, quantitative real-time polymerase chain reaction; ELISA, enzyme-linked immunosorbent assay; NGS, next generation sequencing; MS, mass spectrometry; WB, Western blotting; ECLIA, electrochemiluminescence immunoassay.

sensitivity and specificity of RCa were unable to analyze with only two studies.

DISCUSSION

RCa, BCa, and PCa are the main types of urological tumors; their morbidity and mortality rates have continued to rise in recent years (26). Although prostate-specific antigen (PSA) testing has been used as biomarker in prostate cancer diagnosis, prostate biopsies are still essential to make a definite diagnosis since PSA level is low, and it also leads to overdiagnosis and overtreatment (27, 28). Most RCas are still found during other abdominal tests (29). Although the targeted therapy and immunotherapy have become the main treatment for advanced RCa, the complete responses is still low, and the biomarker-based strategies are still missing (30). Urological tumors still lack the key targeted markers such as epidermal growth factor receptor (EGFR) for lung cancer and human epidermal growth factor receptor 2 (HER2) for breast cancer.

Urinary cytology was one kind of the main non-invasive diagnostic methods for urothelial cancers (including bladder cancer, renal pelvis cancer, ureteral cancer, and urethral cancer), but its sensitivity was proved deficient (7–17%), and its diagnostic accuracy for low-grade urothelial cancer was relatively low (31). Compared to shedded tumor cells which are harder to capture in urine, exosomes are continually released into the urine from tumor cells. Exosomes can carry antigens from tumor-derived cells, so tumor-related exosomes can be purified by tumor antigen-bound magnetic beads to improve diagnostic specificity. Moreover, the nucleic acid cargo in exosomes may directly reflect the molecular characteristics of urological tumors. In addition, the concentration of exosome-related proteins in the first-morning urination and the second-morning urination were quite similar, and the exosomes remain intact during long-term storage or at -80°C (32), suggesting that urinary exosomes were stable enough to be examined their nucleic acid or non nucleic acid cargo.

Urine is easy to obtain and has the advantages of convenience, non-invasive, and repeatability. To systematically evaluate the potential of urinary exosomes as non-invasive markers for urological tumors, we established a meta-analysis including 22 studies from 16 articles with 3224 patients and 1360 healthy controls; the results showed an advanced diagnostic accuracy of urinary exosomes with an AUC of 0.92, a sensitivity of 83%, and a specificity of 88%. The overall PLR value of urological exosome was 6.94, suggesting that the probability of having tumor in a people with a positive test was approximately 7-fold higher than negative controls. Several laboratories including ours have reported some over-expressed proteins in tumor tissues, which are valuable in predicting the prognosis of the urological cancer (33–35). Whether these biomarkers can be detected in urinary exosomes and the use of urinary exosomes for monitoring tumor recurrence are worthy of further investigation.

This meta-analysis study suggests the urinary exosomes may serve as non-invasive biomarkers for urological cancer diagnosis. Several limitations of this study need to be discussed. We also reviewed the study of urinary exosomes in other urological tumors (such as ureteral cancer, renal pelvis cancer, epididymal tumor,

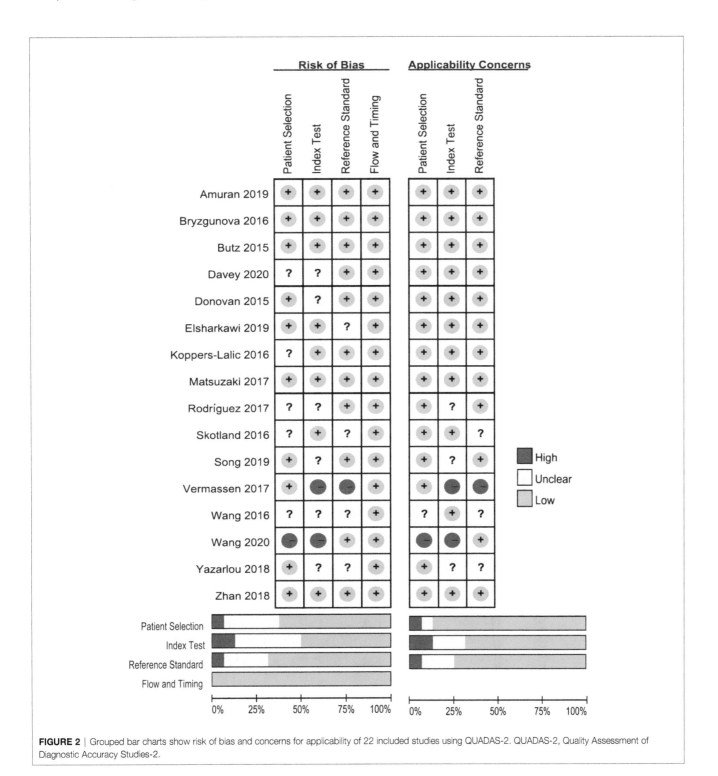

FIGURE 2 | Grouped bar charts show risk of bias and concerns for applicability of 22 included studies using QUADAS-2. QUADAS-2, Quality Assessment of Diagnostic Accuracy Studies-2.

and testis pellet cancer), but no relevant results were found. Thus, there is still a lack of relevant studies for some urological tumors with low incidences. Because of the large number of included studies reporting positive results, it is impossible to rule out the possibility of selection bias. The potential variables, including the type of exosome content, the type of urological cancer, and proportion of patients with urological cancer were not significant factors affecting the heterogeneity, but whether other

factors (such as primers, kits, and quantitative methods) can contribute to bias remains to be evaluated with the enough data.

CONCLUSION

Urinary exosomes has great application potential in the noninvasive diagnosis and monitoring of urological tumors.

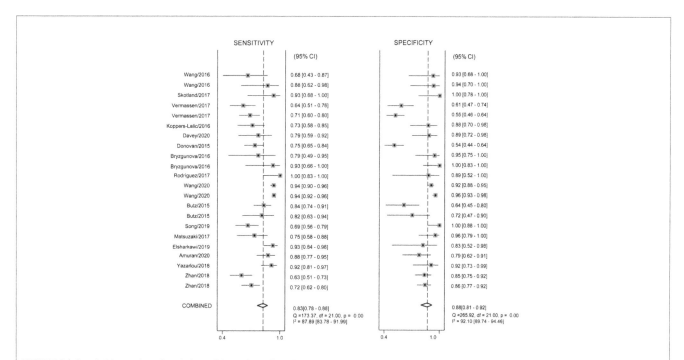

FIGURE 3 | Coupled forest plots of pooled sensitivity and specificity. Numbers are pooled estimates with 95% CI in parentheses. Corresponding heterogeneity statistics are provided at bottom right corners. Horizontal lines indicate 95% CIs. CI, confidence intervals.

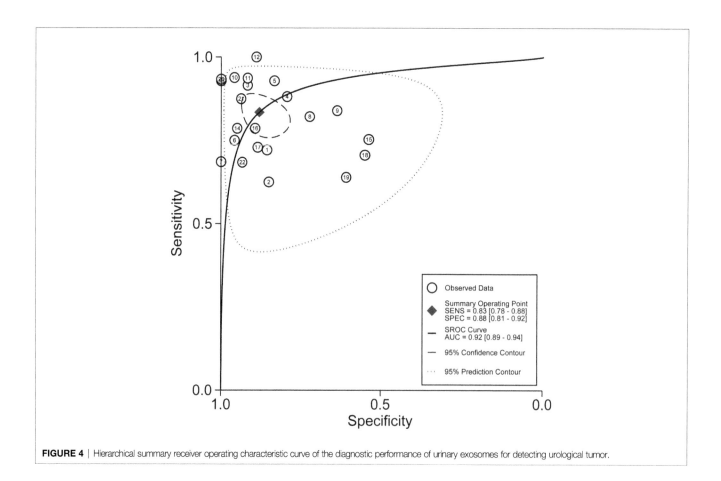

FIGURE 4 | Hierarchical summary receiver operating characteristic curve of the diagnostic performance of urinary exosomes for detecting urological tumor.

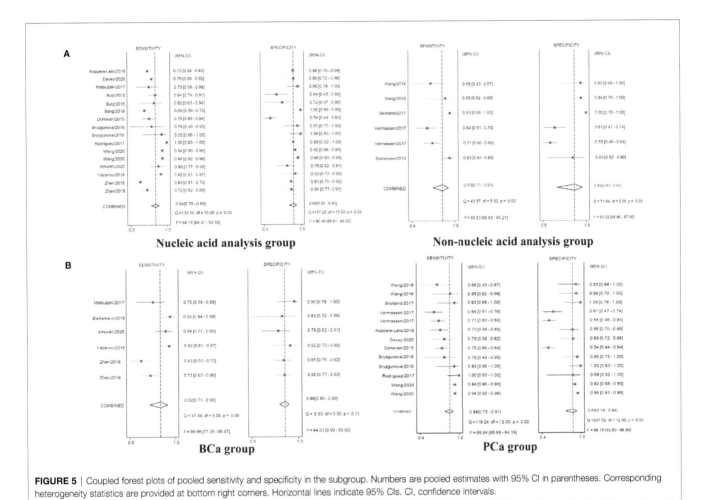

FIGURE 5 | Coupled forest plots of pooled sensitivity and specificity in the subgroup. Numbers are pooled estimates with 95% CI in parentheses. Corresponding heterogeneity statistics are provided at bottom right corners. Horizontal lines indicate 95% CIs. CI, confidence intervals.

Future evolutions will be necessary to validate whether urinary exosomes may serve as a potential non-invasive marker for early diagnosis and treatment response.

AUTHOR CONTRIBUTIONS

Two researchers YX and JL independently assessed the eligibility of each potential study by screening the titles and abstracts. Any disagreements between the two researchers were resolved by discussion with two additional researchers HW and ZW. The manuscript was written by YX, YJ, and HX, and AZ, YX, and GL revised. JL, MY, YG, and YH were responsible for the statistical analysis. All authors contributed to the article and approved the submitted version.

REFERENCES

1. Gerlinger M, Rowan AJ, Horswell S, Math M, Larkin J, Endesfelder D, et al. Intratumor Heterogeneity and Branched Evolution Revealed by Multiregion Sequencing. *N Engl J Med* (2012) 366:883. doi: 10.1056/NEJMoa1113205
2. Bardelli A, Pantel K. Liquid Biopsies, What We Do Not Know (Yet). *Cancer Cell* (2017) 31:172. doi: 10.1016/j.ccell.2017.01.002
3. Adalsteinsson VA, Ha G, Freeman SS, Choudhury AD, Stover DG, Parsons HA, et al. Scalable Whole-Exome Sequencing of Cell-Free DNA Reveals High Concordance With Metastatic Tumors. *Nat Commun* (2017) 8:1324. doi: 10.1038/s41467-017-00965-y
4. Franzen CA, Blackwell RH, Foreman KE, Kuo PC, Flanigan RC, Gupta GN. Urinary Exosomes: The Potential for Biomarker Utility, Intercellular Signaling and Therapeutics in Urological Malignancy. *J Urol* (2016) 195:1331. doi: 10.1016/j.juro.2015.08.115
5. Wortzel I, Dror S, Kenific CM, Lyden D. Exosome-Mediated Metastasis: Communication From a Distance. *Dev Cell* (2019) 49:347. doi: 10.1016/j.devcel.2019.04.011
6. Merchant ML, Rood IM, Deegens JKJ, Klein JB. Isolation and Characterization of Urinary Extracellular Vesicles: Implications for Biomarker Discovery. *Nat Rev Nephrol* (2017) 13:731. doi: 10.1038/nrneph.2017.148
7. Dhondt B, Van Deun J, Vermaerke S, de Marco A, Lumen N, De Wever O, et al. Urinary Extracellular Vesicle Biomarkers in Urological Cancers: From Discovery Towards Clinical Implementation. *Int J Biochem Cell Biol* (2018) 99:236. doi: 10.1016/j.biocel.2018.04.009

8. Liberati A, Altman DG, Tetzlaff J, Mulrow C, Gotzsche PC, Ioannidis JP, et al. The PRISMA Statement for Reporting Systematic Reviews and Meta-Analyses of Studies That Evaluate Healthcare Interventions: Explanation and Elaboration. *BMJ* (2009) 339:b2700. doi: 10.1136/bmj.b2700

9. Whiting PF, Rutjes AW, Westwood ME, Mallett S, Deeks JJ, Reitsma JB, et al. QUADAS-2: A Revised Tool for the Quality Assessment of Diagnostic Accuracy Studies. *Ann Intern Med* (2011) 155:529. doi: 10.7326/0003-4819-155-8-201110180-00009

10. Zhan Y, Du L, Wang L, Jiang X, Zhang S, Li J, et al. Expression Signatures of Exosomal Long Non-Coding RNAs in Urine Serve as Novel Non-Invasive Biomarkers for Diagnosis and Recurrence Prediction of Bladder Cancer. *Mol Cancer* (2018) 17:142. doi: 10.1186/s12943-018-0893-y

11. Yazarlou F, Modarressi MH, Mowla SJ, Oskooei VK, Motevaseli E, Tooli LF, et al. Urinary Exosomal Expression of Long non-Coding RNAs as Diagnostic Marker in Bladder Cancer. *Cancer Manag Res* (2018) 10:6357. doi: 10.2147/CMAR.S186108

12. Gullu Amuran G, Tinay I, Filinte D, Ilgin C, Peker Eyuboglu I, Akkiprik M. Urinary Micro-RNA Expressions and Protein Concentrations May Differentiate Bladder Cancer Patients From Healthy Controls. *Int Urol Nephrol* (2020) 52:461. doi: 10.1007/s11255-019-02328-6

13. Elsharkawi F, Elsabah M, Shabayek M, Khaled H. Urine and Serum Exosomes as Novel Biomarkers in Detection of Bladder Cancer. *Asian Pac J Cancer Prev* (2019) 20:2219. doi: 10.31557/APJCP.2019.20.7.2219

14. Matsuzaki K, Fujita K, Jingushi K, Kawashima A, Ujike T, Nagahara A, et al. MiR-21-5p in Urinary Extracellular Vesicles Is a Novel Biomarker of Urothelial Carcinoma. *Oncotarget* (2017) 8:24668. doi: 10.18632/oncotarget.14969

15. Song S, Long M, Yu G, Cheng Y, Yang Q, Liu J, et al. Urinary Exosome miR-30c-5p as a Biomarker of Clear Cell Renal Cell Carcinoma That Inhibits Progression by Targeting HSPA5. *J Cell Mol Med* (2019) 23:6755. doi: 10.1111/jcmm.14553

16. Butz H, Nofech-Mozes R, Ding Q, Khella HWZ, Szabo PM, Jewett M, et al. Exosomal MicroRNAs Are Diagnostic Biomarkers and Can Mediate Cell-Cell Communication in Renal Cell Carcinoma. *Eur Urol Focus* (2016) 2:210. doi: 10.1016/j.euf.2015.11.006

17. Wang WW, Sorokin I, Aleksic I, Fisher H, Kaufman RPJr, Winer A, et al. Expression of Small Noncoding RNAs in Urinary Exosomes Classifies Prostate Cancer Into Indolent and Aggressive Disease. *J Urol* (2020) 204:466. doi: 10.1097/JU.0000000000001020

18. Rodriguez M, Bajo-Santos C, Hessvik NP, Lorenz S, Fromm B, Berge V, et al. Identification of Non-Invasive miRNAs Biomarkers for Prostate Cancer by Deep Sequencing Analysis of Urinary Exosomes. *Mol Cancer* (2017) 16:156. doi: 10.1186/s12943-017-0726-4

19. Bryzgunova OE, Zaripov MM, Skvortsova TE, Lekchnov EA, Grigor'eva AE, Zaporozhchenko IA, et al. Comparative Study of Extracellular Vesicles From the Urine of Healthy Individuals and Prostate Cancer Patients. *PloS One* (2016) 11:e0157566. doi: 10.1371/journal.pone.0157566

20. Donovan MJ, Noerholm M, Bentink S, Belzer S, Skog J, O'Neill V, et al. A Molecular Signature of PCA3 and ERG Exosomal RNA From Non-DRE Urine Is Predictive of Initial Prostate Biopsy Result. *Prostate Cancer Prostatic Dis* (2015) 18:370. doi: 10.1038/pcan.2015.40

21. Davey M, Benzina S, Savoie M, Breault G, Ghosh A, Ouellette RJ. Affinity Captured Urinary Extracellular Vesicles Provide mRNA and miRNA Biomarkers for Improved Accuracy of Prostate Cancer Detection: A Pilot Study. *Int J Mol Sci* (2020) 21. doi: 10.3390/ijms21218330

22. Koppers-Lalic D, Hackenberg M, de Menezes R, Misovic B, Wachalska M, Geldof A, et al. Noninvasive Prostate Cancer Detection by Measuring miRNA Variants (isomiRs) in Urine Extracellular Vesicles. *Oncotarget* (2016) 7:22566. doi: 10.18632/oncotarget.8124

23. Vermassen T, D'Herde K, Jacobus D, Van Praet C, Poelaert F, Lumen N, et al. Release of Urinary Extracellular Vesicles in Prostate Cancer Is Associated With Altered Urinary N-Glycosylation Profile. *J Clin Pathol* (2017) 70:838. doi: 10.1136/jclinpath-2016-204312

24. Skotland T, Ekroos K, Kauhanen D, Simolin H, Seierstad T, Berge V, et al. Molecular Lipid Species in Urinary Exosomes as Potential Prostate Cancer Biomarkers. *Eur J Cancer* (2017) 70:122. doi: 10.1016/j.ejca.2016.10.011

25. Wang L, Skotland T, Berge V, Sandvig K, Llorente A. Exosomal Proteins as Prostate Cancer Biomarkers in Urine: From Mass Spectrometry Discovery to Immunoassay-Based Validation. *Eur J Pharm Sci* (2017) 98:80. doi: 10.1016/j.ejps.2016.09.023

26. Siegel RL, Miller KD, Jemal A. Cancer Statistics 2020. *CA Cancer J Clin* (2020) 70:7. doi: 10.3322/caac.21590

27. Vickers AJ, Cronin AM, Aus G, Pihl CG, Becker C, Pettersson K, et al. A Panel of Kallikrein Markers Can Reduce Unnecessary Biopsy for Prostate Cancer: Data From the European Randomized Study of Prostate Cancer Screening in Goteborg, Sweden. *BMC Med* (2008) 6:19. doi: 10.1186/1741-7015-6-19

28. Ferro M, Buonerba C, Terracciano D, Lucarelli G, Cosimato V, Bottero D, et al. Biomarkers in Localized Prostate Cancer. *Future Oncol* (2016) 12:399. doi: 10.2217/fon.15.318

29. Vasudev NS, Selby PJ, Banks RE. Renal Cancer Biomarkers: The Promise of Personalized Care. *BMC Med* (2012) 10:112. doi: 10.1186/1741-7015-10-112

30. Larroquette M, Peyraud F, Domblides C, Lefort F, Bernhard JC, Ravaud A, et al. Adjuvant Therapy in Renal Cell Carcinoma: Current Knowledges and Future Perspectives. *Cancer Treat Rev* (2021) 97:102207. doi: 10.1016/j.ctrv.2021.102207

31. Lokeshwar VB, Soloway MS. Current Bladder Tumor Tests: Does Their Projected Utility Fulfill Clinical Necessity? *J Urol* (2001) 165:1067. doi: 10.1016/S0022-5347(05)66428-2

32. Zhou H, Yuen PS, Pisitkun T, Gonzales PA, Yasuda H, Dear JW, et al. Collection, Storage, Preservation, and Normalization of Human Urinary Exosomes for Biomarker Discovery. *Kidney Int* (2006) 69:1471. doi: 10.1038/sj.ki.5000273

33. Sanguedolce F, Russo D, Mancini V, Selvaggio O, Calo B, Carrieri G, et al. Prognostic and Therapeutic Role of HER2 Expression in Micropapillary Carcinoma of the Bladder. *Mol Clin Oncol* (2019) 10:205. doi: 10.3892/mco.2018.1786

34. Netti GS, Lucarelli G, Spadaccino F, Castellano G, Gigante M, Divella C, et al. PTX3 Modulates the Immunoflogosis in Tumor Microenvironment and Is a Prognostic Factor for Patients With Clear Cell Renal Cell Carcinoma. *Aging (Albany NY)* (2020) 12:7585. doi: 10.18632/aging.103169

35. Gigante M, Li G, Ferlay C, Perol D, Blanc E, Paul S, et al. Prognostic Value of Serum CA9 in Patients With Metastatic Clear Cell Renal Cell Carcinoma Under Targeted Therapy. *Anticancer Res* (2012) 32:5447–51.

22

Identification of a Novel UT-B Urea Transporter in Human Urothelial Cancer

Ruida Hou [1,2], Mehrdad Alemozaffar [3], Baoxue Yang [4], Jeff M. Sands [2,5], Xiangbo Kong [1]*
and Guangping Chen [2,5]*

[1] Department of Urology, China-Japan Union Hospital, Jilin University, Changchun, China, [2] Department of Physiology, Emory University School of Medicine, Atlanta, GA, USA, [3] Department of Urology, Emory University School of Medicine, Atlanta, GA, USA, [4] Department of Pharmacology, School of Basic Medical Sciences, Peking University, Beijing, China, [5] Renal Division Department of Medicine, Emory University School of Medicine, Atlanta, GA, USA

*Correspondence:
Xiangbo Kong
Kongxb@jlu.edu.cn
Guangping Chen
gchen3@emory.edu

The urea transporter UT-B is widely expressed and has been studied in erythrocyte, kidney, brain and intestines. Interestingly, UT-B gene has been found more abundant in bladder than any other tissue. Recently, gene analyses demonstrate that SLC14A1 (UT-B) gene mutations are associated with bladder cancer, suggesting that urea transporter UT-B may play an important role in bladder carcinogenesis. In this study, we examined UT-B expression in bladder cancer with human primary bladder cancer tissues and cancer derived cell lines. Human UT-B has two isoforms. We found that normal bladder expresses long form of UT-B2 but was lost in 8 of 24 (33%) or significantly downregulated in 16 of 24 (67%) of primary bladder cancer patients. In contrast, the short form of UT-B1 lacking exon 3 was detected in 20 bladder cancer samples. Surprisingly, a 24-nt in-frame deletion in exon 4 in UT-B1 (UT-B1Δ24) was identified in 11 of 20 (55%) bladder tumors. This deletion caused a functional defect of UT-B1. Immunohistochemistry revealed that UT-B protein levels were significantly decreased in bladder cancers. Western blot analysis showed a weak UT-B band of 40 kDa in some tumors, consistent with UT-B1 gene expression detected by RT-PCR. Interestingly, bladder cancer associate UT-B1Δ24 was barely sialylated, reflecting impaired glycosylation of UT-B1 in bladder tumors. In conclusion, SLC14A1 gene and UT-B protein expression are significantly changed in bladder cancers. The aberrant UT-B expression may promote bladder cancer development or facilitate carcinogenesis induced by other carcinogens.

Keywords: urothelium, tumor, urea transporter, gene expression, sialylation

INTRODUCTION

Urea is the major end product of nitrogen metabolism and is excreted by the kidney. Due to its small molecular size ($\sim$60 Da) and water solubility, urea has been considered to be freely permeable across the cell membrane for over 30 years (Sands, 2003a, 2007). In fact, as a highly polar molecule, urea permeability across lipid bilayers is very low. Urea transport across the cell membrane is mediated by a facilitated urea transporter (Klein et al., 2011; Li et al., 2012a). In mammals, there are two types of urea transporters, UT-A and UT-B, encoded by the solute carrier family SLC14A2 and SLC14A1 genes, respectively. These genes share a high degree of homology and are aligned in tandem at chromosome 18q12.3 in humans. UT-A urea transporters are mainly expressed in kidney epithelial cells while UT-B urea transporters demonstrate a broader tissue distribution including bladder (Timmer et al., 2001; Spector et al., 2004, 2007; Dong et al., 2013). UT-B also serves as a determinant antigen of the Kidd blood group on erythrocytes (Sands, 2003b; Shayakul et al., 2013).

Compared to the kidney UT-A urea transporter, UT-B is under-investigated. Two types of human UT-B are reported. UT-B1 (Genbank NM_001146036) was first cloned from human bone marrow (Olives et al., 1994) and expressed in multiple tissues including brain, heart, kidney, bladder, prostate, etc. (Timmer et al., 2001; Yang et al., 2002). UT-B2, however, was first identified from bovine rumen as bovine UT-B2 (bUT-B2), with an additional 56-amino acid spliced into the N-terminal of the original bovine UT-B1 sequence (Stewart et al., 2005). Both UT-B2 mRNA and protein have been detected in cow rumen (Stewart et al., 2005). The UT-B2 mRNA was initially reported in humans in the caudate nucleus (Genbank NM_001146037) (Stewart, 2011), and recently also in the bladder (Walpole et al., 2014).

In the kidney, urea is reabsorbed by UT-A to establish the medullary osmolarity gradient enabling the concentration of urine (Fenton et al., 2004; Sands, 2007). However, extra-renal urea accumulation in tissues is usually detrimental to cells. High urea exposure can affect cells in many ways, such as destroying protein hydrophobic bonds and causing protein carbamylation (Zou et al., 1998), inducing oxidative stress, DNA damage and apoptosis (Michea et al., 2000; Zhang et al., 2004; Dong et al., 2013). Therefore, urea transporters (mainly UT-B) in non-renal tissues function as scavengers that prevent intracellular urea aggregation and intoxication (Guo et al., 2007; Meng et al., 2009; Li et al., 2012b). Studies in UT-B knockout mice demonstrate that absence of UT-B results in notable urea accumulation, abnormal morphology in the hippocampus and depression-like behavior (Li et al., 2012b). Deletion of the SLC14A1 gene causes urea accumulation in the testis, increases testicular weight and results in early maturation of the male reproductive system (Guo et al., 2007). Dong et al. reported that the urothelium urea concentration is 9 times higher in UT-B knockout mice. This is accompanied by increased cell DNA damage, apoptosis and malfunction of arginine metabolism (Dong et al., 2013). In addition, UT-B suppresses tumor growth; overexpression of UT-B inhibits colony formation of lung cancer cell lines transfected with the SLC14A1 genes (Frullanti et al., 2012).

Bladder urothelium expresses UT-B but not UT-A (Yang et al., 2002; Dong et al., 2013; Walpole et al., 2014). This was confirmed recently by an RNA-sequencing analysis showing high expression of SLC14A1 and the absence of SLC14A2 in bladder tissue (Koutros et al., 2013). Using multiple mouse tissues, Yang et al. reported in 2002 that the bladder expresses the most UT-B mRNA *in vivo* (Yang et al., 2002). However, the physiological significance of bladder UT-B is unknown. Recently, two large-scale genome wide association studies (GWAS) of urothelial bladder cancer by two separate groups discovered that mutations of the SLC14A1 gene are linked to bladder carcinogenesis in humans (Garcia-Closas et al., 2011; Rafnar et al., 2011). This suggests that loss of UT-B function may play an important role in suppressing bladder cancer. Considering that the bladder is a reservoir of urine and

the urothelial cells are constantly in contact with a high urea concentration, it is not very surprising that the bladder needs more urea transporter UT-B than any other organ (Yang et al., 2002).

In this study, we examined UT-B gene and protein expression in human bladder cancer samples. We found that normal bladder expresses UT-B2. However in bladder cancer, UT-B2 gene expression was suppressed. Instead, bladder cancer expresses the short form of the UT-B1 gene: 11 of 20 (55%) of UT-B1 transcripts are tumor specific UT-B1 with a 24-nt in-frame deletion. We also examined UT-B protein expression and found decreased UT-B expression associated with tumor malignancy.

METHODS

Cell Lines and Culture
Normal human urothelial cells (NHU) were kindly provided by Dr. Jennifer Southgate (University of York, UK) and cultured as previously described (Wezel et al., 2013). Primary bladder cancer-derived cell lines including T24 cells (human muscle invasive bladder cancer cell line HTB-4) and 5637 cells (human non-muscle invasive bladder cancer cell line HTB-9) were purchased from the American Type Culture Collection (ATCC, Manassas, VA) and cultured in DMEM (GIBCO, Waltham, MA) supplied with 10% FBS.

Bladder Tumor Specimen Collection
Fresh bladder cancer samples were taken immediately after surgery by the Emory University Hospital Department of Urology and stored at −80°C for further use. All tissue samples were obtained from patients who consented through an IRB approved protocol (IRB: 00055316) at Emory University to have excess pathological specimens for research purposes.

RNA Extraction, cDNA Synthesis, and PCR Amplification
Total RNA was extracted from tissues using TRIzol reagents (Invitrogen, Carlsbad, CA). The RNA integrity was evaluated by RNA electrophoresis and an Agilent Bioanalyzer 2100. Three microgram of total RNA was used for cDNA synthesis. Reverse transcription (RT) was carried out in a 20 µl reaction using SuperScript First-Strand Synthesis System for RT-PCR (Invitrogen 11904-018). One microliter of cDNA was used for PCR using Advantage 2 Polymerase Mix (Clontech 639201100, Mountain View, CA). Two pairs of UT-B primers were designed according to the human UT-B gene (NM_001128588) sequence and used for amplification of UT-B2 or UT-B1 (**Figure 1A**). All amplified products were ligated to TOPO TA vector (Invitrogen K4500-01) and submitted for DNA sequencing.

Quantitative Real-Time PCR Assays
Quantitative real-time PCR (qPCR) was performed as described before (Chen et al., 2010; Qian et al., 2015). Gene specific primers for UT-B1, UT-B2, and GAPDH were designed to generate amplicons of length 100–200 nucleotides by using the Invitrogen Primer program. The sequences of PCR

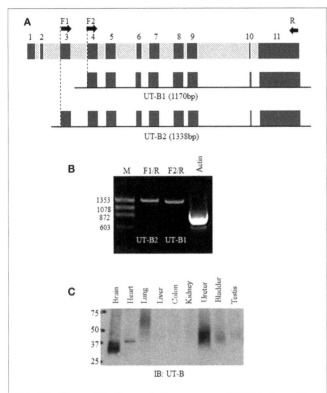

FIGURE 1 | Normal bladder urothelium expresses UT-B2 isoform. (A)
Schematic diagram of human SLC14A1 gene and two pairs of primers for
RT-PCR. **(B)** RT-PCR. PCR amplification of UT-B2 and UT-B1 from normal
bladder tissue cDNA. GAPDH was used as an internal control. **(C)** Western
blot analysis of UT-B protein expression in human tissues. The pre-made
human tissue blot was purchased from Protein Biotechnologies and probed
with UT-B antibody.

primers for real-time PCR used were 5′-ccagtgggagttggtcagat-
3′ (sense) and 5′-gttgaaaccccagagtccaa-3′ for UT-B1, 5′-agga
ccctttggaactaaagc-3′ and 5′-gggctgtccactctaaccatag-3′ for UT-
B2, 5′-cgagatccctccaaaatcaa-3′ and 5′-ttcacacccatgacgaacat-3′ for
GAPDH. Prior to quantitative PCR, a single amplified product
of the predicted size was verified by regular PCR and DNA
sequencing. Real-time PCR was carried out using the Bio-Rad
iCycler Real-Time Detection System with a two-step protocol (3
min at 95°C; followed by 40 cycles of 10 s at 95°C and 45 s at
61°C). Fluorescence of the amplificates was detected with the
Brilliant III Ultra-Fast SYBR Green QPCR Master Mix (Agilent).
The cycle threshold number (Ct) for each sample was determined
at a constant fluorescence threshold by iCycler software 3.0
(Bio-Rad). The experiments were repeated at least twice and all
reactions were performed in triplicate. The gene expression data
were analyzed using the $2^{\Delta Ct}$ formula, which $\Delta Ct = Ct_{UT\text{-}B}$ -
Ct_{GAPDH}. Significance was determined using a two-sample, two
tailed Student's t-test.

Plasmid Construction

The human UT-B2 and UT-B1 cDNAs were PCR amplified from
normal human bladder cDNA (BioChain, C1234010, Newark,
CA). UT-B1Δ24 cDNA was PCR amplified from human bladder
tumor cDNA (BioChain, C1235010). The UT-B cDNAs were

constructed into the mammalian expression vector pcDNA3 or
into an oocyte expression vector pGH19. All constructs were
verified by DNA Sequencing (Beckman Counter Genomics,
Beverly, MA).

Peptide-N-Glycosidase F (PNGase F) Treatment

Human UT-B2, UT-B1, and UT-B1Δ24 in pcDNA3 were
transfected into HEK293 (Stratagene, San Diego, CA) cells using
Lipofectamine2000 (Invitrogen) following the manufacturer's
instructions. After 48 h, cells were solubilized in RIPA buffer (150
mM NaCl, 10 mM Tris·HCl, pH 7.5, 1 mM EDTA, 1%, Triton X-
100, 1% sodium deoxycholate and 0.1% SDS). Lysates were first
denatured with glycoprotein denaturing buffer at 100°C for 10
min, then 10% NP-40 buffer and G7 reaction buffer were added,
and incubated with or without 1 μl PNGase F (500 units/μl, New
England Biolabs, Ipswich, MA) at 37°C for 2 h. UT-B proteins
were examined by western blot analysis.

Protein Extraction and Western Blot

Bladder cancer tissues were lysed in ice-cold RIPA buffer. After
centrifugation at 10,000 rpm at 4°C for 10 min, supernatants
were collected. The protein concentration was determined by
a Bradford method with the Protein Assay reagent (Bio-Rad
Laboratories, Hercules, CA). Proteins (20~50 μg/lane) were size
separated by SDS-PAGE and electroblotted to the nitrocellulose
membrane. The membranes were routinely processed by
blocking with 5% milk/PBS, incubation overnight with primary
rabbit polyclonal anti-UT-B antibody (Doran et al., 2006) and
incubation for 1 h with horseradish peroxidase-conjugated
secondary antibody. Immunoreacting proteins were detected
using an Enhanced Chemiluminescence (ECL) Kit (Amersham,
Pittsburgh, PA).

Immunohistochemistry

Bladder cancer tissue microarray T122, BL803, and BL244
were purchased from US Biomax Inc. (Rockville, MD). Bladder
cancer tissue array TMA-2205 was from Protein Biotechnologies
(Ramona, CA). Bladder cancer tissue array BLC241 was from
Pantomics Inc. (Richmond, CA). The tissue arrays were de-
paraffinized in xylene and rehydrated. For antigen retrieval,
the tissue array slides were immersed in 0.01 M citrate buffer
for 3 min in a microwave oven. Endogenous peroxidase was
blocked with 0.3% hydrogen peroxidase in methanol for 20
min. After blocking with 1% BSA at room temperature for 20
min, the tissues were incubated in a humidified chamber with
UT-B antibody (1:400) at 4°C overnight. After a PBS wash,
tissues were incubated with biotinylated anti-rabbit antibody,
followed by avidin-biotin peroxidase complex (ABC) (Vector
laboratories, Burlingame, CA) at room temperature for 1
h. Antibody localization was detected with diaminobenzidine
(DAB) as a chromogen substrate. Nuclei were counterstained
with hematoxylin. The UT-B protein expression was examined
under a microscope and semi-quantified as 0 ~ 4 scale: 0 = no
appreciable staining or faint staining intensity in <10% of tumor
cells, 1 = faint staining in >10% of tumor cells, 2 = readily

appreciable brown staining, 3 = dark brown staining, or 4 = very strong staining.

Lipid Raft Isolation and Lectin Pulldown Assay

Lipid raft isolation was performed as previously described (Chen et al., 2011). Briefly, fresh bladder cancer tissues or UT-B transfected HEK293 cells were homogenized in ice-cold 0.5% Brij96/TNEV buffer (10 mM Tris·HCl pH 7.5, 150 mM NaCl, 5 mM EDTA and 2 mM Na_3VO_4) on ice for 30 min. Supernatants were loaded in a 5–40% discontinuous sucrose gradient. After centrifugation at 34,000 rpm for 16 h, an equal amount of each fraction (approximately 400 μl) was collected from the top to the bottom. UT-B in the lipid rafts were examined by western blot.

For lectin pulldown assay, equal amounts of lipid raft membrane fractions were incubated with agarose-conjugated lectins at 4°C overnight. Lectin precipitated UT-B were detected by Western blot with anti-UT-B antibody. Agarose-bound concanavalin A (ConA), galanthus nivalis lectin (GNL), wheat germ agglutinin (WGA) and Sambucus nigra lectin (SNA) were purchased from Vector Laboratories (Burlingame, CA).

Water Permeability Experiments in Oocytes

Xenopus laevis oocytes were prepared and maintained in OR3 medium as previously described (Chen et al., 2011). Capped UT-B cRNAs were transcribed from linearized pGH19-UT-B using the mMESSAGE mMACHINE T7 Ultra Kit (Ambion). Two ng of UT-B cRNAs were microinjected into oocytes. Three days later, functional study of oocyte water permeability (Chen et al., 2015) was measured by placing oocytes in a low osmotic solution (one volume of ND96 mixed with one volume of water). The cell rupture time in the hypo-osmolarity solution was counted by visual inspection using a microscope.

Statistical Analysis

The gene expression data collected from qPCR were analyzed using the $2^{\Delta Ct}$ formula, which Δ Ct = Ct $_{UT-B}$ - C-t $_{GAPDH}$. Significance was determined using a two-sample, two tailed Student's t-test. Western blot densities were analyzed with ImageJ. Data collected from Western blot, immunohistochemistry and water permeability experiment in oocytes were performed by one-way analysis of variance (ANOVA) followed by Tukey HSD tests. And values were expressed as means ± SD.

RESULTS

Normal Human Bladder Urothelium Expresses UT-B2

Bladder urothelium expresses urea transporter UT-B (Li et al., 2014; Walpole et al., 2014). However, it remains unclear which forms of UT-B are expressed in human bladder. **Figure 1A** illustrates human SLC14A1 (UT-B) gene with 11 exons. UT-B2 is the large form of UT-B containing exon 3. We designed two pairs of UT-B primers to amplify UT-B2 and UT-B1 from normal human bladder tissue cDNAs purchased from BioChain. Primer location and sequences are shown in **Table 1**. Clearly, UT-B2 (1,338 bp) and UT-B1 (1,170 bp) were successfully amplified

TABLE 1 | Primers for amplification of human UT-B transcripts.

Name	Location and description	Sequence
F1	Exon 3, Forward primer for hUT-B2	5′-CGGGATCCGGATGAATGGACGGTCTTTGATTG-3′
F2	Exon 4, Forward primer for hUT-B1	5′-CGGGATCCATGGAGGACAGCCCCACTATGGTTAG-3′
R	Exon 11, Reverse primer	5′-GCTCTAGATTCTCACAAAGGGCTTTCCACCATTC-3′

from human bladder (**Figure 1B**). The amplified products were verified by DNA sequencing. We then examined UT-B protein expression using a pre-made human tissue blot (Protein biotechnologies). A band around 40–48 kDa was identified in bladder (**Figure 1C**), suggesting that under normal condition, bladder mainly expresses UT-B2. UT-B signals were also detected in human brain, lung, kidney, ureter and testis.

Bladder Cancer Switches to Express UT-B1 Gene

Next, we examined UT-B gene expression in bladder cancer tissues and bladder cancer cell lines. In total 24 fresh bladder cancer tissue samples were collected. The normal human bladder cDNA C1234 and bladder tumor cDNA C1235 from BioChain, normal bladder cell NHU and two bladder cancer derived cell lines (HTB-4 and HTB-9) were used as controls. Using the primers F1/R, UT-B2 (1,338 bp) was amplified in NHU cell and normal human bladder samples (**Figure 2A**). UT-B2 was dramatically suppressed in tumor and tumor cells (**Figure 2A** upper panel). We then investigated UT-B1 transcript expression by primers F2/R in bladder cancer and cancer cells. Interestingly, 16 out of 24 bladder cancer expressed UT-B1 (1,170 bp) which lacks exon 3 (**Figure 2A** middle panel). This indicates that bladder cancer cells somehow switch to express UT-B1 instead of UT-B2. GAPDH (**Figure 2A** lower panel) was used as an internal control. The changes of UT-B1 and UT-B2 mRNA were validated by real-time PCR in 16 bladder cancers and 5 normal human bladder tissues. GAPDH expression was used as reference gene for normalization. **Figure 2B** displays relative quantity of UT-B mRNA in tumor compared to normal bladder tissues. The mRNA levels of UT-B2 were significantly down-regulated in tumor compared to normal bladder ($p < 0.01$). The large SD reflected the heterogeneity of the patient samples individual gene expression levels.

Discovery of a 24-nt Deletion in UT-B1 Gene Only from Bladder Cancer Patients

All PCR products of UT-B1 from bladder cancer patients were purified and sent for DNA sequencing. Surprisingly, in 11 of 20 (55%) samples, gene sequencing showed a 24-nucleotide sequence missing in exon 4 that corresponded to a deletion of 8 amino acids. The 24-nt in-frame deletion was not found in normal bladder samples (commercially purchased) and normal bladder NHU cells. **Figure 2C** illustrates UT-B2, UT-B1, UT-B1Δ24, and the position of 24-nt deletion localized in UT-B1. The deletion starts at the 26th nucleotide downstream of the translation initiation site in UT-B1, and extends over 24

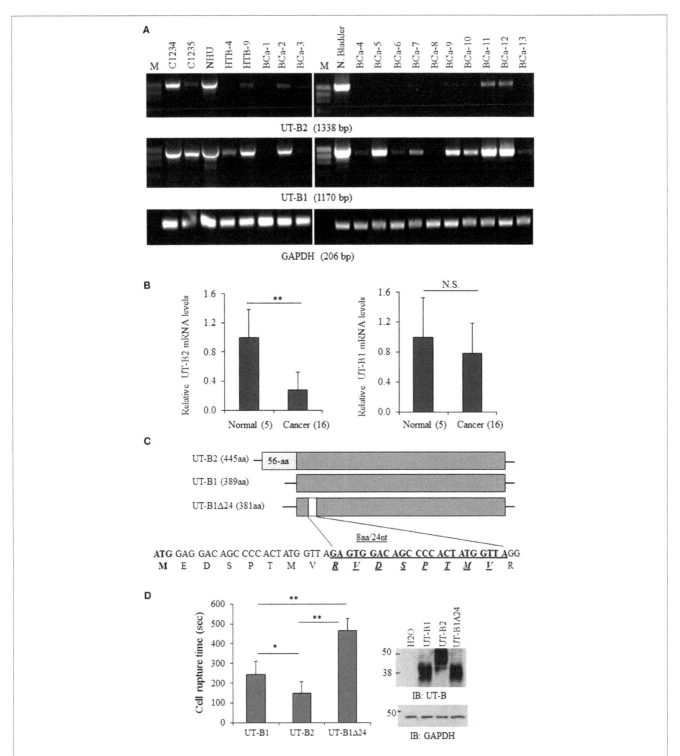

FIGURE 2 | Analysis of UT-B gene expression from bladder cancer patients. (A) Representative RT-PCR amplification of UT-B by two pairs of primers. BCa-1 to Bca-13 are fresh bladder cancer tissues (from total $n = 24$) collected from patients and used for RT-PCR (C1234: normal bladder cDNA, C1235: bladder cancer cDNA, NHU: normal human urothelial cell line, HTB-4 and HTB-9: bladder cancer derived cell lines). **(B)** Quantification of UT-B gene expression by real-time PCR. UT-B gene expression was assessed in normal and cancerous tissues by real-time PCR using gene-specific primers and SYBR Green detection. Gene expression was determined using the $2^{\Delta Ct}$ method with GAPDH as control gene. Relative mRNA levels of UT-B in cancer ($n = 16$) were compared to the normal bladder tissues ($n = 5$), where the expression was set to 1.0 (mean $\pm$ SD, compared to control $^{**}P < 0.01$; NS, no significance). **(C)** Schematic diagram of UT-B2, UT-B1 and UT-B1 $\Delta 24$ and the location of deletion in UT-B1. **(D)** Functional study of UT-B activity. UT-B cRNAs (2ng/cell) were injected into oocytes. Three days later, UT-B activity was assessed by water permeability assay by placing cells in hypo-osmolarity solution. The cell rupture time was counted ($n = 7$–10 cells/group) and the significance was determined by ANOVA ($^{*}p < 0.05$, $^{**}p < 0.01$). UT-B protein expression was examined by western blot with UT-B antibody ($n = 10$ cells/group).

nucleotides. Therefore, bladder cancer expresses tumor specific UT-B1 with a 24-nt deletion (UT-B1Δ24).

UT-B also transports water (Yang and Verkman, 1998). We then evaluated the functional difference of UT-B1, UT-B2, and UT-B1Δ24 by water permeability experiments in oocytes as described before (Chen et al., 2015). The cell rupture time of UT-B1Δ24 in hypo-osmolarity solution was significantly longer than that of UT-B1, reflecting decreased functional activity. The cell rupture time of UT-B2 was shorter than that of UT-B1 (**Figure 2D**). The average cell rupture time for the water-injected control oocytes is around 5,000 s (data not shown).

Decreased UT-B1 Protein Expression in Human Bladder Cancer

We cloned human UT-B2, UT-B1, and UT-B1Δ24 cDNA and transfected them into HEK293 cells. The recombinant protein sizes and glycosylation states were examined (**Figure 3A**). Western blot analysis showed ~40 and ~48 kDa for UT-B2. After de-glycosylation enzyme PNGase F treatment, the two bands were collapsed to ~38 kDa, which is consistent with the previous report (Walpole et al., 2014). UT-B1 showed two bands at ~35 and ~40 kDa, and the deglycosylated form was ~30 kDa. The size of the two glycosylated forms of UT-B1Δ24 was slightly lower than that of UT-B1. After PNGase F treatment, UT-B1Δ24 showed a single band at ~28 kDa.

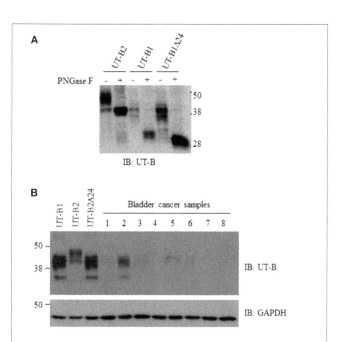

FIGURE 3 | Glycosylation analysis of UT-B2, UT-B1, and UT-B1Δ24 and western blot analysis of UT-B protein expression from bladder cancer patients. (A) PNGase F treatment. The cell lysates of HEK293 cell transfected with UT-B2, UT-B1, and UT-B1Δ24 were treated with or without PNGase F at 37°C for 2 h. **(B)** Fresh bladder cancer tissues were lysed in RIPA buffer. Supernatants were collected. UT-B protein expression was examined by western blot with UT-B antibody. Recombinant UT-B1, UT-B2, and UT-B1Δ24 expressed in HEK293 cells were used as controls. The same membrane was stripped and re-probed with GAPDH antibody.

We collected fresh tumor samples and examined UT-B protein expression in bladder cancer. Most bladder cancer did not express or expressed a low level of UT-B (**Figure 3B**). The size is close to UT-B1, indicating that bladder cancer expresses UT-B1 but not UT-B2 isoform. This is consistent with results of RT-PCR in **Figure 2A**.

Histological Analysis of UT-B Protein Expression in Human Bladder Cancer

To further confirm the finding by western blot showing a decreased level of UT-B in bladder cancer, immunohistochemistry was employed to evaluate UT-B protein expression in situ with human bladder cancer tissues. Six different tissue microarrays of human bladder tumors paired with normal tissues were examined. Excluding adenocarcinoma, 73 cases were patients with urothelial carcinoma. As shown in **Figure 4**, UT-B protein was detected throughout the urothelium in normal bladder tissues and was decreased in bladder cancer. UT-B protein staining was semi-quantified on a scale of 0~4. The average score of UT-B protein staining was 3.67 ± 0.41 (mean ± SD) in normal bladder urothelium, 1.61 ± 0.53 in low grade urothelial carcinoma, and 0.52 ± 0.43 in high grade urothelial carcinoma (**Table 2**), showing a strong association of UT-B protein expression with tumor malignancy.

Hypo-Sialylation Modification of UT-B1 from Bladder Cancer

Glycosylation is a key post-translational modification that can affect the structure and function of glycoproteins. As shown in **Figure 3A**, UT-B is a highly glycosylated protein. A single N-glycosylation site was identified at Asn 211 in the UT-B protein (Shayakul et al., 2013).We previously reported that cell membrane UT-A1 and UT-A3 are localized in lipid raft microdomains and glycosylation facilitates UT-A1 lipid raft distribution in lipid rafts (Chen et al., 2011; Su et al., 2012). We examined bladder cancer UT-B in cell membrane localization using fresh bladder cancer tissues from patients. UT-B2 expressed in HEK293 cells was used as a control. As shown in **Figure 5A**, UT-B1 from bladder cancer was expressed in lipid rafts in the cell membrane, although the total UT-B1 protein level was low.

We then collected lipid raft fractions and profiled the glycan structure of UT-B1 from bladder cancer patients by lectin pulldown. Lectin is a group of proteins specifically recognizing carbohydrates. As shown in **Figure 5B**, the 40–48 kDa UT-B2 band was mainly bound by WGA and SNA, which recognize N-acetylglucosamine and α-2,6 sialic acid, respectively (Chen et al., 2011; Su et al., 2012). The lower band of UT-B2 contained mannose, which was pulled down by GNL. Interestingly, the UT-B1 from bladder cancer contains N-acetylglucosamine pulled down by WGA. However, bladder cancer UT-B1 was not pulled down by SNA, indicating an impaired glycan sialylation of UT-B1 from bladder cancer.

DISCUSSION

Bladder cancer is one of the most common cancers in the United States with 74,000 estimated cases and 16,000 estimated

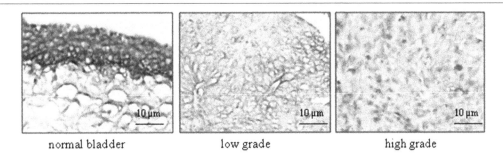

FIGURE 4 | Immunohistochemical analysis of UT-B expression with bladder cancer tissues. Human bladder cancer tissue arrays paired with normal tissues were processed for immunostaining with UT-B antibody (1:400), followed by biotinylated anti-rabbit antibody, and ABC (Vector laboratories). Color was developed by DAB. The nuclei were counterstained with hematoxylin. Representative pictures of UT-B staining in bladder cancer are shown from total 63 cases ($n = 73$) (magnification: x200).

TABLE 2 | Semi-quantification of UT-B expression in bladder cancer.

Grade	N	IHC score
Control	73	3.67 ± 0.41
Low grade	45	1.61 ± 0.53^a
High grade	28	$0.52 \pm 0.43^{a,b}$

[a]Compared to control $p < 0.01$; [b]Compared to low grade $p < 0.01$.

deaths in 2015 (Siegel et al., 2015). Despite significant progress in the cancer research field overall, little has been achieved in bladder cancer in the same time and the molecular mechanism of bladder tumorigenesis and cancer progression remains poorly understood. In this study, we found that the SLC14A1 gene, which encodes urea transporter UT-B and mediates urea transport across the cell membrane, was suppressed or aberrantly expressed in bladder cancer. We, for the first time, identified a tumor specific UT-B1Δ24 with a 24-nt in-frame deletion in exon 4 from bladder cancer patients. Consistently, UT-B protein was significantly decreased in bladder cancer in our study and others (Li et al., 2014). Thus, a significant alteration of the UT-B gene/protein in bladder tumors supports the potential tumor suppressive role of UT-B in bladder cancer carcinogenesis.

The bladder is a unique urine storage organ dealing with highly concentrated urea. The "urogenous contact hypothesis" proposed by Braver (Braver et al., 1987) in 1987 is still prevalent in the etiology of bladder cancer. Environmental exposures, particularly tobacco smoking, are important risk factors in bladder cancer. However, one important factor we may have ignored in bladder carcinogenesis is urea. High intracellular urea concentration damages cells in many ways. The urea concentration in urine is 20–100 times higher than in blood in humans (Yang and Bankir, 2005; Spector et al., 2007). Bladder urothelium is inevitably and constantly insulted by a higher concentration of urea than any other tissue/organ. This could be the reason why urothelium expresses the most abundant UT-B when compared to any other tissue (Yang et al., 2002). It is not very surprising that genomic analysis from two groups discovered UT-B gene mutations as bladder cancer

susceptibility genes (Garcia-Closas et al., 2011; Rafnar et al., 2011).

UT-B has two isoforms, UT-B1 with 389 aa and UT-B2 with 445 aa. UT-B2 is the longer form. UT-B1, which lacks exon 3, has been identified in multiple tissues. UT-B2 with an extra 56 aa in the N-terminus is only reported in the human caudate nucleus (Stewart, 2011), mouse thymus (Yang et al., 2002), and bovine rumen (Tickle et al., 2009). In this study, we found that normal bladder urothelium expresses UT-B2. We also found that, for an unknown reason, UT-B2 expression was suppressed in bladder tumors. Instead, tumor cells switched to expression of the short form of UT-B1.

Gene deletion and mutation are frequently involved in the development of human urothelial carcinoma, such as the deletion in chromosome 9 (Schulz, 2006; Knowles, 2008), point mutations of the fibroblast growth factor receptor-3 (FGFR3) (Iyer and Milowsky, 2013; Pandith et al., 2013), and alterations in tumor suppressor gene TP53 and RB1 (Mitra et al., 2006) and FHIT (Baffa et al., 2000). In this study, we found a 24-nt in-frame deletion in UT-B1 (UT-B1Δ24) in a high incidence (55%) from bladder cancer patients. This deletion has never been reported before. The cause of this deletion currently is unknown. Notably, the SLC14A1 (18q12.1-18q21.1) gene happens to be localized at one of the common fragile sites on chromosome 18(18q12.2, 18q21.3) (Durkin and Glover, 2007). Interestingly, the in-frame deletion starts from nt 26 and is not in a triple reading frame. However, this does not interrupt the blueprint of protein translation except for an 8-aa missing. The in-frame deletion has been reported in multi gene mutations. Chloride channel CFTR ΔF508 has a 3-bp in-frame deletion in exon 10 and causes a single amino acid deletion at F508. CFTR ΔF508 is the most common cystic fibrosis causing genetic mutation (Kalin et al., 1999; Lukacs and Verkman, 2012). Greater than 90% of EGFR tyrosine kinase domain mutations are short in-frame deletions in exon 19 with different deletion sizes (9, 12, 15, 18, and 24 bp; Bethune et al., 2010; Brevet et al., 2010). Evaluation of EGFR mutation has been employed to predict lung adenocarcinoma response to EGFR kinase inhibitors in clinic (Brevet et al., 2010). It is also interesting whether assessment of

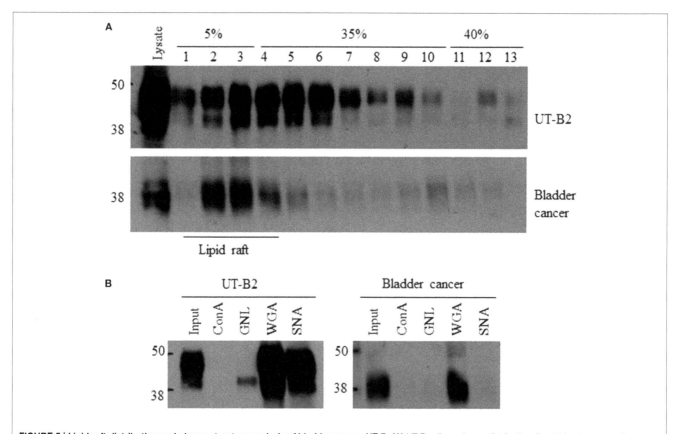

FIGURE 5 | Lipid raft distribution and glycan structure analysis of bladder cancer UT-B. (A) UT-B cell membrane distribution. Fresh bladder cancer tissues were lysed in 0.5% Brij96/TNEV. Supernatants were loaded in a 5–40% sucrose gradient for ultracentrifugation. Fractions were collected and UT-B was examined by western blot. UT-B2 expressed in HEK293 cells was used as a control. **(B)** Lectin pulldown assay. Lipid raft fractions 2–5 were collected from the samples above and incubated with different lectins. Lectin precipitated UT-B was examined by western blot. Representative figures are shown from 5 independent experiments. ConA, Concanavalin A; GNL, Galanthus nivalis lectin; WGA, Wheat germ agglutinin; SNA, Sambucus nigra lectin.

UT-BΔ24 could guide the selection of bladder cancer treatment in the future.

Sialylation modification of glycoproteins plays crucial roles in many biological processes of human health and disease (Park et al., 2012). The alteration of cell membrane protein sialylation is often involved in the development of cancer and tumor metastasis (Pinho and Reis, 2015; Vajaria et al., 2015). Using specific lectin SNA, we found that UT-B1 from bladder cancer has defective alpha-2,6-sialylation. This is consistent with a study by Antony et al. showing that tumor-specific DNA methylation of the ST6GAL1 promoter occurs in human bladder cancer (Antony et al., 2014).The ST6GAL1 gene encodes the alpha-2,6-sialyltransferase, which catalyzes glycan alpha-2,6 sialylation. Presumably, the impaired sialylation of UT-B might be due to inactivation of ST6GalI in bladder cancer. Therefore, in bladder cancer, not only is UT-B protein decreased, but UT-B sialylation is also affected.

Additionally, a unique feature of bladder cancer is that up to 70% of these patients will experience relapse within 5 years after the first standard transurethral resection of the bladder tumor (TURBT), the highest rate of recurrence of any cancer (Al-Sukhun and Hussain, 2003; Chamie et al., 2013). Considering

that the bladder urothelium is bathed in fluid with a high urea concentration, loss of UT-B protection exposes the urothelium to constant attack by urea. Therefore, dysfunction of UT-B may contribute to high rates of bladder cancer recurrence.

In summary, the significant amount of UT-B expressed in bladder (Yang et al., 2002) suggests that UT-B is important for the bladder cells to balance intracellular urea and protect them from damage caused by the high urine urea concentration. In this study, we found that the normal UT-B2 gene is suppressed in bladder cancer. Bladder cancer cells aberrantly express UT-B1 with a 24-nt deletion. Protein analysis confirmed a decrease of UT-B protein expression in bladder cancer and the level of UT-B protein is inversely associated with tumor malignancy. We also found abnormal sialylation of UT-B protein glycan in bladder cancer. Since the bladder is a unique organ holding high urea-containing urine, its urothelium is constantly in contact with a high concentration of urea. Aberrant (gene mutation) or absent expression of UT-B inevitably causes intracellular urea accumulation and subsequently may activate a carcinogenic pathway and/or enhance the bladder cell susceptibility to carcinogen exposure. The novel bladder cancer associated UT-B1Δ24 could be a new biomarker for bladder cancer diagnosis and prognosis. Future work is required to elucidate the mechanism about how UT-B gene expression switches from UT-B2 to UT-B1 and how the 24-nt deletion in UT-B1 occurs in bladder cancers.

Data Deposition

The sequence of the new UT-B1 gene has been deposited in Genbank with the accession number KY706499.

AUTHOR CONTRIBUTIONS

GC, RH, MA, BY, JS, and XK conception, design, data analysis, and interpretation; RH and MA – sample and data collection; RH, and GC –experimental execution; GC, RH, MA, and JS – manuscript writing; GC – final approval of manuscript. All authors have read and approved the manuscript.

ACKNOWLEDGMENTS

We thank Otor Al-Khalili and Dr. Douglas Eaton for help with real-time PCR.

REFERENCES

1. Al-Sukhun, S., and Hussain, M. (2003). Current understanding of the biology of advanced bladder cancer. *Cancer* 97, 2064–2075. doi: 10.1002/cncr.11289

2. Antony, P., Rose, M., Heidenreich, A., Knuchel, R., Gaisa, N. T., and Dahl, E. (2014). Epigenetic inactivation of ST6GAL1 in human bladder cancer. *BMC Cancer* 14:901. doi: 10.1186/1471-2407-14-901

3. Baffa, R., Gomella, L. G., Vecchione, A., Bassi, P., Mimori, K., Sedor, J., et al. (2000). Loss of FHIT expression in transitional cell carcinoma of the urinary bladder. *Am. J. Pathol.* 156, 419–424. doi: 10.1016/S0002-9440(10)64745-1

4. Bethune, G., Bethune, D., Ridgway, N., and Xu, Z. (2010). Epidermal growth factor receptor (EGFR) in lung cancer: an overview and update. *J. Thorac. Dis.* 2, 48–51.

5. Braver, D. J., Modan, M., Chetrit, A., Lusky, A., and Braf, Z. (1987). Drinking, micturition habits, and urine concentration as potential risk factors in urinary bladder cancer. *J. Natl. Cancer Inst.* 78, 437–440.

6. Brevet, M., Arcila, M., and Ladanyi, M. (2010). Assessment of EGFR mutation status in lung adenocarcinoma by immunohistochemistry using antibodies specific to the two major forms of mutant EGFR. *J. Mol. Diagn.* 12, 169–176. doi: 10.2353/jmoldx.2010.090140

7. Chamie, K., Litwin, M. S., Bassett, J. C., Daskivich, T. J., Lai, J., Hanley, J. M., et al. (2013). Recurrence of high-risk bladder cancer: a population-based analysis. *Cancer* 119, 3219–3227. doi: 10.1002/cncr.28147

8. Chen, G., Howe, A. G., Xu, G., Frohlich, O., Klein, J. D., and Sands, J. M. (2011). Mature N-linked glycans facilitate UT-A1 urea transporter lipid raft compartmentalization. *FASEB J.* 25, 4531–4539. doi: 10.1096/fj.11-185991

9. Chen, G., Yang, Y., Frohlich, O., Klein, J. D., and Sands, J. M. (2010). Suppression subtractive hybridization analysis of low-protein diet- and vitamin D-induced gene expression from rat kidney inner medullary base. *Physiol. Geomics* 41, 203–211. doi: 10.1152/physiolgenomics.00129.2009

10. Chen, M., Cai, H., Klein, J. D., Laur, O., and Chen, G. (2015). Dexamethasone increases aquaporin-2 protein expression in *ex vivo* inner medullary collecting duct suspensions. *Front. Physiol.* 6:310. doi: 10.3389/fphys.2015.00310

11. Dong, Z., Ran, J., Zhou, H., Chen, J., Lei, T., Wang, W., et al. (2013). Urea transporter UT-B deletion induces DNA damage and apoptosis in mouse bladder urothelium. *PLoS ONE* 8:e76952. doi: 10.1371/journal.pone.0076952

12. Doran, J. J., Klein, J. D., Kim, Y. H., Smith, T. D., Kozlowski, S. D., Gunn, R. B., et al. (2006). Tissue distribution of UT-A and UT-B mRNA and protein in rat. *Am. J. Physiol. Regul. Integr. Comp. Physiol.* 290, R1446–R1459. doi: 10.1152/ajpregu.00352.2004

13. Durkin, S. G., and Glover, T. W. (2007). Chromosome fragile sites. *Annu. Rev. Genet.* 41, 169–192. doi: 10.1146/annurev.genet.41.042007.165900

14. Fenton, R. A., Chou, C. L., Stewart, G. S., Smith, C. P., and Knepper, M. A. (2004). Urinary concentrating defect in mice with selective deletion of phloretin- sensitive urea transporters in the renal collecting duct. *Proc. Natl. Acad. Sci. U.S.A.* 101, 7469–7474. doi: 10.1073/pnas.0401704101

15. Frullanti, E., Colombo, F., Falvella, F. S., Galvan, A., Noci, S., De Cecco, L., et al. (2012). Association of lung adenocarcinoma clinical stage with gene expression pattern in noninvolved lung tissue. *Int. J. Cancer* 131, E643–E648. doi: 10.1002/ijc.27426

16. Garcia-Closas, M., Ye, Y., Rothman, N., Figueroa, J. D., Malats, N., Dinney, C. P., et al. (2011). A genome-wide association study of bladder cancer identifies a new susceptibility locus within SLC14A1, a urea transporter gene on chromosome 18q12.3. *Hum. Mol. Genet.* 20, 4282–4289. doi: 10.1093/hmg/ddr342

17. Guo, L., Zhao, D., Song, Y., Meng, Y., Zhao, H., Zhao, X., et al. (2007). Reduced urea flux across the blood-testis barrier and early maturation in the male reproductive system in UT-B-null mice. *Am. J. Physiol. Cell Physiol.* 293, C305–C312. doi: 10.1152/ajpcell.00608.2006

18. Iyer, G., and Milowsky, M. I. (2013). Fibroblast growth factor receptor-3 in urothelial tumorigenesis. *Urol. Oncol.* 31, 303–311. doi: 10.1016/j.urolonc.2011.12.001

19. Kalin, N., Claass, A., Sommer, M., Puchelle, E., and Tummler, B. (1999). DeltaF508 CFTR protein expression in tissues from patients with cystic fibrosis. *J. Clin. Invest.* 103, 1379–1389. doi: 10.1172/JCI5731

20. Klein, J. D., Blount, M. A., and Sands, J. M. (2011). Urea transport in the kidney. *Compr. Physiol.* 1, 699–729. doi: 10.1002/cphy.c100030

21. Knowles, M. A. (2008). Molecular pathogenesis of bladder cancer. *Int. J. Clin. Oncol.* 13, 287–297. doi: 10.1007/s10147-008-0812-0

22. Koutros, S., Baris, D., Fischer, A., Tang, W., Garcia-Closas, M., Karagas, M. R., et al. (2013). Differential urinary specific gravity as a molecular phenotype of the bladder cancer genetic association in the urea transporter gene, SLC14A1. *Int. J. Cancer* 133, 3008–3013. doi: 10.1002/ijc.28325

23. Li, C., Xue, H., Lei, Y., Zhu, J., Yang, B., and Gai, X. (2014). Clinical significance of the reduction of UT-B expression in urothelial carcinoma of the bladder. *Pathol. Res. Pract.* 210, 799–803. doi: 10.1016/j.prp.2014.09.012

24. Li, X., Chen, G., and Yang, B. (2012a). Urea transporter physiology studied in knockout mice. *Front. Physiol.* 3:217. doi: 10.3389/fphys.2012.00217

25. Li, X., Ran, J., Zhou, H., Lei, T., Zhou, L., Han, J., et al. (2012b). Mice lacking urea transporter UT-B display depression-like behavior. *J. Mol. Neurosci.* 46, 362–372. doi: 10.1007/s12031-011-9594-3

26. Lukacs, G. L., and Verkman, A. S. (2012). CFTR: folding, misfolding and correcting the DeltaF508 conformational defect. *Trends Mol. Med.* 18, 81–91. doi: 10.1016/j.molmed.2011.10.003

27. Meng, Y., Zhao, C., Zhang, X., Zhao, H., Guo, L., Lu, B., et al. (2009). Surface electrocardiogram and action potential in mice lacking urea transporter UT-B. *Sci. China C. Life Sci.* 52, 474–478. doi: 10.1007/s11427-009-0047-y

28. Michea, L., Ferguson, D. R., Peters, E. M., Andrews, P. M., Kirby, M. R., and Burg, M. B. (2000). Cell cycle delay and apoptosis are induced by high salt and urea in renal medullary cells. *Am. J. Physiol. Renal Physiol.* 278, F209–F218.

29. Mitra. A. P., Datar, R. H., and Cote, R. J. (2006). Molecular pathways in invasive bladder cancer, new insights into mechanisms, progression, and target identification. *J. Clin. Oncol.* 24, 5552–5564. doi: 10.1200/JCO.2006.08.2073

30. Olives, B., Neau, P., Bailly, P., Hediger, M. A., Rousselet, G., Cartron, J. P., et al. (1994). Cloning and functional expression of a urea transporter from human bone marrow cells. *J. Biol. Chem.* 269, 31649–31652.

31. Pandith, A. A., Shah, Z. A., and Siddiqi, M. A. (2013). Oncogenic role of fibroblast growth factor receptor 3 in tumorigenesis of urinary bladder cancer. *Urol. Oncol.* 31, 398–406. doi: 10.1016/j.urolonc.2010.07.014

32. Park, J. J., Yi, J. Y., Jin, Y. B., Lee, Y. J., Lee, J. S., Lee, Y. S., et al. (2012). Sialylation of epidermal growth factor receptor regulates receptor activity and chemosensitivity to gefitinib in colon cancer cells. *Biochem. Pharmacol.* 83, 849–857. doi: 10.1016/j.bcp.2012.01.007

33. Pinho, S. S., and Reis, C. A. (2015). Glycosylation in cancer: mechanisms and clinical implications. *Nat. Rev. Cancer* 15, 540–555. doi: 10.1038/nrc3982

34. Qian, X., Li, X., Ilori, T. O., Klein, J. D., Hughey, R. P., Li, C. J., et al. (2015). RNA-seq analysis of glycosylation related gene expression in STZ-induced diabetic rat kidney inner medulla. *Front. Physiol.* 6:274. doi: 10.3389/fphys.2015.00274

35. Rafnar, T., Vermeulen, S. H., Sulem, P., Thorleifsson, G., Aben, K. K., Witjes, J. A., et al. (2011). European genome-wide association study identifies SLC14A1 as a new urinary bladder cancer susceptibility gene. *Hum. Mol. Genet.* 20, 4268–4281. doi: 10.1093/hmg/ddr303

36. Sands, J. M. (2003a). Mammalian urea transporters. *Annu. Rev. Physiol.* 65, 543–66. doi: 10.1146/annurev.physiol.65.092101.142638

37. Sands, J. M. (2003b). Molecular mechanisms of urea transport. *J. Membr. Biol.* 191, 149–163. doi: 10.1146/annurev.physiol.65.092101.142638

38. Sands, J. M. (2007). Critical role of urea in the urine-concentrating mechanism. *J. Am. Soc. Nephrol.* 18, 670–671. doi: 10.1681/ASN.2006121314

39. Schulz, W. A. (2006). Understanding urothelial carcinoma through cancer pathways. *Int. J. Cancer* 119, 1513–1518. doi: 10.1002/ijc.21852

40. Shayakul, C., Clemencon, B., and Hediger, M. A. (2013). The urea transporter family (SLC14), physiological, pathological and structural aspects. *Mol. Aspects Med.* 34, 313–322. doi: 10.1016/j.mam.2012.12.003

41. Siegel, R. L., Miller, K. D., and Jemal, A. (2015). Cancer statistics CA. *Cancer J. Clin.* 65, 5–29. doi: 10.3322/caac.21254

42. Spector, D. A., Yang, Q., Liu, J., and Wade, J. B. (2004). Expression, localization, and regulation of urea transporter B in rat urothelia. *Am. J. Physiol. Ren. Physiol.* 287, F102–F108. doi: 10.1152/ajprenal.00442.2003

43. Spector, D. A., Yang, Q., and Wade, J. B. (2007). High urea and creatinine concentrations and urea transporter B in mammalian urinary tract tissues. *Am. J. Physiol. Ren. Physiol.* 292, F467–F474. doi: 10.1152/ajprenal.001 81.2006

44. Stewart, G. (2011). The emerging physiological roles of the SLC14A family of urea transporters. *Br. J. Pharmacol.* 164, 1780–1792. doi: 10.1111/j.1476-5381.2011. 01377.x

45. Stewart, G. S., Graham, C., Cattell, S., Smith, T. P., Simmons, N. L., and Smith, C. P. (2005). UT-B is expressed in bovine rumen: potential role in ruminal urea transport. *Am. J. Physiol. Regul. Integr. Comp. Physiol.* 289, R605–R12. doi: 10.1152/ajpregu.00127.2005

46. Su, H., Carter, C. B., Frohlich, O., Cummings, R. D., and Chen, G. (2012). Glycoforms of UT-A3 urea transporter with poly-N-acetyllactosamine glycosylation have enhanced transport activity. *Am. J. Physiol. Ren. Physiol.* 303, F201–F208. doi: 10.1152/ajprenal.00140.2012

47. Tickle, P., Thistlethwaite, A., Smith, C. P., and Stewart, G. S. (2009). Novel bUT-B2 urea transporter isoform is constitutively activated. *Am. J. Physiol. Regul. Integr. Comp. Physiol.* 297, R323–R329. doi: 10.1152/ajpregu.00199.2009

48. Timmer, R. T., Klein, J. D., Bagnasco, S. M., Doran, J. J., Verlander, J. W., Gunn, R. B., et al. (2001). Localization of the urea transporter UT-B protein in human and rat erythrocytes and tissues. *Am. J. Physiol. Cell Physiol.* 281, C1318–C1325.

49. Vajaria, B. N., Patel, K. R., Begum, R., and Patel, P. S. (2015). Sialylation: an avenue to target cancer cells. *Pathol. Oncol. Res.* 22, 443–7. doi: 10.1007/s12253-015-0033-6

50. Walpole, C., Farrell, A., McGrane, A., and Stewart, G. S. (2014). Expression and localization of a UT-B urea transporter in the human bladder. *Am. J. Physiol. Ren. Physiol.* 307, F1088–F1094. doi: 10.1152/ajprenal.00284.2014

51. Wezel, F., Pearson, J., Kirkwood, L. A., and Southgate, J. (2013). Differential expression of Oct4 variants and pseudogenes in normal urothelium and urothelial cancer. *Am. J. Pathol.* 183, 1128–1136. doi: 10.1016/j.ajpath.2013.06.025

52. Yang, B., and Bankir, L. (2005). Urea and urine concentrating ability: new insights from studies in mice. *Am. J. Physiol. Ren. Physiol.* 288, F881–F896. doi: 10.1152/ajprenal.00367.2004

53. Yang, B., Bankir, L., Gillespie, A., Epstein, C. J., and Verkman, A. S. (2002). Urea-selective concentrating defect in transgenic mice lacking urea transporter UT-B. *J. Biol. Chem.* 277, 10633–10637. doi: 10.1074/jbc.M200207200

54. Yang, B., and Verkman, A. S. (1998). Urea transporter UT3 functions as an efficient water channel. Direct evidence for a common water/urea pathway. *J. Biol. Chem.* 273, 9369–9372. doi: 10.1074/jbc.273.16.9369

56. Zhang, Z., Dmitrieva, N. I., Park, J. H., Levine, R. L., and Burg, M. B. (2004). High urea and NaCl carbonylate proteins in renal cells in culture and *in vivo*, and high urea causes 8-oxoguanine lesions in their DNA. *Proc. Natl. Acad. Sci. U.S.A.* 101, 9491–9496. doi: 10.1073/pnas.0402961101

57. Zou, Q., Habermann-Rottinghaus, S. M., and Murphy, K. P. (1998). Urea effects on protein stability, hydrogen bonding and the hydrophobic effect. *Proteins* 31, 107–115.

23

Quantitative Evaluation of Encrustations in Double-J Ureteral Stents with Micro-Computed Tomography and Semantic Segmentation

Shaokai Zheng[1]*, Pedro Amado[1], Bernhard Kiss[2], Fabian Stangl[2,3], Andreas Haeberlin[4], Daniel Sidler[5], Dominik Obrist[1], Fiona Burkhard[2] and Francesco Clavica[1]

[1] ARTORG Center for Biomedical Engineering Research, University of Bern, Bern, Switzerland, [2] Department of Urology, Inselspital, Bern University Hospital, University of Bern, Bern, Switzerland, [3] Department of Urology, Cantonal Hospital Olten, Olten, Switzerland, [4] Department of Cardiology, Inselspital, Bern University Hospital, University of Bern, Bern, Switzerland, [5] Department of Nephrology and Hypertension, Inselspital, Bern University Hospital, University of Bern, Bern, Switzerland

*Correspondence:
Shaokai Zheng
shaokai.zheng@outlook.com

Accurate evaluation of stent encrustation patterns, such as volume distribution, from different patient groups are valuable for clinical management and the development of better stents. This study quantitatively compares stent encrustation patterns from stone and kidney transplant patients. Twenty-seven double-J ureteral stents were collected from patients with stone disease or who underwent kidney transplantation. Encrustations on stent samples were quantified by means of micro–Computed Tomography and semantic segmentation using a Convolutional Neural Network model. Luminal encrustation volume per stent unit was derived to represent encrustation level, which did not differ between patient groups in the first six weeks. However, stone patients showed higher encrustation levels over prolonged indwelling times (p = 0.02). Along the stent shaft body, the stone group showed higher encrustation levels near the ureteropelvic junction compared to the ureterovesical junction (p = 0.013), whereas the transplant group showed no such difference. Possible explanations were discussed regarding vesicoureteral reflux. In both patient groups, stent pigtails were more susceptible to encrustations, and no difference between renal and bladder pigtail was identified. The segmentation method presented in this study is also applicable to other image analysis tasks in urology.

Keywords: Double J, ureteral stent, encrustation, stone, renal transplantation, micro CT, segmentation, deep learning

INTRODUCTION

Double-J ureteral stents are commonly used to bypass obstruction and alleviate pain in acute obstruction as well as in preparations prior to endoscopic stone treatment, or to stent the ureterovesical anastomosis after kidney transplantation to avoid obstruction due to edema in the early postoperative phase. In spite of various material upgrades and design modifications, encrustation remains a major problem causing stent associated complications with a significant impact on patients' quality of life (1, 2). Encrusted stents can become blocked and cause obstructive pyelonephritis. Foreign bodies in the urinary tract also tend to be colonized by bacteria that cause urinary tract infections. Severely encrusted stents can no longer be retrieved endoscopically and require more invasive approaches to be removed. As a result, indwelling stents have to be replaced in regular intervals. For stone patients, indwelling times longer than six weeks have been associated with significantly higher encrustation rates (2–4). For transplant patients, indwelling times from two to six weeks after transplantation have been recommended based on urinary tract infection (UTI) rates and stent-related complications such as pain, hematuria, encrustation and migration (5–8).

In this study, we are interested in clarifying the encrustation level over indwelling time in both stone and transplant patient groups, with a specific focus on the localization of the encrustations in each group. Therefore, evaluation of the encrustation volume is crucial. Earlier approaches were mainly qualitative, relying on visual examination of Scanning Electron Microscopy (9) or kidney-ureter-bladder (KUB) radiography images (10, 11). Extracting quantitative information from KUB images had been attempted by measuring the projected area of encrustations (12). Unfortunately, the inherent uncertainty is not negligible as encrustations are three-dimensional. Another established approach proposed to measure the level of encrustation by weighing the stent sample before and after oxidative acid treatment to dissolve the encrustations (13). The spatial distribution of encrustations, however, is destroyed during the process, and encrustations in the stent lumen (luminal encrustations) and on the external surfaces cannot be distinguished. In addition, encrustations on external stent surfaces can be affected during stent removal and consequently introduce significant uncertainties to quantitative results. It is therefore desirable to isolate the luminal encrustations, which are less affected by stent removal and critical to the drainage capacity of indwelling stents.

In a recent publication, micro-computed tomography (μ-CT) was applied to quantify stent encrustation volumes in order to assess the anti-encrustation efficacy of two commercially available stents (14). The authors performed morphological segmentation on the μ-CT images, and managed to distinguish between luminal and external encrustations. Based on their results, more than 90% of the stent had luminal encrustations, which appeared more in the shaft body (the straight part of the stent) than in the renal and bladder pigtails, respectively. Nonetheless, one limitation associated with the method was that the volume of the individual stent remained unknown, so the encrustation volume might be biased according to the actual stent material volumes. Moreover, treating the entire stent shaft body as a unified section inherently ignores any heterogeneity of the encrustation volume distribution along the shaft, which might overlook some key characteristics along the shaft body.

In this study, we compared patterns of luminal stent encrustation volumes in stone and transplant patients. A semantic segmentation approach was first evaluated and implemented by means of Convolutional Neural Network (CNN)

to simultaneously quantify the volume of luminal encrustations and of the stent. Luminal encrustation volume per stent unit was derived, representing the normalized encrustation level, such that the inter-subject changes of stent volume were accounted for. Further, luminal encrustation levels along the stent were assessed to evaluate the heterogeneity along the stent, and comparisons were made between stone and transplant patients.

MATERIALS AND METHODS

The retrospective study is reported in accordance with guidelines from the STROBE statement (15). The stone and transplant cohorts consisted of double-J stents removed endoscopically from patients who underwent stone treatment and kidney transplantation, respectively, between January 2020 and June 2021 at the Department of Urology of Bern University Hospital (n = 24) and the Cantonal Hospital Olten (n = 3) in Switzerland. Samples were selected by matching age, gender, presence of UTI, and stent indwelling time were matched between the two cohorts (p > 0.05). Stents placed for external obstructions such as pregnancy and urothelial carcinoma, and stents with unknown indwelling times were excluded.

All stents were collected as by-products of regular urological treatment and the personally identifiable information were anonymized. Under the Human Research Act (Swiss Federal Act on Research involving Human Beings, Art. 2, The Federal Assembly of the Swiss Confederation), approval of the local ethics committee was exempted, and informed consent was waived. Written general consent was obtained from all patients. All methods were carried out in accordance with relevant guidelines and regulations.

Each collected stent was dried in an oven at 60°C for three hours to remove residual urine, which helps solidify the sample and prevent contamination during the following processes. To assess the encrustation volume in different sections of the stent, four sections of each stent were separated, i.e., the renal pigtail, the proximal straight part (near the ureteropelvic junction), the distal straight part (near the ureterovesical junction), and the bladder pigtail (see **Figure 1A**). This was done under the assumption that the two junctions are critical regions for the development of encrustations as they are the entrance and exit of the ureter, where urine flows are regulated by the physiologically narrowing tract.

Subsequently, each section was scanned using a μ-CT scanner (SCANCO Medical AG, Bruettisellen, CH) operated at 90 kVp and 200 μA with an integration time of 200 ms, optimized based on preliminary experiments. The final resolution was 11.4 μm in all three dimensions. The acquired images were segmented using a CNN model known as the U-Net (16), available in the Dragonfly software (v2020.1, Object Research Systems Inc. Quebec, CA). The segmentation results allowed evaluation of the luminal encrustations including the luminal space of the side holes (SHs) without losing their spatial distribution (see **Figures 1B–E**), thus offering a more reliable representation of the encrustations. Full technical details on μ-CT, discussion on accuracy, and examples can be found in the **Supplementary Material**.

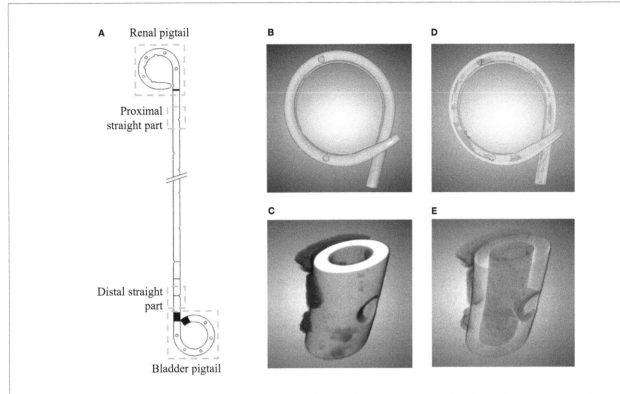

FIGURE 1 | Illustration of the four separated sections from a ureteral stent **(A)**. Three dimensional μ-CT images from the pigtail and straight part before **(B, C)** and after **(D, E)** segmentations, respectively. Luminal encrustations from the segmentation results are shown in orange, where stents are rendered semi-transparent for better visualization.

After the segmentation, volumes of the encrustations and of the stent were extracted, respectively. By defining the encrustation volume ratio (EVR) as the encrustation volume normalized by the corresponding stent volume, which gives the encrustation volume per stent unit, the bias introduced by the different volumes of individual stent samples was eliminated. The total encrustation volume ratio (TEVR) was defined by summing the EVR over the four stent sections, which indicates the overall susceptibility to encrustations of a stent. To study the relative level of encrustations at different stent sections, we defined the encrustation risk level (ERL) by dividing EVR over TEVR. As such, the inter-subject variability between samples is removed, as the ERL of each stent sums to one (100%). The stent section with highest ERL would be likely to attract more encrustations.

To compare the encrustation level over time, stents from stone patients were divided into two groups: group one with indwelling time < 42 d, and group two with indwelling time ≥ 42 d. The choice of 42 days was based on the fact that an indwelling time over six weeks is commonly associated with significantly higher encrustation levels (2–4). Since optimal removal time in transplant patients has been reported to range between two and six weeks and no consensus has been reached, subgroups with indwelling times < 28 d or ≥ 28 d (four weeks) were chosen for comparison.

For statistical comparisons, the two-sided Mann-Whitney U-test was used for continuous data, while the Fisher's exact test was used for the categorical data in **Table 1**. P-values from multiple comparisons were corrected using the Bonferroni-Holm method, and $p < 0.05$ was considered significant in this study.

RESULTS

A total of 27 stents were analyzed, as summarized in **Table 1**. Stent indwelling times were 11-99 days for stone patients and 22-47 days for kidney transplant patients, with no significant difference between the groups ($p = 0.4$). All retrieved stents were made of polyurethane manufactured by PURE Medical Device SA (Geneva, CH) and Optimed Medical Instruments GmbH (Ettlingen, DE).

Encrustations Near Side Holes

Segmented images from stents at different indwelling times are shown in **Figure 2** for each patient group. The amount of luminal encrustations (orange) in the stone group seems to increase over time, which is not observed in the transplant group. The increasing encrustation in the stone group is more apparent on the renal pigtail and proximal straight part of the stent. Aggregates of encrustations were mostly found near the SHs, whose locations along the pigtails are marked (arrows) in **Figure 2**. The example with indwelling time of 90 days showed complete blockage in the proximal lumen, as evidenced by the cross-sectional inset in **Figure 2**.

TABLE 1 | Characteristics of patients and stents.

	Stone patients	Transplant patients	p value
Patients, *n*	16	10	
Female, *n* (%)	6 (37.5%)	5 (50%)	0.7
Median age, yr (IQR)	60.5 (48.5-75)	57 (40-73)	0.7
Presence of UTI, *n* (%)	3/16 (18.8%)	4/10 (40%)	0.4
Ureter units, *n*	17	10	
Stone location, *n* (%)			
Nephrolithiasis	10/17 (58.8%)	NA	
Ureterolithiasis	6/17 (35.3%)	NA	
Nephro- & Ureterolithiasis	1/17 (5.9%)	NA	
Collected stents, *n*	17	10	
Stent size, Fr/cm	6/26 (*n*=15)	6/10 (*n*=9)	
	4.5/26 (*n*=2)	4.8/10 (*n*=1)	
Median indwelling time, d (IQR)	36 (24.5-66)	29.5 (26-37)	0.4

IQR, interquartile range; UTI, urinary tract infection; yr, year; d, day.

P values are calculated using the Mann-Whitney U-test for continuous data (age, indwelling time), and the Fisher's exact test for categorical data (gender, UTI).

Encrustation Over Time

The total encrustation volume ratios (TEVRs) from stone patients were significantly different (p = 0.02) between indwelling times < 42 d (median: 0.45, IQR: 0.10-0.80) and ≥ 42 d (median: 5.9, IQR: 3.8-26). Further comparisons of the encrustation volume ratios (EVRs) in each section (**Figure 3A**) revealed that encrustations increased significantly in the renal pigtail (p = 0.002) and the distal straight part (p = 0.01). The EVR in the proximal straight part also showed considerable increase over six weeks but did not reach statistical significance (p = 0.1). In the transplant group no significant difference was found between short indwelling time (< 28 d) and long indwelling time (≥ 28 d) groups, although the median EVRs were higher in both pigtails (**Figure 3B**). The comparison was also made between stents from stone and transplant groups with indwelling times < 42 d (**Figure 3C**) and no differences were found in EVR (p > 0.05 in all sections) or TEVR (p = 0.2).

Most Encrusted Stent Region

Subsequent comparisons of encrustation risk levels (ERLs) were made between stone and transplant groups for each stent section (**Figure 3D**). In both patient groups, the highest median ERLs were found in the pigtails with no significant difference between renal and bladder. Interestingly, in stone patients, the ERL of the proximal straight part was higher than that of the distal part (p = 0.013). In transplant patients, however, no significant difference was found between the two straight parts. The ERLs of the pigtails were significantly higher than in the proximal (p = 0.022) and distal (p = 0.014) straight parts, respectively. Comparison of ERLs between stone and transplant groups revealed a significant difference in the proximal straight part, with the higher ERL in the stone patients (p = 0.007). Further data can be found in the **Supplementary Material**.

DISCUSSION

The segmentation method based on the CNN model U-Net (16) allowed us to evaluate luminal encrustation and stent volumes simultaneously with unparalleled accuracy. Once trained, the model can be applied to subsequent data sets without further tuning, and therefore reduces random error or bias imposed during the quantitative analyses. Moreover, to the best of the authors' knowledge, this study is the first to measure both the encrustation volume and the stent volume. As such, the encrustation volume per stent unit was derived, which is more representative than directly comparing the encrustation volumes, as was done in several previous studies (13, 14).

One observation in our study was that SHs were often the anchoring sites of encrustations even for stents with short indwelling times regardless of the patient group (**Figure 2**). The initial deposits of encrustations near SHs might be explained by recent *in vitro* experiments such that SHs facilitate local urine flow stasis and promote particle accumulation in the neighboring regions (17–19). These initial deposits exacerbate the local encrustation process, causing severe stone burden near SHs, which has been previously reported in clinical studies (11, 20). The stony encrustation could compromise the stent tensile strength at the SHs, and eventually deteriorate into fractures (11, 20). In spite of the negative effects, stents with SHs should not be simply advised against as they are crucial in exchanging urine flow between the stent lumen and extraluminal spaces (between the stent and the ureter wall) in case of obstruction. Further studies are required to fully evaluate their efficacy in order to give clinical suggestions.

Another observation was that that encrustation levels did not differ between patient groups in the first six weeks (**Figure 3C**), but stone patients had a higher tendency to build up encrustations over prolonged indwelling time than transplant patients (**Figures 3A, B**). The higher tendency could be explained by the fact that stone patients have supersaturated urine. The similar encrustation levels in the first six weeks, however, would require further studies to fully clarify, as the early stages of encrustation involve biological processes such as the formation of conditioning film and biofilms, which might have an impact on the encrustation levels in both patient groups in the long term.

The highest median ERLs were observed in the pigtails in both patient groups, suggesting higher risks of excessive encrustations per stent unit. The pigtails at both ends exhibited high median in ERL and did not differ from each other, so the risk seemed

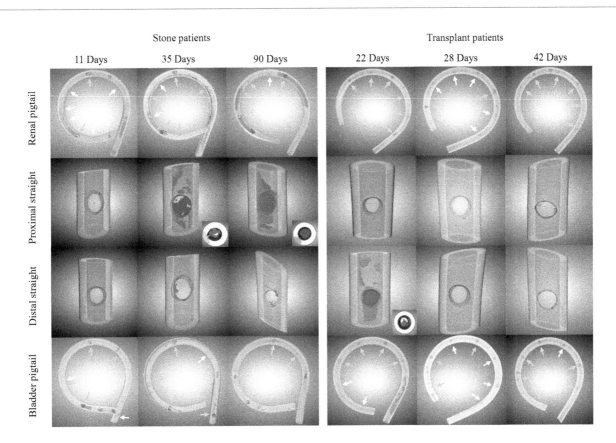

FIGURE 2 | Examples of luminal encrustations (orange) in the renal pigtail, proximal straight part, distal straight part, and bladder pigtail of the stents from stone and transplant patient groups. Stents are rendered semi-transparent for better visualization. Side hole locations on the pigtails are marked by arrows, where yellow arrows indicate clear evidence of encrustations and white arrows suggest otherwise. Cross sectional insets are given for visually significant encrustations to show the blockage level in the stent lumen.

equivalent in the renal and bladder ends. Since our results were based on encrustation volume per stent unit, it seems that shorter pigtails are preferrable to alleviate encrustations. The shorter length may also reduce other stent associated complications since stents crossing the bladder midline has been reported to cause more pain and urinary symptoms (21).

Nonetheless, the double pigtail or multi-coil stents are less prone to migration, which is also a significant complication of indwelling stent (22). The risks of encrustation and migration with shorter pigtail must be balanced. Further assessment on the encrustation level and urinary symptoms against pigtail length may offer valuable perspectives on the clinical choice of stents.

In practice, proximal stone burden has been associated with multiple surgical complications (23), and accurate determination of the stent section most susceptible to encrustations has been an active topic of discussion. Previous studies on stent encrustation patterns mainly focused on stone patients. While some suggested the renal pigtail as the most susceptible section followed by the bladder pigtail (4, 11, 13), others reported that the two pigtails were most and equally susceptible (9), or that the distal part of stent (12) was most encrusted. The recent study using μ-CT (14)

also suggested the stent's shaft body (the entire straight part) as the most susceptible region. For one thing, the disputed conclusions can be attributed to the lack of quantitative tools to accurately measure the encrustation volumes. For another, the fact that there were no significant differences between certain comparisons (as demonstrated in **Figure 3**) should also be acknowledged, such that qualitative observations can be biased. By identifying the most encrusted stent region, we hope to guide further studies to address the most problematic regions of current stents, offering possible ideas for subsequent optimizations. The encrustation volume per stent unit presented in the current study might be adopted for subsequent works, which offers more meaningful insights than direct comparison of encrustation volumes.

In contrast to stone patients, quantitative evaluation of stent encrustation patterns in transplant patients are lacking. Following kidney transplantation, stents are usually placed to prevent strictures or urine leakage. These prophylactic stents are much shorter than those in stone patients since the allograft ureter is kept short to ensure a good blood supply. Consequently, higher grades of vesicoureteral reflux (VUR) in transplant patients are common as urine reaches up to the renal pelvis

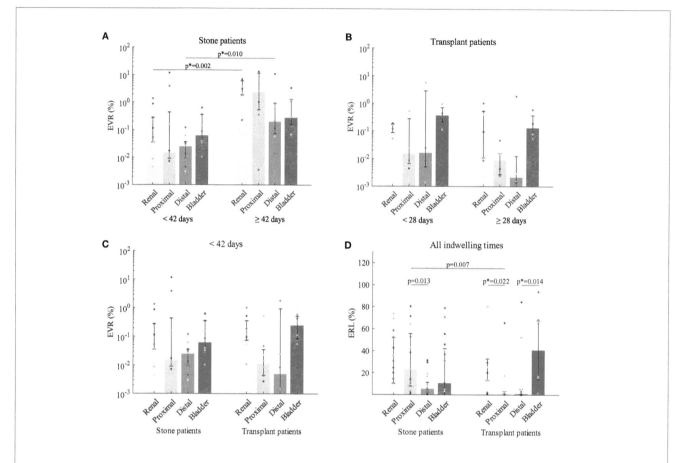

FIGURE 3 | Encrustation volume ratios (EVR) compared with respect to indwelling time for stone patients **(A)** and transplant patients **(B)**. **(C)** EVR compared between patient groups with stent indwelling time < 42 days. **(D)** Encrustation risk levels (ERL) from stone and transplant patients for each stent section. The median (bar) and interquartile range (error bars) are presented. Raw data from the same stent are coded by color (filled circles). P-values corrected by the Bonferroni-Holm method is indicated by the asteroid (*). Further data can be found in the **Supplementary Material**.

more easily (24). This retrograde flow might create a flushing effect, periodically stirring the deposits in the stent lumen, whereas in stone patients the VUR would not reach up to renal pelvis as easily since the stents are often longer. This might explain the higher encrustation level in the proximal straight part in stone patients (**Figure 3D**).

Moreover, stent implantation significantly impedes the peristalsis of the ureter (25), and thus the urine transport from kidney to bladder is largely passive. The openings at each end of the stent lumen (usually with internal diameter of 1mm) create significant hydraulic resistance to the urine flow so local stasis are expected in the pigtails. In the stent shaft, since the hydraulic resistance is proportional to the tube length, the shorter stent in transplant patients could better facilitate urine flows in the stent lumen, either from kidney to bladder or in the presence of VUR. As such, on the basis that encrustations are regulated by the local fluid mechanical characteristics (17, 26), the luminal encrustation levels along the stent are influenced by both the forward and retrograde urine flows, co-creating the different patterns presented in **Figure 3**.

Limitations of this study include the limited sample size, which did not allow for further subgroup analysis. Discussions regarding the biological aspects of the encrustation process were therefore missing. An extended study focusing on the correlation between specific complications and degree of encrustation would be highly desirable. Also, by separating the stent into four parts, the central part of the stent shaft was omitted. It might be interesting to assess the distribution of encrustations along the entire stent body. Nevertheless, the current study offers the first data connecting urinary flow dynamics and quantitative encrustation levels. Further studies on the specific urine flow conditions at each part of the stent could help elucidate the process of encrustations in stented native or allograft ureters.

As a closing remark, the semantic segmentation approach delivered accurate and intuitive results and is applicable to other image analysis tasks in urology. Our results highlighted the similarities and differences in stent encrustation patterns between stone and renal transplant groups, and possible explanations were discussed. Further investigations in both engineering and clinical disciplines are necessary to fully understand the dynamics of encrustations in order to develop the "perfect stent".

AUTHOR CONTRIBUTIONS

Conception and design: FB, FC, DO, and SZ. Acquisition of data: PA, FB, BK, FS, and SZ. Analysis and interpretation of data: PA and SZ. Figure preparation: PA, SZ. Drafting of the manuscript: SZ. Statistical analysis: AH and SZ. All authors contributed to the article and approved the submitted version.

ACKNOWLEDGMENTS

SZ acknowledges Mr. Michael Indermaur from the Musculoskeletal Biomechanics group at the University of Bern for his support in operating the Micro-CT scanner, and Mr. Emile Talon for his contribution in the preliminary study.

REFERENCES

1. Bibby LM, Wiseman OJ. Double JJ Ureteral Stenting: Encrustation and Tolerability. *Eur Urol Focus* (2020) 7(1):7–8. doi: 10.1016/j.euf.2020.08.014
2. Tomer N, Garden E, Small A, Palese M. Ureteral Stent Encrustation: Epidemiology, Pathophysiology, Management and Current Technology. *J Urol* (2021) 205(1):68–77. doi: 10.1097/JU.0000000000001343
3. El-Faqih SR, Shamsuddin AB, Chakrabarti A, Atassi R, Kardar AH, Osman MK, et al. Polyurethane Internal Ureteral Stents in Treatment of Stone Patients: Morbidity Related to Indwelling Times. *J Urol* (1991) 146 (6):1487–91. doi: 10.1016/S0022-5347(17)38146-6
4. Kawahara T, Ito H, Terao H, Yoshida M, Matsuzaki J. Ureteral Stent Encrustation, Incrustation, and Coloring: Morbidity Related to Indwelling Times. *J Endourol* (2011) 26(2):178–82. doi: 10.1089/end.2011.0385
5. Tavakoli A, Surange RS, Pearson RC, Parrott NR, Augustine T, Riad HN. Impact of Stents on Urological Complications and Health Care Expenditure in Renal Transplant Recipients: Results of a Prospective, Randomized Clinical Trial. *J Urol* (2007) 177(6):2260–4. doi: 10.1016/j.juro.2007.01.152
6. Thompson ER, Hosgood SA, Nicholson ML, Wilson CH. Early Versus Late Ureteric Stent Removal After Kidney Transplantation. *Cochrane Database Syst Rev* (2018) 1:1–27. doi: 10.1002/14651858.CD011455.pub2
7. Visser IJ, van der Staaij JPT, Muthusamy A, Willicombe M, Lafranca JA, Dor FJMF. Timing of Ureteric Stent Removal and Occurrence of Urological Complications After Kidney Transplantation: A Systematic Review and Meta-Analysis. *J Clin Med* (2019) 8(5):1–15. doi: 10.3390/jcm8050689
8. Wilson CH, Rix DA, Manas DM. Routine Intraoperative Ureteric Stenting for Kidney Transplant Recipients. *Cochrane Database Syst Rev* (2013) 6:1–24. doi: 10.1002/14651858.CD004925.pub3
9. Arkusz K, Pasik K, Halinski A, Halinski A. Surface Analysis of Ureteral Stent Before and After Implantation in the Bodies of Child Patients. *Urolithiasis* (2020) 49:83–92. doi: 10.1007/s00240-020-01211-9
10. Acosta-Miranda AM, Milner J, Turk TMT. The FECal Double-J: A Simplified Approach in the Management of Encrusted and Retained Ureteral Stents. *J Endourol* (2009) 23(3):409–15. doi: 10.1089/end.2008.0214
11. Singh I, Gupta NP, Hemal AK, Aron M, Seth A, Dogra PN. Severely Encrusted Polyurethane Ureteral Stents: Management and Analysis of Potential Risk Factors. *Urology* (2001) 58(4):526–31. doi: 10.1016/S0090-4295(01)01317-6
12. Rana AM, Sabooh A. Management Strategies and Results for Severely Encrusted Retained Ureteral Stents. *J Endourol* (2007) 21(6):628–32. doi: 10.1089/end.2006.0250
13. Sighinolfi MC, Sighinolfi GP, Galli E, Micali S, Ferrari N, Mofferdin A, et al. Chemical and Mineralogical Analysis of Ureteral Stent Encrustation and Associated Risk Factors. *Urology* (2015) 86(4):703–6. doi: 10.1016/j.urology.2015.05.015
14. Yoshida T, Takemoto K, Sakata Y, Matsuzaki T, Koito Y, Yamashita S, et al. A Randomized Clinical Trial Evaluating the Short-Term Results of Ureteral Stent Encrustation in Urolithiasis Patients Undergoing Ureteroscopy: Micro-Computed Tomography Evaluation. *Sci Rep* (2021) 11(1):10337. doi: 10.1038/s41598-021-89808-x
15. Vandenbroucke JP, von Elm E, Altman DG, Gøtzsche PC, Mulrow CD, Pocock SJ, et al. Strengthening the Reporting of Observational Studies in Epidemiology (STROBE): Explanation and Elaboration. *PloS Med* (2007) 4 (10):e297. doi: 10.1371/journal.pmed.0040297
16. Ronneberger O, Fischer P, Brox T, eds. U-Net: Convolutional Networks for Biomedical Image Segmentation. In: *18th International Conference on Medical Image Computing and Computer-Assisted Intervention (MICCAI 2015)*, 2015 October 5-9. Munich, Germany: Springer International Publishing (2015). doi: 10.1007/978-3-319-24574-4_28
17. Mosayyebi A, Yue QY, Somani BK, Zhang X, Manes C, Carugo D. Particle Accumulation in Ureteral Stents Is Governed by Fluid Dynamics: *In Vitro* Study Using a "Stent-On-Chip" Model. *J Endourol* (2018) 32(7):639–46. doi: 10.1089/end.2017.0946
18. Clavica F, Zhao X, ElMahdy M, Drake MJ, Zhang X, Carugo D. Investigating the Flow Dynamics in the Obstructed and Stented Ureter by Means of a Biomimetic Artificial Model. Proceedings of the 18th International Conference on Miniaturized Systems for Chemistry and Life Sciences, MicroTAS. *PloS One* (2014) 9(2):e87433. doi: 10.1371/journal.pone.0087433
19. D Carugo, X Zhang, JM Drake, F Clavica, eds. Formation and Characteristics of Laminar Vortices in Microscale Environments Within an Obstructed and Stented Ureter: A Computational Study. In: *Proceedings of the 18th International Conference on Miniaturized Systems for Chemistry and Life Sciences, MicroTAS*. San Antonio, Texas, USA: MicroTAS.
20. Zisman A, Siegel YI, Siegmann A, Lindner A. Spontaneous Ureteral Stent Fragmentation. *J Urol* (1995) 153(3):718–21. doi: 10.1016/S0022-5347(01)67697-3
21. Taguchi M, Yoshida K, Sugi M, Matsuda T, Kinoshita H. A Ureteral Stent Crossing the Bladder Midline Leads to Worse Urinary Symptoms. *Cent Eur J Urol* (2017) 70(4):412–7. doi: 10.5173/ceju.2017.1533
22. Saltzman B. Ureteral Stents: Indications, Variations, and Complications. *Urol Clin N Am* (1988) 15(3):481–91. doi: 10.1016/S0094-0143(21)01594-9
23. Weedin JW, Coburn M, Link RE. The Impact of Proximal Stone Burden on the Management of Encrusted and Retained Ureteral Stents. *J Urol* (2011) 185 (2):542–7. doi: 10.1016/j.juro.2010.09.085
24. Ness D, Olsburgh J. UTI in Kidney Transplant. *World J Urol* (2020) 38(1):81–8. doi: 10.1007/s00345-019-02742-6
25. Mosli Hisham A, Farsi Hasan MA, Al-Zimaity Mohammed F, Saleh Tarik R, Al-Zamzami Mokhtar M. Vesicoureteral Reflux in Patients With Double Pigtail Stents. *J Urol* (1991) 146(4):966–9. doi: 10.1016/S0022-5347(17)37976-4
26. Zheng S, Carugo D, Mosayyebi A, Turney B, Burkhard F, Lange D, et al. Fluid Mechanical Modeling of the Upper Urinary Tract. *WIREs Mech Dis* (2021) 13 (6):e01523. doi: 10.1002/wsbm.1523

24

Design and Evaluation of a Virtual Urology Sub-Internship During the COVID-19 Pandemic

Amelia A. Khoei[1], Blair T. Stocks[2], Jerry Zhuo[2], Wesley A. Mayer[2], Michael Coburn[2], Caroline Hubbard[2] and Jennifer M. Taylor[2]*

[1] School of Medicine, Baylor College of Medicine, Houston, TX, United States, [2] Scott Department of Urology, Baylor College of Medicine, Houston, TX, United States

*Correspondence:
Jennifer M. Taylor
jennifer.taylor@bcm.edu

Objective: To offer learning opportunities to medical students during the pandemic and address technical challenges for operating room involvement, the Scott Department of Urology at the Baylor College of Medicine designed and evaluated a 2-week virtual elective course.

Materials and Methods: A manual for a virtual sub-internship was created by members of the Society of Academic Urologists, structured around core competencies. Our curriculum incorporated the manual to design a virtual experience. The course combined live surgical case streaming, one-on-one didactics, and virtual participation during in-person clinic sessions. The surgical streaming was enabled through a nominal investment of $150 for equipment. A post-course evaluation was distributed to participating students.

Results: The course evaluation received a 91% response rate from 11 enrolled fourth-year medical students. There was a very high level of satisfaction with the quality of the educational experience (M=5.8 +/-0.4). Open comments on course strengths highlighted the surgical streaming aspect of the experience, and 80% of evaluation respondents reported that one-on-one time with physicians was a strength of the virtual format.

Conclusions: Our curriculum effectively engaged medical students during a 2-week virtual urology elective. The surgical video streaming format is unique even among virtual rotations nationwide and may be adapted for any learners within or beyond an institution. Our curriculum provides an example for programs to incorporate these inexpensive streaming techniques and for students to gain exposure in their surgical areas of interest.

Keywords: urology, medical students, COVID-19, undergraduate medical education (UME), distance education

1 INTRODUCTION

The current novel coronavirus (COVID-19) pandemic is an unprecedented global crisis which has had significant ramifications upon worldwide economies and healthcare burdens (1). The pandemic has consequently affected education for medical students, residents, and fellows (2–4). In March 2020, both the Association of American Colleges (AAMC) and Liaison Committee of Medical

Education (LCME) issued recommendations to limit direct patient care for medical students in clinical learning environments (5). The recommendations were made for the purpose of reducing personal protective equipment usage (PPE) and reducing risk of coronavirus transmission (6). Overnight, students pivoted to alternative learning modalities.

In addition, the LCME discouraged in-person clerkships, and the Accreditation Council for Graduate Medical Education (ACGME) discouraged visiting student rotations (5, 7). This recommendation disrupted many fourth-year medical students' clinical experience and curricular plans. In many specialties, students rely on the visiting sub-internship as a component of their residency applications (8). For surgical specialties such as Urology, the visiting sub-internship is an important component for both the applicants and the resident program. Visiting sub-internships are a critical opportunity for medical students to learn and demonstrate clinical knowledge and skills, network with institutions throughout the country, and explore their fields of interest. The rotations further generate useful feedback regarding an applicant's candidacy in the field. The visiting rotation may provide invaluable clinical education and specific access to a subspecialty like Urology (9–12).

In response to the pandemic and travel restrictions, The Society of Academic Urologists (SAU), a national society of chairs and program directors, quickly assembled a taskforce to develop a manual to help institutions implement a virtual sub-internship in Urology (13). Our residency program created a 2-week virtual elective curriculum that utilized Zoom™ to facilitate didactic sessions, simulated patient modules, journal clubs, virtual conferences, virtual participation in live clinic visits, livestreaming of surgical cases, and inpatient census discussion with resident teams.

To our knowledge, a virtual elective with the extensive technical aspects of the Scott Department of Urology at the Baylor College of Medicine's (BCMSDU) offering has not been previously described. While a few urology programs also executed virtual electives, many experienced technical challenges and limited virtual operating room experiences (14). Our program targeted these challenges and designed a

technologically innovative solution for virtual student engagement in the operating room. Our hypothesis was that our virtual urology elective could sufficiently represent the breadth of an in-person urology rotation, showcasing the surgical experience in particular.

2 METHODS AND COMPETENCIES

2.1 Methods

2.1.1 Core Competencies and Principles

Due to the recommendations of professional medical organizations, BCM suspended all in-person clinical rotations in March 2020. Two faculty (WAM and MC) members from BCMSDU worked on the SAU curricular taskforces and helped design the SAU manual with content areas based on the ACGME Core Competencies and Milestones for Urology. **Table 1** provides a reference for the intersection between the ACGME Core Competencies and the course components. There were novel opportunities in the virtual format to include more of the core competencies explicitly in the course structure.

The BCMSDU course director (JMT) and program director (WAM) met with key stakeholders within the urology department, at each clinical site, the Office of the Registrar, and the Curriculum Committee to determine necessary steps and components for a Non-Clinical Advanced Elective. Following course approval, we designed specific daily activities considering varying capabilities at each clinical site to integrate students virtually in clinical activities. As the students were registered as visiting students at our institution, their activities were protected under medical education policies. Our institutional license of Zoom, utilized for transmission of clinical activities, is fully compliant with federal HIPAA policies and Texas state privacy laws. Orientation for the students enrolled in the virtual elective included standard required trainings, including privacy modules, for visiting students at our institution. Multiple residents and faculty members within the department committed to scheduled didactic sessions during each 2-week rotation. The reduced clinical activity and volume due to pandemic restrictions

---

TABLE 1 | Curricular elements which met ACGME core competencies.

ACGME Core Competencies	BCM Curricular Structure
Patient Care	One-on-one clinic with faculty
	Surgical case streaming and participation
	Case discussions with resident educator
Medical Knowledge	Didactic teaching sessions
	Suggested pre-requisite reading
	Department conferences
Interpersonal and Communication Skills	Daily Huddle with resident physicians
	Patient interviews in clinic encounters
	Guided discussion of handoff (iPASS) and serious news counseling with resident educator
Professionalism	Independent learning
Practice-Based Learning and Improvement	Interactive standardized patient case discussions
	Reflective Writing
	Grand Rounds
	Critical appraisal of research articles
Systems-Based Practice	Independent learning using SAU-created videos on healthcare systems, quality & patient safety

allowed for greater educator availability, and residents fulfilled alternative educational plans by participating in the course design and implementation. At least one clinical site acquired new equipment to implement the virtual format at a relatively nominal cost of $150 USD.

2.1.2 Execution and Learning Environment
The course availability was advertised through multiple channels including the SAU website, the BCMSDU website, our Twitter account, and a website created by current fourth-year students applying into Urology (uroresidency.com). Students applied *via* the Visiting Student Application System (VSAS) to the 2-week virtual elective in Urology. Accepted Virtual Away Students (VASs) participated in scheduled content from Monday to Friday over the 2-week experience. VASs spent one dedicated week at one of our public hospital practice sites and one dedicated week at one of our private hospital practice sites. Public practice sites included the Michael E. DeBakey Veterans Administration Medical Center (MEDVAMC) and Ben Taub Hospital (BTH). The private practice sites included Baylor St. Luke's Medical Center (BSLMC) and Texas Children's' Hospital (TCH).

This weekly structure mirrored previous years' in-person visiting sub-internship with exposure and experience spanning across our many residency training sites. The proportion of time at each site was determined by logistics of virtual connectivity and clinical volume, with some sites experiencing reductions in clinic and case volume due to the pandemic surge. All students were enrolled as visiting students at BCM, and most students received course credit *via* their home institutions. Prerequisite resources needed by learners included a personal computer with audio/video conferencing capabilities, installation of Zoom™ Video Communications software (San Jose, California), and a dedicated high-speed internet connection. Facilitators included BCMSDU faculty and residents with access to similar technology.

2.1.3 Curricular Design, Pedagogical Format, and Learning Objectives
The learning objectives were approved with assessment measures as follows:

1) Objective: Student will demonstrate knowledge of common conditions in Urology and their management.
   Assessment Method: Didactics; Student Assessment Form.

2) Objective: Student will describe indications, anatomy, basic technical steps, and potential complications for common urological surgeries.
   Assessment Method: Didactics, Surgical case review; Student Assessment Form.

3) Objective: Student will locate, appraise, and assimilate evidence from scientific studies related to patients' urologic problems.

   Assessment Method: Reflective Writing Assessment Tool.
   Each morning, VASs logged into secure Zoom™ video meetings and proceeded to interact with faculty and residents throughout the day. After a one-hour orientation session at the start of the two-week rotation, typical sessions included the following:

1) Surgical Case streaming: Real-time participation in surgical cases.
   As described in detail in the next section, VASs interacted with faculty and residents *via* live audio/video feeds of ongoing urologic surgeries.

2) Clinic Encounters: Dedicated one-on-one clinic time with faculty.
   In these sessions, faculty members would include VASs in live clinic encounters *via* audio/video conference enabled laptops. The VAS was allowed to interview the patient individually and then present to the attending physician and accompany the attending physician for further discussion, or the student was connected live while the attending interviewed and examined the patient.

3) Didactic teaching sessions with department educators: Small-group didactic sessions scheduled with BCMSDU faculty, chief resident, or fellow on a variety of topics, including guidelines and clinical management of common conditions.

4) Interactive case discussions: Small-group standardized patient scenarios moderated by residents.
   Cases were adapted from the SAU Virtual Sub-Internship manual and included the evaluation and surgical management of patients presenting with conditions such as testicular torsion, male factor infertility, gross hematuria, and metabolic stone disease.

5) Critical Appraisal of Literature: Small group journal clubs with residents and faculty.
   VASs presented and critically evaluated peer-reviewed journal articles focusing on clinical topics.

6) Daily huddle with residents: Each VAS would have time at the end of the clinical day with residents at one site to discuss the inpatient census, consults, and cases. This also provided time to ask questions informally.

7) Independent learning: Scheduled blocks in which the VASs could prepare for the above sessions as well review assigned online content, including quality improvement, patient safety, interprofessional communication, and the business of medicine. This online content was adapted from the SAU Virtual Sub-Internship manual.

8) Reflective writing: Each VAS was given an assignment and the writing was reviewed with a faculty member in an individual virtual session.

9) Department conferences: Participation in weekly Grand Rounds, Resident Educational Conference, Preoperative Case Conference, and/or site-specific Tumor Board.

ACGME Core Competencies are also referenced in the short course description: "This course will engage the student in observation and participation in clinical scenarios specific to Urologic practice, with a distribution of experiences across ACGME core competencies (in parentheses). Through this 2-week rotation, the student will participate in virtual experiences to include: group didactics with an attending physician (Medical Knowledge), critical appraisal of sentinel literature (Evidence-Based Medicine), facilitated case discussion with residents (Medical Knowledge, Practice-Based Learning), self-directed learning through reading and video assignments (Practice-Based Learning), surgical case review and discussion (Patient Care and Procedural Skills), and self-reflection (Professionalism, Practice-Based Learning)" (**Table 1**).

At the conclusion of the two-week course, VASs attended a wrap-up session with the course director and residency program director. VASs were also invited to participate in an open forum with BCMSDU residents pertaining to resident life, living in Houston, the interview process, or any topic of their choosing.

Feedback was formative and provided face-to-face by the attending physician. Each student had a performance assessment form completed by the Course Director, based on compiling feedback from the faculty and resident educators, that was submitted to their home institution. All students were graded Pass/Fail given the Non-Clinical structure of the course.

2.1.4 Technological Considerations
Critical to the success of the BCMSDU Virtual Elective Student Rotation was the integration of live video and audio streams from within our surgical suites. Streamed surgical cases included robotic, laparoscopic, percutaneous, endoscopic, and microsurgical cases.

For the MEDVAMC rotation, faculty and residents worked closely with onsite system engineers from Karl Storz Endoscopy-America, Inc (El Segundo, California) to leverage the Karl Storz StreamConnect software platform, which already provided internal streaming of video input from several operating rooms. As a result, we were able to stream live video and audio content from the DaVinci Si/Xi Surgical System (Intuitive, Sunnyvale, California) or the endoscopic suite to secure Zoom™ Video meetings attended by VASs.

At BSLMC, we partnered with surgical and IT staff to stream live video and audio from operating rooms not equipped with this integrated software. Specifically, we created a mobile and cost-effective solution for other surgical programs and/or subspecialities wishing to creative a virtual operating room experience. Both the Intuitive DaVinci Surgical System and Karl Storz Endoscopic surgical platforms transmit high-definition video *via* uncompressed Digital Visual Interface (DVI) connections. Accordingly, we utilized an available "DVI Video Out" connection on these platforms to capture live robotic or endoscopic video feeds. For our needs, we purchased a 10-foot long male DVI to male High-Definition Multimedia Interface (HMDI) cable (~$10 - **Figure 1A**). However, as most personal computers do not have a graphics card with dedicated video input, an external video capture card was required. We utilized a female HDMI to male USB HMDI Video Capture Card (~$20 – **Figure 1B**). Ultimately, the set up was as follows: Female DVI-OUT (as found on the robotic console or endoscopic tower) to our male DVI/male HDMI cable, to our female HDMI/male USB video capture card, to a personal laptop or desktop computer in the operating room, which was logged into Zoom™ with a high-speed internet connection. Once connected, facilitators were able to select "USB Camera" as a video input source that the Zoom™ Software streamed to VASs in high definition. Students were able to communicate with the surgical team through a two-way audio-video stream. In some cases, the attending physician

wore a Bluetooth-enabled headset to allow discussion that was less intrusive to the case.

To augment the live operating room experience to show both the video image and the operating room interior perspective, we installed "gooseneck" smartphone stands (~$20 - **Figure 1C**) within the operating room to provide a bird's eye view of the operating surgeons and patients. A facilitator placed a Zoom™-enabled smartphone in the stand with camera pointed over the operating table. Additionally, we paired a Bluetooth enabled audio-conferencing speakerphone with noise-reducing technology (~$90 – **Figure 1D**) to the smartphone in order to dampen OR cacophony, which provided surgeons and VASs clear communication.

2.1.5 Course Evaluation Design
At the conclusion of the virtual elective, our program requested students to complete a course evaluation in a deidentified fashion. The electronic questionnaires were designed in SurveyHero (Zurich, Switzerland) to evaluate satisfaction with the course, effectiveness of faculty and resident teaching in the virtual format, satisfaction with learning opportunities, and success in achieving learning objectives. The evaluation also solicited qualitative feedback. Outcomes were measured on a 6-point Likert scale (1=strongly disagree, 6=strongly agree).

3 RESULTS

3.1 Demographics
Our curriculum was implemented as a virtual elective for 11 virtual fourth-year medical students. We hosted a total of 5 rotation blocks, which ran consecutively from August 3, 2020, to October 9, 2020. Participants were 36% female and attended medical schools from the following geographic regions: Mid-Atlantic, Southeast, Southwest, Midwest, and West. Evaluation responses were collected from 10 of the 11 participants using the electronic questionnaire via SurveyHero.

3.2 Overall Outcomes
In the course evaluation (**Table 2**), students reported a high level of satisfaction with the quality of the educational experience provided by the virtual elective (M=5.8 out of 6, SD=0.4). Students felt the elective was well organized (M=6, SD=0.0). With regards to learning, students felt that the elective provided sufficient opportunities to meet the stated knowledge objectives (M=5.7, SD=0.45), attending physicians provided effective teaching during the rotation (M=5.7, SD=0.64), and residents and fellows provided effective teaching during the rotation (M=5.9, SD=0.3).

3.3 Qualitative Appraisal
The majority of respondents (80%) reported that a major strength of the virtual format was one-on-one time with residents and attendings. Within the comments, students highlighted that they experienced more meaningful and dedicated discussions with faculty through the scheduled

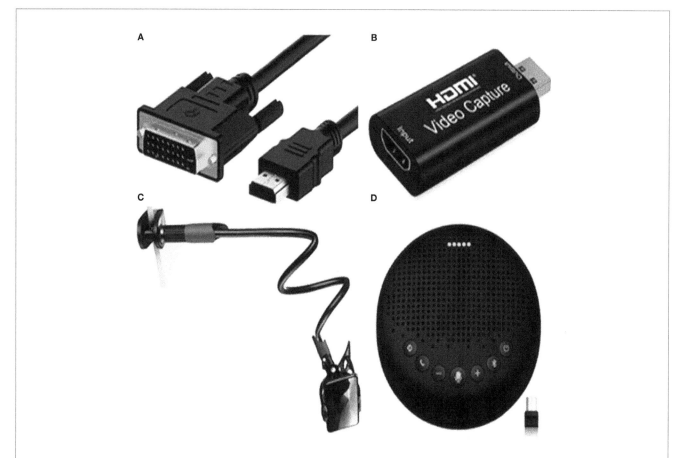

FIGURE 1 | Video Equipment used for Virtual Away Student Live OR Streaming Experience. **(A)** Male DVI to Male HDMI cable ($~10 – preferably 10 feet or longer). **(B)** Female HDMI to Male USB external video capture card (~$20). **(C)** Smartphone gooseneck stand (~$20). **(D)** Bluetooth enabled noise-reducing audio conferencing speakerphone (~$90).

TABLE 2 | Course evaluation components and results.

Evaluation Component	Mean Score (+/- SD)
"The elective was well organized."	6 (+/- 0.0)
"The elective provided sufficient learning opportunities to meet the learning objectives."	5.7 (+/- 0.5)
"Faculty provided effective teaching during this elective."	5.7 (+/- 0.6)
"Residents and/or fellows provided effective teaching during this elective."	5.9 (+/- 0.3)
"Rate the overall quality of the educational experience provided by this elective."	5.8 (+/- 0.4)

virtual format than they would have experienced in-person. One student noted, "I felt the biggest strength of this elective was having one-on-one sessions with faculty and residents. This allowed for an uninterrupted learning experience that was valuable in learning more about urology and the program in general. I was able to ask any questions I wanted in a non-hostile setting." Another student noted, "This is dedicated time that likely would not be possible in an in-person away rotation, and this is what made the rotation so special."

Many students (40%) also noted the virtual urology clinic component as a strength, as they were able to follow patients through the electronic medical record, complete a history and physical exam, and present an assessment and plan to their attending physician. A couple of students also noted as a strength

that our institution was equipped with streaming and recording equipment prior to the start of the pandemic. One student noted, "I loved having time in the operating room, [especially] streaming in the operating room when headphones were attached to the attending physician." Other strengths noted include the research/journal club assignments (40%) and faculty mentorship (100%).

3.4 Feedback for Future Improvements

When asked about potential improvements to the virtual rotation, two respondents (20%) noted that differences in time-zones made evening sign-out difficult to attend. One respondent noted a desire for more educational information on in-patient hospital management of urology patients. This student recommended the option of following a hospital patient *via* electronic medical record with virtual discussion of the patient's hospital course with the team. Other recommendations include purchasing headsets with longer battery life for operation streams, including more institution-specific educational videos, and more scheduled time at the affiliated county hospital, BTH.

4 DISCUSSION

Our curriculum was successful in providing a virtual format for a 2-week rotation in urology. Students were highly satisfied with the rotation. Strengths of the program included video streaming capabilities in the operating room, dedicated time in the urology clinic with attending physicians, one-on-one time with residents and faculty, and journal club assignments. Given the positive evaluation feedback, we believe that our curricular structure in a virtual format can be adapted to multiple institutions and specialties.

A major goal of our rotation included addressing the challenge of student integration into operating room experiences while in a virtual format. While other virtual urology rotations existed, a unique strength of our institution's adaptation was inexpensive video streaming capabilities. Prior examples of virtual rotations in surgical subspecialties have been shorter (15, 16) or do not incorporate virtual operating room experiences (14). For the cost of roughly $150, our partnering institutions became equipped to integrate our virtual students directly into the operating room.

Although this rotation was designed for off-site away-rotation students, the procedural video streaming format is largely unique and may be further adapted for any interested learners in any setting. In addition, the standardized virtual one-on-one didactic sessions allowed residents and faculty to measure and comparatively evaluate students' knowledge and participation. This presents an opportunity for virtual surgical rotations to continue even after the COVID-19 pandemic subsides, as the option may offer more personal and dedicated time with faculty than an in-person rotation. In addition, the virtual rotation can create availability for students who were not selected for in-person rotations.

Benefits of this virtual rotation included efficiency for students to be involved with patients and faculty at multiple hospital sites in the span of a single day and reduced cost for students participating in away-rotations. The urology match cost a median of $9,725 for applicants in 2020 (17). The mean estimated cost to participate in an in-person away rotation prior to the COVID-19 pandemic was $958 per rotation (18). In comparison, the cost for students who participated in our rotation only included the Visiting Student Application Service (VSAS) application fee, which is $15 per application. The virtual option will further allow programs to market their strengths and weaknesses for interested students who may not have direct access. Many leaders in medical education note the cost of traveling for in-person rotations bring potential disparities in opportunities for students to light (18). Providing a meaningful and educational experience in a virtual format may create opportunities for students from a spectrum of geographic and socioeconomic backgrounds.

There is an additional concern over the loss of in-person exposure to a student translating to a decreased ability to evaluate a student's performance. A clear disadvantage of the virtual rotation is the inability to assess a student's collaborative efforts on the inpatient team or perform a direct observation of the student's skills with patient examination or surgical techniques. However, standardizing the virtual curriculum ensured a consistency to the rotation and provided more objective experiences by which to evaluate students comparatively. The virtual format presented opportunities to develop content in core competencies, such as Interpersonal and Communication Skills, Problem Based Learning, and Improvement. It is notable that one of the students who participated in the virtual elective matched to our program for residency, signaling an experience that gave the student familiarity with the program and its strengths.

A limitation of this report is the lack of pre- versus post-measures assessing the impact on participants' subjective knowledge, attitudes, and/or behavior changes. Future iterations of this rotation may include pre- and post-session evaluations to assess participants' planned behaviors. In addition, while our program explored the novel technological facets of a virtual operating room, and this contributed to overall user satisfaction scores, the evaluation design did not specifically track technological satisfaction. These results may not be generalizable to all medical schools or hospital sites in the US as this iteration included 11 students rotating at several clinical sites at a single institution.

In terms of future directions, the video-based teaching strategies may be applied for in-person students participating at various clinic sites with the addition of active narration. In addition, the unique one-on-one didactic sessions may be further adapted for in-person and on-site medical students; we utilized the format already this year for synchronous learning activities with several students at various clinical sites. Furthermore, this virtual curriculum lends to more standardized learning opportunities for all participating students.

Our curriculum is effective and feasible for integrating medical students virtually into a surgical visiting elective rotation. Our curriculum offers other medical institutions and specialties a model for operating room integration, didactic education, and medical student mentoring in a virtual format. We hope that our promising results inspire education leadership to incorporate technological equipment to design future successful virtual electives in surgical specialties.

5 CONSTRAINTS

The virtual program was made possible by significant time investments from BCMSDU residency program faculty and trainees during COVID-19 restrictions, and the resource of time may be difficult to secure in traditional, non-restricted schedules. When considering a virtual rotation in subsequent years, it was challenging to reproduce the availability of the teaching faculty and teaching residents; the unique context of the pandemic created additional time for teaching, which was not as easily secured in the standard non-pandemic context.

AUTHOR CONTRIBUTIONS

Study conception and design, JT, WM, MC, CH, BS, and JZ. Acquisition of data, AK, JT, and WM. Analysis and interpretation of data, AK, JT, and WM. Drafting of manuscript, AK, JT, WM, MC, CH, BS, and JZ. Critical

REFERENCES

1. Sohrabi C, Alsafi Z, O'Neill N, Khan M, Kerwan A, Al-Jabir A. World Health Organization Declares Global Emergency: A Review of the 2019 Novel Coronavirus (COVID-19). *Int J Surg* (2020) 76:71–6. doi: 10.1016/j.ijsu.2020.02.034
2. Rose S. Medical Student Education in the Time of COVID-19. *JAMA* (2020) 323(21):2131. doi: 10.1001/jama.2020.5227
3. Akers A, Blough C, Iyer MS. COVID-19 Implications on Clinical Clerkships and the Residency Application Process for Medical Students. *Cureus* (2020) 12(4):525e–57e. doi: 10.7759/cureus.7800
4. Donohue JM, Miller E. COVID-19 and School Closures. *JAMA* (2020) 324 (9):845. doi: 10.1001/jama.2020.13092
5. Barzansky B, Catanese VM. *LCME Update on Medical Students, Patients, and COVID-19: Approaches to the Clinical Curriculum* (2020). Available at: https://lcme.org/wp-content/uploads/filebase/March-20-2020-LCME-Approaches-to-Clinical-Curriculum.pdf (Accessed May 23, 2021).
6. Whelan A, Prescott J, Young G, Catanese VM, McKinney R. *Guidance on Medical Students' Participation in Direct In-Person Patient Contact Activities* (2020). Available at: https://www.aamc.org/system/files/2020-08/meded-August-14-Guidance-on-Medical-Students-on-Clinical-Rotations.pdf.
7. The Coalition for Physician Accountability's Work Group on Medical Students in the Class of 2021 Moving Across Institutions for Post Graduate Training. *Final Report and Recommendations for Medical Education Institutions of LCME-Accredited, U.S. Osteopathic, and Non-U.S. Medical School Applicants.* Available at: https://www.aamc.org/system/files/2020-05/covid19_Final_Recommendations_Executive%20Summary_Final_05112020.pdf (Accessed May 23, 2021).
8. Nikonow TN, Lyon TD, Jackman SV, Averch TD. Survey of Applicant Experience and Cost in the Urology Match: Opportunities for Reform. *J Urol* (2015) 194(4):1063–7. doi: 10.1016/j.juro.2015.04.074
9. Viers BR. COVID-19 Adjustments Impact Urology Residency Training, in: *Mayo Clinic* (2020). Available at: https://www.mayoclinic.org/medical-professionals/urology/news/covid-19-adjustments-impact-urology-residency-training/mqc-20504203 (Accessed May 23, 2021).
10. Theoret C, Ming X. Our Education, Our Concerns: The Impact on Medical Student Education of COVID-19. *Med Educ* (2020) 54(7):591–2. doi: 10.1111/medu.14181
11. Williams C, Familusi OO, Ziemba J, Lee D, Mittal S, Mucksavage P. Adapting to the Educational Challenges of a Pandemic: Development of a Novel Virtual Urology Subinternship During the Time of COVID-19. *Urology* (2021) 148:70–6. doi: 10.1016/j.urology.2020.08.071
12. Kenigsberg AP, Khouri RK, Kuprasertkul A, Wong D, Ganesan V, Lemack GE. Urology Residency Applications in the COVID-19 Era. *Urology* (2020) 143:55–61. doi: 10.1016/j.urology.2020.05.072
13. Mikhail D, Margolin EJ, Sfakianos J, Clifton M, Sorensen M, Thavaseelan S. Changing the Status Quo: Developing a Virtual Sub-Internship in the Era of COVID-19. *J Surg Educ* (2021) 78(5):1544–55. doi: 10.1016/j.jsurg.2021.03.007
14. Margolin EJ, Gordon RJ, Anderson CB, Badalato GM. Reimagining the Away Rotation: A 4-Week Virtual Subinternship in Urology. *J Surg Educ* (2021) 78 (5):1563–73. doi: 10.1016/j.jsurg.2021.01.008
15. Farlow JL, Marchiano EJ, Fischer IP, Moyer JS, Thorne MC, Bohm LA. Addressing the Impact of COVID-19 on the Residency Application Process Through a Virtual Subinternship. *Otolaryngol Head Neck Surg* (2020) 163 (5):926–8. doi: 10.1177/0194599820934775
16. Dean RA, Reghunathan M, Hauch A, Reid CM, Gosman AA, Lance SH. Establishing a Virtual Curriculum for Surgical Subinternships. *Plast Reconstr Surg* (2020) 146(4):525e–57e. doi: 10.1097/prs.0000000000007267
17. Tabakin AL, Srivastava A, Polotti CF, Gupta NK. The Financial Burden of Applying to Urology Residency in 2020. *Urology* (2021) 154:62–7. doi: 10.1016/j.urology.2021.01.013
18. Winterton M, Ahn J, Bernstein J. The Prevalence and Cost of Medical Student Visiting Rotations. *BMC Med Educ* (2016) 16(1):291. doi: 10.1186/s12909-016-0805-z

ACKNOWLEDGMENTS

revision, AK, JT, WM, MC, CH, BS, and JZ. All authors contributed to the article and approved the submitted version.

aders and faculty volunteers. We acknowledge the contributions of other valued members of the intervention implementation teams, including the case discussion resident educator le
Our team also formally acknowledges the SAU taskforce for creating the manual, and Lee Richstone, MD who chaired the effort nationally.

25

Adherence to Urological Therapies for Lower Urinary Tract Symptoms due to Benign Prostatic Enlargement During COVID-19 Lockdown

Giuseppe Morgia[1,2], Arturo Lo Giudice[2], Maria Giovanna Asmundo[2], Ilenia Rapallo[2], Maurizio Carrino[3], Francesco Persico[3], Carlo Terrone[4], Rafaela Malinaric[4], Alessandro Tedde[5], Massimo Madonia[5], Salvatore Voce[6], Giulio Reale[6], Gaetano Larganà[6], Andrea Cocci[7], Lorenzo Masieri[7], Francesca Zingone[1], Daniela Carcò[8] and Giorgio Ivan Russo[2*]

[1] Department of Urology, Mediterranean Institute of Oncology (IOM), Catania, Italy, [2] Urology Section, Department of Surgery, University of Catania, Catania, Italy, [3] Department of Urology, AORN Cardarelli, Naples, Italy, [4] Department of Urology, University of Genoa, Genova, Italy, [5] Department of Urology, University of Sassari, Sassari, Italy, [6] Department of Urology, S. M. Delle Croci, Ravenna, Italy, [7] Department of Urology, University of Florence, Florence, Italy, [8] Laboratory of Clinical Pathology, Mediterranean Institute of Oncology (IOM), Catania, Italy

*Correspondence:
Giorgio Ivan Russo
giorgioivan.russo@unict.it

Background: Due to the pandemic emergency caused by COVID-19, many countries were forced to apply a variety of measures such as quarantine and full national lockdown in order to contain the contagion. Medication adherence to chronic diseases may have been negatively influenced by restrictions due to the COVID-19 pandemic. The purpose of this study is to investigate adherence to urological therapies of patients with lower urinary tract symptoms (LUTSs) secondary to benign prostatic hyperplasia (BPH) during the COVID-19 lockdown period.

Methods: In this cohort study, we included a total of 151 male patients who were prescribed medications for LUTSs/benign prostatic enlargement (BPE) between January 2019 and December 2020. The prescriptive data of the following medications were collected: alpha-blockers (AB), 5-alpha reductase inhibitors (5-ARIs), 5-phosphodiesterase inhibitors (PDE5-i), antimuscarinics, and phytotherapy (i.e., *Serenoa repens*). According to adherence or discontinuation of therapy, patients were divided into two groups: those who took their medications for a minimum of 6 months during the index period were considered in the "Medication adherence group" and those whose treatment was considered "discontinued" if it was interrupted for a 1-month period.

Results: Overall, the median age was 69.0 (interquartile range [IQR]: 63.0–74.0), the median International Prostate Symptom Score (IPSS) before the lockdown was 15.0 (IQR: 11.0–18.0), and the median IPSS–quality of life (IPSS-QoL) before the lockdown was 2.0 (IQR: 2.0–3.0). During the lockdown, 19 patients (12.58%) stopped taking their medications due to the pandemic situation: six (31.58%) stopped phytotherapy, two stopped AB+phytotherapy (10.53%), five stopped AB (26.32%), three stopped 5-ARIs (15.79%), one stopped antimuscarinics (5.26%), and two stopped other combination therapies (p < 0.01). Among the patients who stopped therapy, five (26.31%) reported the presence of worsening symptoms (score ≥ 3), while 14 (73.69%) reported the absence of worsening symptoms (score < 3). During the lockdown, five (3.31%) patients required hospitalization: three (1.99%) for acute urinary retention and two (1.32%) for urinary tract infection.

Conclusions: The rate of medication adherence for LUTSs/BPE during COVID-19 was 86.75%, but 13.25% of the patients had their treatments interrupted due to the pandemic situation. This rate determined a slight increase in symptoms with a potential impact on hospitalization. These results should be taken into account in order to develop adequate strategies in telehealth to maintain medication adherence for chronic diseases.

Keywords: COVID-19, BPH (benign prostatic hyperplasia), drug, therapy, adherence, compliance, persistence

INTRODUCTION

The novel severe acute respiratory syndrome caused by severe acute respiratory syndrome coronavirus 2 (SARS-CoV-2) quickly spread throughout the whole world since its very first detection in Wuhan, China, on December 1, 2019 (1). COVID-19 was soon declared a pandemic, and on April 2, one million cases were confirmed (2).

Due to the pandemic emergency, many countries were forced to apply a variety of measures such as quarantine and full national lockdown in order to contain the contagion. In fact, on March 9, the Italian government imposed a stay-at-home order that moved toward a full lockdown, with workplaces, schools, shops, and bars closed and the application of smart-working systems. The interruption of the lockdown statement on May 1, 2020, determined the start of "phase 2" of the pandemic (3).

Hospitals and health authorities took unprecedented stringent measures to curb the wave of COVID-19 patients; in fact, many hospitals were converted into dedicated facilities that had the specific task to manage these patients. However, despite that preventive measures were applied, it was unavoidable that doctors and nurses who assisted patients affected by COVID-19 were infected by the virus too. This moment became critical, as it imposed enormous difficulties and challenges on urology health professionals globally.

The global pandemic led many urologists to make unprecedented decisions to strike a balance between providing optimal and high-quality urological care to their patients and mitigating the risk of infection.

The European Association of Urology (EAU) provided an update of its guidelines with the aim to reduce the risk of contagion and optimize the resources during pandemic emergencies (4).

In this context, medication adherence to chronic diseases may have been negatively influenced by restrictions due to the COVID-19 pandemic. In particular, it was reported that approximately 51% of the patients reported a medication-related problem, with 19.6% reporting problems in obtaining medications and 31.7% reporting forgetting or not taking their medications (5).

Among chronic urological diseases, lower urinary tract symptoms (LUTSs) secondary to benign prostatic enlargement (BPE) are very common in adult men, and they are related to age as well as genetic factors and family history (6). LUTSs/BPE is defined as a variety of storage, voiding, and post-voiding urination symptoms (7).

A study conducted by McNicholas et al. reported that α1-blockers are the most frequently prescribed medications in men who suffer from LUTSs/BPE (8); however, phytotherapy surprisingly accounted for 27% of all monotherapies and 54% of all combination therapies. A similar prescription profile was reported between general practitioners and urologists who represent 92% and 3.7% of total prescribers, respectively. In 95.4% of cases, the first approach is a medical treatment consisting mainly of α1-blockers (AB) (60.3%), phytotherapy (31.8%), or 5 alpha-reductase inhibitors (5-ARIs) (7.9%), although modification of treatments within 12 months from the beginning may occur at an extremely high rate (8.7%, 14.6%, and 12.9%, respectively) (9).

The purpose of this study is to investigate LUTS/BPE patients' adherence to urological therapies during the COVID-19 lockdown period.

MATERIALS AND METHODS

In this cohort study, we included a total of 151 male patients who were prescribed medications for LUTSs/BPE between January 2019 and December 2020. Data were collected through Google form sent by email using hospital records.

The prescriptive data of the following medications were collected: AB, 5-ARIs, 5-phosphodiesterase inhibitors (PDE5-i), antimuscarinics, and phytotherapy (i.e., *Serenoa repens*).

According to adherence or discontinuation of therapy, patients were divided into two groups: those who took their medications for a minimum of 6 months during the index period were considered in the "Medication adherence group" and those whose treatment was considered "discontinued" if it was interrupted for a 1-month period. The presence or absence of worsening symptoms was considered only in patients who discontinued their therapy.

Data collection forms included baseline data, consisting of the International Prostate Symptom Score (IPSS) questionnaire, which referred to the period before and after lockdown.

The second part of the form included questions regarding the interruption of LUTS/BPE therapy: which main or association medications were discontinued, the reason the therapy was abandoned, if after discontinued therapy any worsening of urinary symptoms occurred, and a potential hospitalization for urological LUTS/BPE-related condition. Finally, the reasons for medical therapy discontinuation were categorized into "reasons related to pandemic and lockdown" and "other reasons". Moreover, any self-reported worsening of urological symptoms was objectified by a numerical scale graduated from 0 to 5, where "0" means "absence of worsening" and "5" means "very high worsening". Patients were divided into two groups according to continuation or interruption of LUTS/BPE treatment.

Statistical Analysis

Continuous variables are presented as the median and interquartile range (IQR) and were compared by Student's independent t-test or the Mann–Whitney U test based on their normal or non-normal distribution, respectively (normality of variables' distribution was tested by the Kolmogorov–Smirnov test). Categorical variables were tested with the χ^2 test. Data analysis was performed under the guidance of our statistics expert, using SPSS version 17 (Statistical Package for the Social Sciences, SPSS Inc., released 2008; SPSS Statistics for Windows, Version 17.0) (SPSS Inc.).

RESULTS

Overall, the median age was 69.0 (IQR: 63.0–74.0), median IPSS before the lockdown was 15.0 (IQR: 11.0–18.0), and median IPSS–quality of life (IPSS-QoL) before the lockdown was 2.0 (IQR: 2.0–3.0). **Figure 1** shows the type of medications taken by our cohort before the pandemic. During the lockdown, 19

patients (12.58%) stopped taking their medications due to the pandemic situation: six (31.58%) stopped phytotherapy, two stopped AB+phytotherapy (10.53%), five stopped AB (26.32%), three stopped 5-ARIs (15.79%), one stopped antimuscarinics (5.26%), and two stopped other combination therapies (p < 0.01) (**Figure 1**). Among the patients who stopped therapy, five (26.31%) reported the presence of worsening symptoms (score ≥ 3), while 14 (73.69%) reported the absence of worsening symptoms (score < 3).

Table 1 shows the characteristics of patients according to discontinuation of therapy.

During the lockdown, five (3.31%) patients required hospitalization: three (1.99%) for acute urinary retention (AUR) and two (1.32%) for urinary tract infection (UTI). Among these patients, two (40.0%) were under AB+phytotherapy, two (40.0%) were under AB+5-ARIs, and one (20.0%) stopped therapy (p = 0.38).

After lockdown, 147 patients (97.35%) continued to take their medication for LUTSs/BPE, while only four (2.65%) stopped taking their medication. **Figure 1** shows the type of medications taken by our cohort after the pandemic.

The median IPSS after lockdown was 14.0 (IQR: 9.0–18.0) (p < 0.01), while the median IPSS-QoL was 2.0 (IQR: 2.0–3.0) (p = 0.12). Only one patient (0.66%) was hospitalized for AUR after the lockdown.

DISCUSSION

Herein we demonstrated that the medication adherence for LUTSs/BPE during the COVID-19 pandemic was 86.75%, but 13.25% interrupted their medications due to lockdown. Although the rate of hospitalization was low due to the short period of observation, we observed a statistically significant reduction of IPSS after lockdown.

A study by Assenza et al. about the impact of COVID-19 lockdown on the treatment of patients with epilepsy

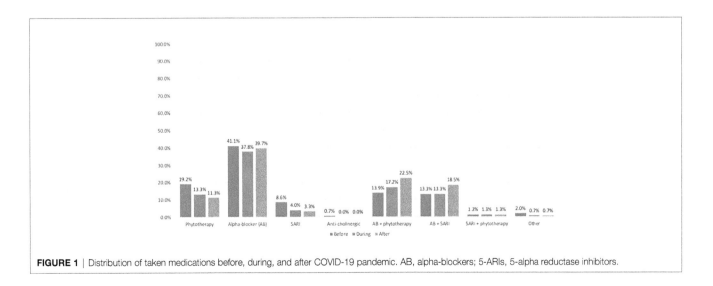

FIGURE 1 | Distribution of taken medications before, during, and after COVID-19 pandemic. AB, alpha-blockers; 5-ARIs, 5-alpha reductase inhibitors.

TABLE 1 | Characteristics of patients according to the discontinuation of therapy.

	Group 1 (n = 132)	Group 2 (n = 19)	P-value
Age (years), median (IQR)	70.0 (64.0–74.0)	67.0 (61.0–73.0)	0.24
IPSS pre-lockdown, median (IQR)	14.0 (9.0–18.0)	14.0 (9.0–18.0)	1.0
IPSS-QoL pre-lockdown, median (IQR)	2.0 (2.0–3.0)	2.0 (2.0–3.0)	1.0
IPSS post-lockdown, median (IQR)	14.0 (9.0–18.0)	15.0 (11.0–18.0)	0.01
IPSS-QoL lockdown, median (IQR)	2.0 (2.0–3.0)	2.5 (2.5–3.5)	0.65
Complications, n (%)			0.27
AUR	3 (2.27)	0 (0.0)	
UTI	1 (0.76)	1 (5.26)	

IQR, interquartile range; IPSS, International Prostate Symptom Score; QoL, quality of life; AUR, acute urinary retention; UTI, urinary tract infection.

demonstrated that during the COVID-19 pandemic, 32 (7%) people who reported inadequate adherence to therapy attributed it primarily to forgetfulness (70%), demotivation (15%), and adverse events (10%) (10). Further, Midao et al. reported that during the pandemic, 8.2% of participants reported that their adherence improved, 5.9% had worsened adherence results, widowers were 3 times more prone to be less adherent, and comorbid patients were 1.8 times more prone to be less adherent (11).

Literature data demonstrated that more prescriptions were filled in March 2020 than in any prior month, followed by a significant drop in monthly dispensing (12). A patient's likelihood of discontinuing some medications increased after the spread of COVID compared to the pre-COVID era (12).

A study by Cindolo et al. was conducted in 2015 on 1.5 million men aged ≥40 years treated with alpha-blockers (ABs) and 5-alpha reductase inhibitors (5-ARIs) alone or in combination (CT) for their LUTSs/BPE. The authors reported that the 1-year adherence was 29% in patients exposed to at least 6-month therapy and that patients on CT had a higher discontinuation rate in the first 2 years as compared to those on monotherapy (p < 0.0001). Interestingly, the overall hospitalization rates for BPE and BPE surgery were 9.04 and 12.6 per 1,000 patient-years, respectively. Finally, discontinuation of medication treatment was an independent risk factor for hospitalization for benign prostatic hyperplasia (BPH) and BPH surgery (HR 1.65 and 2.80; p < 0.0001) regardless of the therapeutic group (13).

These findings highlight the importance of medication adherence for LUTSs/BPE in order to reduce the rate of hospitalization and disease progression in these patients.

Based on these premises, telehealth could be an important tool in caring services while keeping patients and health providers safe during the COVID-19 outbreak (14). In particular, phone calls and electronic health records can be used for screening or treating patients without the need for in-person visits and can be helpful in case of urgent care (15). Furthermore, elderly people can access health services using electronic devices (16).

Before concluding, we would like to underline some limitations. Firstly, we did not include a great number of patients. Secondly, the short follow-up of the lockdown could have limited the rate of complications and hospitalization in patients with a lack of adherence to medical therapy. Finally, we did not consider the potential influence of COVID-19 infection in our cohort.

CONCLUSIONS

The rate of medication adherence for LUTSs/BPE during COVID-19 was 86.75%, but 13.25% of the patients interrupted medications due to the pandemic situation. This rate determined a slight increase in symptoms with a potential impact on hospitalization.

These results should be taken into account in order to develop adequate strategies in telehealth to maintain medication adherence for chronic diseases.

AUTHOR CONTRIBUTIONS

GM and GIR designed the study. ALG, MC, FP, CT, RM, AT, MM, SV, GR, GL, AC, LM, FZ, and DC collected the data. AL, MA, and GIR drafted the manuscript. All authors approved the manuscript.

REFERENCES

1. Huang C, Wang Y, Li X, Ren L, Zhao J, Hu Y, et al. Clinical Features of Patients Infected With 2019 Novel Coronavirus in Wuhan, China. *Lancet (London England)* (2020) 395:497–506. doi: 10.1016/S0140-6736(20)30183-5

2. Sharma A, Ahmad Farouk I, Lal SK. COVID-19: A Review on the Novel Coronavirus Disease Evolution, Transmission, Detection, Control and Prevention. *Viruses* (2021) 13:202. doi: 10.3390/v13020202

3. Signorelli C, Scognamiglio T, Odone A. COVID-19 in Italy: Impact of Containment Measures and Prevalence Estimates of Infection in the General Population. *Acta BioMed* (2020) 91:175–9. doi: 10.23750/abm.v91i3-S.9511

4. Ribal MJ, Cornford P, Briganti A, Knoll T, Gravas S, Babjuk M, et al. An Organisation-Wide Collaborative Effort to Adapt the European Association of Urology Guidelines Recommendations to the Coronavirus Disease 2019 Era. *Eur Urol* (2020) 78:21–8. doi: 10.1016/j.eururo.2020.04.056

Adherence to Urological Therapies for Lower Urinary Tract Symptoms due to Benign Prostatic Enlargement...

231

5. Ismail H, Marshall VD, Patel M, Tariq M, Mohammad RA. The Impact of the COVID-19 Pandemic on Medical Conditions and Medication Adherence in People With Chronic Diseases. *J Am Pharm Assoc* (2003) 62(3):834-9. doi: 10.1016/j.japh.2021.11.013

6. Langan RC. Benign Prostatic Hyperplasia. *Prim Care Clin Off Pract* (2019) 46:223-32. doi: 10.1016/j.pop.2019.02.003

7. Abrams P, Cardozo L, Fall M, Griffiths D, Rosier P, Ulmsten U, et al. The Standardisation of Terminology in Lower Urinary Tract Function: Report From the Standardisation Sub-Committee of the International Continence Society. *Urology* (2003) 61(1):37-49. doi: 10.1016/S0090-4295(02)02243-4

8. McNicholas T, Kirby R. Benign Prostatic Hyperplasia and Male Lower Urinary Tract Symptoms (LUTS). *BMJ Clin Evid* (2011) 86(4):359-60.

9. Lukacs B, Cornu J-N, Aout M, Tessier N, Hodée C, Haab F, et al. Management of Lower Urinary Tract Symptoms Related to Benign Prostatic Hyperplasia in Real-Life Practice in France: A Comprehensive Population Study. *Eur Urol* (2013) 64:493–501. doi: 10.1016/j.eururo.2013.02.026

10. Assenza G, Lanzone J, Brigo F, Coppola A, Di Gennaro G, Di Lazzaro V, et al. Epilepsy Care in the Time of COVID-19 Pandemic in Italy: Risk Factors for Seizure Worsening. *Front Neurol* (2020) 11:737. doi: 10.3389/fneur.2020.00737

11. Midão L, Almada M, Carrilho J, Sampaio R, Costa E. Pharmacological Adherence Behavior Changes During COVID-19 Outbreak in a Portugal Patient Cohort. *Int J Environ Res Public Health* (2022) 19:1135. doi: 10.3390/ijerph19031135

12. Clement J, Jacobi M, Greenwood BN. Patient Access to Chronic Medications During the Covid-19 Pandemic: Evidence From a Comprehensive Dataset of US Insurance Claims. *PloS One* (2021) 16:e0249453. doi: 10.1371/journal.pone.0249453

13. Cindolo L, Pirozzi L, Fanizza C, Romero M, Tubaro A, Autorino R, et al. Drug Adherence and Clinical Outcomes for Patients Under Pharmacological Therapy for Lower Urinary Tract Symptoms Related to Benign Prostatic Hyperplasia: Population-Based Cohort Study. *Eur Urol* (2015) 68:418–25. doi: 10.1016/j.eururo.2014.11.006

14. Portnoy J, Waller M, Elliott T. Telemedicine in the Era of COVID-19. *J Allergy Clin Immunol Pract* (2020) 8:1489–91. doi: 10.1016/j.jaip.2020.03.008

15. Reeves JJ, Hollandsworth HM, Torriani FJ, Taplitz R, Abeles S, Tai-Seale M, et al. Rapid Response to COVID-19: Health Informatics Support for Outbreak Management in an Academic Health System. *J Am Med Inf Assoc* (2020) 27:853–9. doi: 10.1093/jamia/ocaa037

16. Nicol GE, Piccirillo JF, Mulsant BH, Lenze EJ. Action at a Distance: Geriatric Research During a Pandemic. *J Am Geriatr Soc* (2020) 68:922–5. doi: 10.1111/jgs.16443

Permissions

All chapters in this book were first published by Frontiers; hereby published with permission under the Creative Commons Attribution License or equivalent. Every chapter published in this book has been scrutinized by our experts. Their significance has been extensively debated. The topics covered herein carry significant findings which will fuel the growth of the discipline. They may even be implemented as practical applications or may be referred to as a beginning point for another development.

The contributors of this book come from diverse backgrounds, making this book a truly international effort. This book will bring forth new frontiers with its revolutionizing research information and detailed analysis of the nascent developments around the world.

We would like to thank all the contributing authors for lending their expertise to make the book truly unique. They have played a crucial role in the development of this book. Without their invaluable contributions this book wouldn't have been possible. They have made vital efforts to compile up to date information on the varied aspects of this subject to make this book a valuable addition to the collection of many professionals and students.

This book was conceptualized with the vision of imparting up-to-date information and advanced data in this field. To ensure the same, a matchless editorial board was set up. Every individual on the board went through rigorous rounds of assessment to prove their worth. After which they invested a large part of their time researching and compiling the most relevant data for our readers.

The editorial board has been involved in producing this book since its inception. They have spent rigorous hours researching and exploring the diverse topics which have resulted in the successful publishing of this book. They have passed on their knowledge of decades through this book. To expedite this challenging task, the publisher supported the team at every step. A small team of assistant editors was also appointed to further simplify the editing procedure and attain best results for the readers.

Apart from the editorial board, the designing team has also invested a significant amount of their time in understanding the subject and creating the most relevant covers. They scrutinized every image to scout for the most suitable representation of the subject and create an appropriate cover for the book.

The publishing team has been an ardent support to the editorial, designing and production team. Their endless efforts to recruit the best for this project, has resulted in the accomplishment of this book. They are a veteran in the field of academics and their pool of knowledge is as vast as their experience in printing. Their expertise and guidance has proved useful at every step. Their uncompromising quality standards have made this book an exceptional effort. Their encouragement from time to time has been an inspiration for everyone.

The publisher and the editorial board hope that this book will prove to be a valuable piece of knowledge for researchers, students, practitioners and scholars across the globe.

List of Contributors

Santiago Vallasciani
Division of Urology, Department of Surgery, Sidra Medicine, Doha, Qatar

Anna Bujons Tur
Division of Pediatric Urology, Puigvert Foundation, Barcelona, Spain

John Gatti
Division of Pediatric Urology, Children's Mercy Hospital, Kansas City, MO, United States

Marcos Machado
Division of Pediatric Urology, University of São Paulo, São Paulo, Brazil

Christopher S. Cooper
Department of Urology, University of Iowa Hospitals and Clinics, Iowa City, IA, United States

Marie Klaire Farrugia
Division of Pediatric Urology, Chelsea and Westminster Hospital NHS Foundation Trust, London, United Kingdom

Mohammed El Anbari
Division of Clinical Informatics, Sidra Medicine, Doha, Qatar

Pedro-José Lopez
Hospital Exequiel Gonzalez Cortes & Clinica Alemana, Santiago, Chile
University of Chile, Santiago, Chile

Recep Has and Tugba Sarac Sivrikoz
Division of Perinatology, Department of Obstetrics and Gynecology, Istanbul Faculty of Medicine, Istanbul University, Istanbul, Turkey

Lauren C. Smail
Department of Psychology, Neuroscience & Behaviour, McMaster University, Hamilton, ON, Canada
Office of Education Science, McMaster University, Hamilton, ON, Canada

Kiret Dhindsa
Department of Surgery, McMaster University, Hamilton, ON, Canada
Research and High Performance Computing, McMaster University, Hamilton, ON, Canada
Vector Institute for Artificial Intelligence, Toronto, ON, Canada

Luis H. Braga
Division of Urology, Department of Surgery, McMaster University, Hamilton, ON, Canada
Division of Urology, Department of Surgery, McMaster Children's Hospital, Hamilton, ON, Canada
McMaster Pediatric Surgery Research Collaborative, McMaster University, Hamilton, ON, Canada
Department of Health Research, Methods, Evidence & Impact, McMaster University, Hamilton, ON, Canada

Suzanna Becker
Department of Psychology, Neuroscience & Behaviour, McMaster University, Hamilton, ON, Canada
Vector Institute for Artificial Intelligence, Toronto, ON, Canada
Centre for Advanced Research in Experimental and Applied Linguistics, McMaster University, Hamilton, ON, Canada

Ranil R. Sonnadara
Department of Psychology, Neuroscience & Behaviour, McMaster University, Hamilton, ON, Canada
Office of Education Science, McMaster University, Hamilton, ON, Canada
Department of Surgery, McMaster University, Hamilton, ON, Canada
Research and High Performance Computing, McMaster University, Hamilton, ON, Canada
Vector Institute for Artificial Intelligence, Toronto, ON, Canada
Centre for Advanced Research in Experimental and Applied Linguistics, McMaster University, Hamilton, ON, Canada

Ilmay Bilge
Division of Pediatric Nephrology, Department of Pediatrics, School of Medicine, Koc University, Istanbul, Turkey

Niccolo Maria Passoni and Craig Andrew Peters
University of Texas Southwestern Medical Center, Dallas, TX, United States

Yuenshan Sammi Wong, Kristine Kit Yi Pang and Yuk Him Tam
Division of Paediatric Surgery and Paediatric Urology, Department of Surgery, Prince of Wales Hospital, The Chinese University of Hong Kong, Shatin, Hong Kong

Xiangpan Kong, Zhenpeng Li, Mujie Li, Xing Liu and Dawei He
Department of Urology, Children's Hospital of Chongqing Medical University, Chongqing, China
Ministry of Education Key Laboratory of Child Development and Disorders, International Science and Technology Cooperation Base of Child Development and Critical Disorders, National Clinical Research Center for Child Health and Disorders, Chongqing Key Laboratory of Pediatrics, Chongqing Key Laboratory of Children Urogenital Development and Tissue Engineering, Chongqing, China

Marco Castagnetti and Massimo Iafrate
Section of Paediatric Urology, Department of Surgical, Oncological, and Gastrointestinal Sciences, University Hospital of Padova, Padua, Italy

Ciro Esposito
Department of Paediatrics, Federico II University of Naples, Naples, Italy

Ramnath Subramaniam
Department of Paediatric Urology, Leeds Teaching Hospitals NHS Trust, University of Leeds, Leeds, United Kingdom
Department of Paediatric Urology, University of Ghent, Ghent, Belgium

Pin Li, Tian Tao, Xiaoguang Zhou, Lifei Ma and Zhichun Feng
Department of Pediatric Urology, Bayi Children's Hospital, Affiliated of the Seventh Medical Center of People's Liberation Army General Hospital, Beijing, China

Huixia Zhou
Department of Pediatric Urology, Bayi Children's Hospital, Affiliated of the Seventh Medical Center of People's Liberation Army General Hospital, Beijing, China
The Second School of Clinical Medicine, Southern Medical University, Guangzhou, China

Hualin Cao
Department of Pediatric Urology, Bayi Children's Hospital, Affiliated of the Seventh Medical Center of People's Liberation Army General Hospital, Beijing, China
Department of Urology, Nan Xi Shan Hospital of Guangxi Zhuang Autonomous Region, Guilin, China

Tao Guo and Weiwei Zhu
Medical School of Chinese People's Liberation Army, Beijing, China

Yang Zhao
Medical School of Chinese People's Liberation Army, Beijing, China
Department of Pediatrics, The Third Medical Center of People's Liberation Army General Hospital, Beijing, China

Yunjie Yang
The Second School of Clinical Medicine, Southern Medical University, Guangzhou, China
Department of Urology, The Affiliated Nanhai Hospital of the Southern Medical University, Foshan, China

Fengming Ji, Li Chen, Chengchuang Wu, Jinrong Li, Yu Hang and Bing Yan
Kunming Children's Hospital, Kunming, China

Ali Avanoglu
Division of Pediatric Urology, Department of Pediatric Surgery, Ege University, Izmir, Turkey

Sibel Tiryaki
Gaziantep Maternity and Children's Hospital, Pediatric Urology, Gaziantep, Turkey

Ayse Kalyoncu Ucar
Istanbul Kanuni Sultan Suleyman Training and Research Hospital, Istanbul, Turkey

Sebuh Kurugoglu
Istanbul University Cerrahpasa Faculty of Medicine, Istanbul, Turkey

U. M. J. E. Samaranayake
Department of Anatomy, Faculty of Medicine, Sabaragamuwa University of Sri Lanka, Ratnapura, Sri Lanka
Department of Anatomy, Faculty of Medicine, University of Colombo, Colombo, Sri Lanka

Y. Mathangasinghe
Department of Anatomy, Faculty of Medicine, University of Colombo, Colombo, Sri Lanka
Proteostasis and Neurodegeneration Laboratory, Australian Regenerative Medicine Institute, Monash University, Clayton, VIC, Australia

U. A. Liyanage and A. P. Malalasekera
Department of Anatomy, Faculty of Medicine, University of Colombo, Colombo, Sri Lanka

M. V. C. de Silva
Department of Pathology, Faculty of Medicine, University of Colombo, Colombo, Sri Lanka

M. C. Samarasinghe
Department of Surgery, Faculty of Medicine, University of Colombo, Colombo, Sri Lanka

S. Abeygunasekera and A. K. Lamahewage
Lady Ridgeway Hospital for Children, Colombo, Sri Lanka

Abdurrahman Onen
Section of Pediatric Urology, Department of Pediatric Surgery, Faculty of Medicine, Dicle University, Diyarbakir, Turkey

Hamdan Al-Hazmi and Khalid Fouda Neel
Department of Pediatric Urology, Robert-Debré University Hospital, Assistance Publique - Hôpitaux de Paris (APHP), Paris, France
College of Medicine and King Saud University Medical City, King Saud University, Riyad, Saudi Arabia

Elisabeth Carricaburu, Annabel Paye-Jaouen and Liza Ali
Department of Pediatric Urology, Robert-Debré University Hospital, Assistance Publique - Hôpitaux de Paris (APHP), Paris, France
National Reference Center of Rare Urinary Tract Malformations (MARVU), Paris, France

Matthieu Peycelon, Christine Grapin and Alaa El-Ghoneimi
Department of Pediatric Urology, Robert-Debré University Hospital, Assistance Publique - Hôpitaux de Paris (APHP), Paris, France
National Reference Center of Rare Urinary Tract Malformations (MARVU), Paris, France
University of Paris, Paris, France

Gianantonio Manzoni
Department of Pediatric Urology, Robert-Debré University Hospital, Assistance Publique - Hôpitaux de Paris (APHP), Paris, France
Department of Pediatric Urology Fondazione Cà Granda Ospedale Maggiore Policlinico, Milan, Italy

Bruce Li
Michael G. DeGroote School of Medicine, McMaster University, Hamilton, ON, Canada

Melissa McGrath
McMaster Pediatric Surgical Research Collaborative, McMaster University, Hamilton, ON, Canada
Division of Urology, McMaster University, Hamilton, ON, Canada
McMaster Children's Hospital Foundation, Hamilton, ON, Canada

Forough Farrokhyar
McMaster Children's Hospital Foundation, Hamilton, ON, Canada
Department of Health Research, Methods, Evidence & Impact, McMaster University, Hamilton, ON, Canada

Yuqi Xia, Xiangjun Zhou, Zehua Ye, Weimin Yu, Jinzhuo Ning, Yuan Ruan, Run Yuan, Fangyou Lin, Peng Ye, Di Zheng, Ting Rao and Fan Cheng
Department of Urology, Renmin Hospital of Wuhan University, Wuhan, China

Chih-Chien Sung, Min-Hsiu Chen, Sung-Sen Yang and Shih-Hua Lin
Division of Nephrology, Department of Medicine, National Defense Medical Center, Tri-Service General Hospital, Taipei, Taiwan

Yi-Chang Lin
Division of Cardiovascular Surgery, Department of Surgery, National Defense Medical Center, Tri-Service General Hospital, Taipei, Taiwan

Yu-Chun Lin and Yi-Jia Lin
Deparment of Pathology, National Defense Medical Center, Tri-Service General Hospital, Taipei, Taiwan

Libo Yang, Yang Qin, Guoying Zhang, Bin Zhao and Yong Yang
Department of Urology, The Third Affiliated Hospital of Kunming Medical University, Kunming, China

Chunyan Li
Second Department of Head and Neck Surgery, The Third Affiliated Hospital of Kunming Medical University, Kunming, China

Ziyuan Wang and Youguang Huang
Department of Yunnan Tumor Research Institute, The Third Affiliated Hospital of Kunming Medical University, Kunming, China

Zhuolun Sun
Department of Urology, Third Affiliated Hospital, Sun Yat-sen University, Guangzhou, China

Changying Jing
School of Medicine, Technical University of Munich, Munich, Germany

Xudong Guo, Feng Kong, Shaobo Jiang and Hanbo Wang
Department of Urology, Shandong Provincial Hospital Affiliated to Shandong First Medical University, Jinan, China

Mingxiao Zhang and Zhenqing Wang
Department of Urology, The First Affiliated Hospital of Sun Yat-sen University, Guangzhou, China

Yipeng Xu, Hua Wang and Zongping Wang
Department of Urology, Cancer Hospital of University of Chinese Academy of Sciences, Zhejiang Cancer Hospital, Hangzhou, China

Jianmin Lou, Mingke Yu and Yueyu Huang
Zhejiang Chinese Medical University, Hangzhou, China

Yingjun Jiang
Hangzhou Traditional Chinese Medicine Hospital, Zhejiang Chinese Medical University, Hangzhou, China

Han Xu
Central Research Laboratory, Children's Hospital of Nanchang University, Nanchang, China

Yun Gao and An Zhao
Experimental Research Center, Cancer Hospital of University of Chinese Academy of Sciences, Zhejiang Cancer Hospital, Hangzhou, China
Institute of Cancer and Basic Medicine (ICBM), Chinese Academy of Sciences, Hangzhou, China

Guorong Li
Department of Urology, North Hospital, CHU of Saint-Etienne, University of Jean-Monnet, Saint-Etienne, France
Inserm U1059, Faculty of Medicine, University of Jean-Monnet, Saint-Etienne, France

Xiangbo Kong
Department of Urology, China-Japan Union Hospital, Jilin University, Changchun, China

Ruida Hou
Department of Urology, China-Japan Union Hospital, Jilin University, Changchun, China
Department of Physiology, Emory University School of Medicine, Atlanta, GA, USA

Mehrdad Alemozaffar
Department of Urology, Emory University School of Medicine, Atlanta, GA, USA

Baoxue Yang
Department of Pharmacology, School of Basic Medical Sciences, Peking University, Beijing, China

Jeff M. Sands and Guangping Chen
Department of Physiology, Emory University School of Medicine, Atlanta, GA, USA
Renal Division Department of Medicine, Emory University School of Medicine, Atlanta, GA, USA

Shaokai Zheng, Pedro Amado, Dominik Obrist and Francesco Clavica
ARTORG Center for Biomedical Engineering Research, University of Bern, Bern, Switzerland

Bernhard Kiss and Fiona Burkhard
Department of Urology, Inselspital, Bern University Hospital, University of Bern, Bern, Switzerland

Fabian Stangl
Department of Urology, Cantonal Hospital Olten, Olten, Switzerland

Andreas Haeberlin
Department of Cardiology, Inselspital, Bern University Hospital, University of Bern, Bern, Switzerland

Daniel Sidler
Department of Nephrology and Hypertension, Inselspital, Bern University Hospital, University of Bern, Bern, Switzerland

Amelia A. Khoei
School of Medicine, Baylor College of Medicine, Houston, TX, United States

Blair T. Stocks, Jerry Zhuo, Wesley A. Mayer, Michael Coburn, Caroline Hubbard and Jennifer M. Taylor
Scott Department of Urology, Baylor College of Medicine, Houston, TX, United States

Francesca Zingone
Department of Urology, Mediterranean Institute of Oncology (IOM), Catania, Italy

Giuseppe Morgia
Department of Urology, Mediterranean Institute of Oncology (IOM), Catania, Italy
Urology Section, Department of Surgery, University of Catania, Catania, Italy

Arturo Lo Giudice, Maria Giovanna Asmundo, Ilenia Rapallo and Giorgio Ivan Russo
Urology Section, Department of Surgery, University of Catania, Catania, Italy

Maurizio Carrino and Francesco Persico
Department of Urology, AORN Cardarelli, Naples, Italy

Carlo Terrone and Rafaela Malinaric
Department of Urology, University of Genoa, Genova, Italy

Alessandro Tedde and Massimo Madonia
Department of Urology, University of Sassari, Sassari, Italy

Salvatore Voce, Giulio Reale and Gaetano Larganà
Department of Urology, S. M. Delle Croci, Ravenna, Italy

Andrea Cocci and Lorenzo Masieri
Department of Urology, University of Florence, Florence, Italy

Daniela Carcò
Laboratory of Clinical Pathology, Mediterranean Institute of Oncology (IOM), Catania, Italy

Index

Printed in the USA
CPSIA information can be obtained
at www.ICGtesting.com
JSHW051407091023
49903JS00006B/309

9 781646 475506